THE **OFFICIAL** GUIDE TO LEVEL 3, REVISED 6E

Professional

Hairdressing

Revised 6th Edition

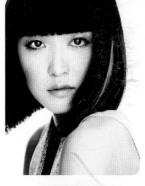

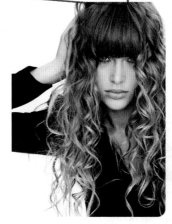

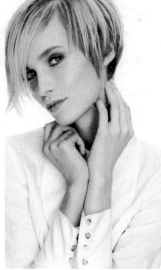

SCOTT SMURTHWAITE @ CREAM

Hairdressing

Student textbooks

Begin Hairdressing: The Official Guide to Level 1 1e *Martin Green*

Hairdressing – The Foundations: The Official Guide to Level 2 5e *Leo Palladino and Martin Green*

Professional Hairdressing: The Official Guide to Level 3 5e *Martin Green and Leo Palladino*

The Official Guide to the City and Guilds Certificate in Salon Services 1e *John Armstrong with Anita Crosland, Martin Green and Lorraine Nordmann*

The Colour Book: The Official Guide to Colour for NVQ Levels 2 and 3 1e *Tracey Lloyd with Christine McMillan-Bodell*

eXtensions: The Official Guide to Hair Extensions 1e *Theresa Bullock*

Salon Management *Martin Green*

Men's Hairdressing: Traditional and Modern Barbering 2e *Maurice Lister*

African-Caribbean Hairdressing 2e *Sandra Gittens*

The World of Hair Colour 1e *John Gray*

The Cutting Book: The Official Guide to Cutting at S/NVQ Levels 2 and 3 *Jane Goldsbro and Elaine White*

Professional Hairdressing titles

Trevor Sorbie: The Bridal Hair Book 1e *Trevor Sorbie and Jacki Wadeson*

The Art of Dressing Long Hair 1e *Guy Kremer and Jacki Wadeson*

Patrick Cameron: Dressing Long Hair 1e *Patrick Cameron and Jacki Wadeson*

Patrick Cameron: Dressing Long Hair 2 1e *Patrick Cameron and Jacki Wadeson*

Bridal Hair 1e *Pat Dixon and Jacki Wadeson*

Professional Men's Hairdressing: The art of cutting and styling 1e *Guy Kremer and Jacki Wadeson*

Essensuals, The Next Generation Toni and Guy: Step by Step 1e *Sacha Mascolo, Christian Mascolo and Stuart Wesson*

Mahogany Hairdressing: Steps to Cutting, Colouring and Finishing Hair 1e *Martin Gannon and Richard Thompson*

Mahogany Hairdressing: Advanced Looks 1e *Martin Gannon and Richard Thompson*

The Total Look: The Style Guide for Hair and Make-Up Professionals 1e *Ian Mistlin*

Trevor Sorbie: Visions in Hair 1e *Trevor Sorbie, Kris Sorbie and Jacki Wadeson*

The Art of Hair Colouring 1e *David Adams and Jacki Wadeson*

Beauty therapy

Beauty Basics: The Official Guide to Level 1 1e *Lorraine Nordmann*

Beauty Therapy – The Foundations: The Official Guide to Level 2 3e *Lorraine Nordmann*

Professional Beauty Therapy – The Official Guide to Level 3 2e *Lorraine Nordmann*

The Official Guide to the City and Guilds Certificate in Salon Services 1e *John Armstrong with Anita Crosland, Martin Green and Lorraine Nordmann*

The Complete Guide to Make-Up 1e *Suzanne Le Quesne*

The Complete Make-Up Artist 2e *Penny Delamar*

The Encyclopedia of Nails 1e *Jacqui Jefford and Anne Swain*

The Art of Nails: A Comprehensive Style Guide to Nail Treatments and Nail Art 1e *Jacqui Jefford*

Nail Artistry 1e *Jacqui Jefford*

The Complete Nail Technician 2e *Marian Newman*

Manicure, Pedicure and Advanced Nail Techniques 1e *Elaine Almond*

The Official Guide to Body Massage 2e *Adele O'Keefe*

An Holistic Guide to Massage 1e *Tina Parsons*

Indian Head Massage 2e *Muriel Burnham-Airey and Adele O'Keefe*

Aromatherapy for the Beauty Therapist 1e *Valerie Worwood*

An Holistic Guide to Reflexology 1e *Tina Parsons*

An Holistic Guide to Anatomy and Physiology 1e *Tina Parsons*

The Essential Guide to Holistic and Complementary Therapy 1e *Helen Beckmann and Suzanne Le Quesne*

The Spa Book 1e *Jane Crebbin-Bailey, Dr John Harcup and John Harrington*

SPA: The Official Guide to Spa Therapy at Levels 2 and 3 *Joan Scott and Andrea Harrison*

Nutrition: A Practical Approach 1e *Suzanne Le Quesne*

Hands on Sports Therapy 1e *Keith Ward*

Encyclopedia of Hair Removal: A Complete Reference to Methods, Techniques and Career Opportunities *Gill Morris and Janice Brown*

The Anatomy and Physiology Workbook: For Beauty and Holistic Therapies Levels 1-3 *Tina Parsons*

The Anatomy and Physiology CD-Rom

Beautiful Selling: The Complete Guide to Sales Success in the Salon *Ruth Langley*

THE **OFFICIAL** Guide to Level 3, Revised 6e

Professional

Hairdressing

Revised 6th Edition

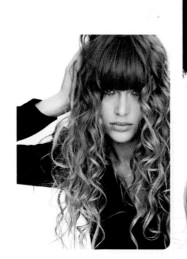

Martin Green and Leo Palladino

SCOTT SMURTHWAITE @ CREAM

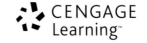
CENGAGE
Learning™

Australia • Brazil • Japan • Korea • Mexico • Singapore • Spain • United Kingdom • United States

CENGAGE
Learning™

Professional Hairdressing - The Official Guide to Level 3, Revised 6e

Martin Green and Leo Palladino

Publishing Director: Linden Harris

Publisher: Lucy Mills

Content Project Editor: Lucy Arthy

Production Controller: Richard Gogarty

Marketing Executive: Lauren Redwood

Typesetter: MPS Limited, a Macmillan Company

Cover design: HCT Creative

Text design: Design Deluxe

For product information and technology assistance,
contact **emea.info@cengage.com**.

For permission to use material from this text or product,
and for permission queries,
email **emea.permissions@cengage.com**.

The Author has asserted the right under the Copyright, Designs and Patents Act 1988 to be identified as the Author of this book.

British Library Cataloguing-in-Publication Data
A catalogue record for this book is available from the British Library.

ISBN: 978-1-4080-3981-6

Cengage Learning EMEA
Cheriton House, North Way, Andover, Hampshire, SP10 5BE
United Kingdom

Cengage Learning products are represented in Canada by Nelson Education Ltd.

For your lifelong learning solutions, visit **www.cengage.co.uk**

Purchase your next print book, e-book or e-chapter at
www.cengagebrain.com

Printed in China by RR Donnelley
2 3 4 5 6 7 8 9 10 – 13 12 11

Contents

xiii Foreword
xiv Acknowledgements
xvi Introduction
xvii Level 3 NVQ Diploma in Hairdressing or Barbering
xxiv About this book
xxvii Essential Knowledge mapping

Part**one**

2 **Customer-centred services**

Chapter**one**

4 **Consultation and advice: Unit G21 Provide hairdressing consultation services**

4 Consultation: quick overview
4 What do I need to do for G21.1?
4 What do I need to do for G21.2?
4 What do I need to do for G21.3?
5 What do I need to do for G21.4?
5 What do I need to do for G21.5?
5 What aspects do I need to cover for G21.1, G21.2, G21.3, G21.4 and G21.5?
5 What do I need to know for G21.1, G21.2, G21.3, G21.4 and G21.5?
6 Introduction
6 About you – the senior stylist
7 **G21.1 Identify clients' needs and wishes**
8 Good, effective communication
8 Body language
11 Questioning techniques
13 Avoid misunderstandings
14 Leading the consultation
15 **G21.2 Analyse the hair, skin and scalp**
15 Structure of hair and skin
20 Hair and skin tests

TRACEY DEVINE @ ANGELS

23 Hair and scalp diseases, conditions and defects
28 Influencing factors and features
29 Hair growth patterns
30 Face and head shape
32 Lifestyle, personality and age
33 Using visual aids in consultation
35 **G21.3 Make recommendations to clients**
36 Keep abreast of current fashions
36 Referrals
37 **G21.4 Advise clients on hair maintenance and management**
37 What is the client already doing with their hair?
38 Advise them on the correct product regimen to maintain their hair at home
38 Tell them how to maintain their hair between salon visits
39 **G21.5 Agree services with your client**
40 Final notes
42 Checkerboard
43 Revision questions

Chapter**two**

44 **Promote services and products: Unit G18 Promote additional services or products to clients**

44 Promoting services/products: quick overview
44 What do I need to do for G18.1?
44 What do I need to do for G18.2?
44 What do I need to do for G18.3?
45 What aspects do I need to cover for G18.1, G18.2 and G18.3?
45 What do I need to know for G18.1, G18.2 and G18.3?
45 Introduction
46 **G18.1 Identify additional services or products that are available**

46 Promoting ourselves first
46 Salon services and products
46 Products are not wallpaper!
47 Features and benefits
47 **G18.2 Inform clients about services or products**
48 How do we inform clients?
48 Implementation stages of product or service promotion
49 Common senses
50 Promotional materials
50 Window displays
50 Website
50 **G18.3 Gain client commitment to using additional services or products**
50 Recognising interest – buying signals
51 Communication
53 Consumer legislation
53 Checkerboard
54 Revision questions

Chapter**three**

55 **Customer services: Unit G19 Support client service improvements**

55 Improving services: quick overview
55 What do I need to do for G19.1?
55 What do I need to do for G19.2?
55 What do I need to do for G19.3?
56 What aspects do I need to cover for G19.1, G19.2 and G19.3?
56 What do I need to know for G19.1, G19.2 and G19.3?
56 Introduction
56 Why change services at all?
57 What is different about your salon's offerings?
57 **G19.1 Use feedback to identify potential client service improvements**
58 Customer feedback
59 Collecting information from the client
60 Informal information collection
60 Formal collection of information
62 What are your competitors doing?
64 **G19.2 Implement change in client service**
64 Sharing the information
64 Identifying possible changes to services
65 Presenting and sharing your ideas
66 Be positive and explain changes
66 **G19.3 Assist with the evaluation of changes in client service**
67 Negative comments

67 Salon and legal requirements
68 Checkerboard
69 Revision questions

Part**two**

70 **Hairdressing technical services**

Chapter**four**

72 **Creative cutting: Unit GH16 Creatively cut hair using a combination of techniques**

72 Creative cutting: quick overview
72 What do I need to do for GH16.1?
72 What do I need to do for GH16.2?
73 What do I need to do for GH16.3?
73 What aspects do I need to cover for GH16.1, GH16.2 and GH16.3?
73 What aspects do I need to know for GH16.1, GH16.2 and GH16.3?
73 Introduction
73 Building on from the basics
74 **GH16.1 Maintain effective and safe methods of working when cutting**
74 Preparing the client
75 Your personal hygiene
76 Preparing the tools and equipment
77 Preventing infection
77 Your work position
77 Working efficiently, safely and effectively
78 Your working position and posture
79 Consultation
79 General styling limitations
80 Head, face and body physical features
81 Reason or purpose for hairstyle
81 Quality, quantity and distribution of hair
82 Style suitability
84 Cutting tools
87 **GH16.2 Creatively restyle women's hair**
87 Accurate sectioning
87 Cut hair with natural fall
88 Controlling the shape
89 Cross-checking the cut
89 Dealing with cutting problems
90 Cutting and styling techniques

95   Sources for more information on cutting
95   Checklists
96   Step-by-steps
100   GH16.3   Provide aftercare advice
100   Talk through the style as you work
101   Show and recommend the products/equipment that you use
101   Explain how routine styling tools can have detrimental effects
101   Demonstrate the techniques that you use
102   Checkerboard
103   Revision questions

Chapterfive

104   Creative barbering: Unit GB8 Creatively cut hair using a combination of barbering techniques

104   Creative barbering: quick overview
104   What do I need to do for GB8.1?
104   What do I need to do for GB8.2?
105   What do I need to do for GB8.3?
105   What aspects do I need to cover for GB8.1, GB8.2 and GB8.3?
105   What aspects do I need to know for GB8.1, GB8.2 and GB8.3?
105   Introduction
106   Beyond basic barbering
106   GB8.1   Maintain effective and safe methods of working when cutting hair
106   Protect the client
108   Disposal of waste and sharps
109   Prevent infection
109   Remove product build-up before attempting to cut
110   Consultation
111   Influencing factors affecting style choice
113   Examination of hair and scalp
114   Hair growth patterns
115   Finding out what the client wants
116   Cutting tools and equipment
119   Cutting tools and techniques
120   GB8.2   Creatively restyle men's hair
120   Cutting rules
121   Outline shapes
121   Common cutting problems
123   Finishing products for men
125   Step-by-steps
126   GB8.3   Provide aftercare advice

127   Checkerboard
128   Revision questions

Chaptersix

129   Styling beards and moustaches: Unit GB7 Design and create a range of facial hair shapes

129   Beards and moustaches: quick overview
129   What do I need to do for GB7.1?
129   What do I need to do for GB7.2?
130   What do I need to do for GB7.3?
130   What aspects do I need to cover for GB7.1, GB7.2 and GB7.3?
130   What aspects do I need to know for GB7.1, GB7.2 and GB7.3?
130   Introduction
130   Facial hair barbering
131   GB7.1   Maintain effective and safe methods of working when cutting facial hair
131   Preparing the client
132   Your working position and posture
132   Your personal hygiene
132   Working efficiently, safely and effectively
132   Prevent infection
133   Safe disposal of sharps
133   Prepare the client's facial hair
133   Consultation
134   Aspects to consider
137   Tools and equipment
139   GB7.2   Create a range of facial hair shapes
139   Designing an outline shape
139   Facial hair cutting techniques
141   Removing unwanted hair outside the desired style line
142   Step-by-step
142   GB7.3   Provide aftercare advice
143   How long will it last?
143   Products and skin care
144   Checkerboard
145   Revision questions

Chapterseven

146   Shaving: Unit GB6 Provide shaving services

146   Shaving: quick overview
146   What do I need to do for GB6.1?

146 What do I need to do for GB6.2?
147 What do I need to do for GB6.3?
147 What do I need to do for GB6.4?
147 What aspects do I need to cover for GB6.1, GB6.2, GB6.3 and GB6.4?
147 What aspects do I need to know for GB6.1, GB6.2, GB6.3 and GB6.4?
147 Introduction
148 The barber's shave
148 **GB6.1 Maintain effective and safe methods of working when shaving**
148 Tool preparation and maintenance
149 Shaving tools and equipment
150 Honing (setting) fixed blade razors
151 Stropping
152 **GB6.2 Prepare the hair and skin for shaving**
152 Client preparation
153 Contra-indications to shaving
153 Lathering
154 **GB6.3 Shave hair**
154 First time over
155 Second time over
155 Finishing
155 Sponge shaving
156 Shaving problems
156 Disposal of waste materials
157 **GB6.4 Provide aftercare advice**
157 Recommended re-shaving intervals
157 Aftercare advice
158 Checkerboard
159 Revision questions

Chapter**eight**

160 **Creatively style and dress hair: Unit GH19 Creatively style and dress hair**
160 Style and dress Hair: quick overview
160 What do I need to do for GH19.1?
160 What do I need to do for GH19.2?
161 What do I need to do for GH19.3?
161 What aspects do I need to cover for GH19.1, GH19.2 and GH19.3?
161 What do I need to know for GH19.1, GH19.2 and GH19.3?
161 Introduction
162 **GH19.1 Maintain effective and safe methods of working when styling hair**
163 Preparing the tools and equipment for setting and dressing hair
164 Styling materials and tools
172 **GH19.2 Creatively style and dress hair**
172 Consultation
173 The principles of heat styling
175 Setting techniques
178 Blow-drying hair
180 Dressing hair
182 Heated styling equipment
184 **GH19.3 Provide aftercare advice**
185 Checkerboard
186 Revision questions

Chapter**nine**

187 **Creatively dress long hair: Unit GH20 Creatively dress long hair**
187 Dressing long hair: quick overview
187 What do I need to do for GH20.1?
187 What do I need to do for GH20.2?
188 What do I need to do for GH20.3?
188 What aspects do I need to cover for GH20.1, GH20.2 and GH20.3?
188 What do I need to know for GH20.1, GH20.2 and GH20.3?
188 Introduction
189 **GH20.1 Maintain effective and safe methods of working when dressing long hair**
190 Preparing the tools and equipment for setting and dressing hair
191 Service timings
191 Styling materials and tools
193 Added hair and hair pieces
195 Brushes
195 Styling products
197 **GH20.2 Creatively dress long hair**
197 Consultation
198 Agree the effect before you start
198 General rules for style suitability
199 Building enough structure and support in to the look
201 Vertical roll (French pleat)
202 Plaiting hair
203 Weaving
204 Step-by-steps
211 **GH20.3 Provide aftercare advice**
212 Checkerboard
213 Revision questions

Chapter**ten**

214 **Hair extensions: Unit GH23 Provide creative hair extensions services**

214 Hair extensions: quick overview
214 What do I need to do for GH23.1?
214 What do I need to do for GH23.2?
215 What do I need to do for GH23.3?
215 What do I need to do for GH23.4?
215 What do I need to do for GH23.5?
215 What do I need to do for GH23.6?
215 What aspects do I need to cover for GH23.1, GH23.2, GH23.3, GH23.4, GH23.5 and GH23.6?
216 What do I need to know for GH23.1, GH23.2, GH23.3, GH23.4, GH23.5 and GH23.6?
216 Introduction
216 **GH23.1 Maintain effective and safe methods of working when adding hair extensions**
217 Potential risks with different hair extension methods
218 General health and safety considerations
219 Products and equipment for hair extensions
222 **GH23.2 Plan and prepare to add hair extensions**
222 Consultation
223 Contra-indications for hair extensions
224 Hair tests for extension services
225 Choosing extension hair
226 Maintenance appointments
226 How long will it take?
226 Consultation: Points to remember
227 Finalising the consultation and completing the records
227 Selecting and blending extensions and colours together
229 **GH23.3 Attach hair extensions**
229 Adding hair extensions
230 Step-by-steps
234 Planning and placement
238 **GH23.4 Cut and finish hair with extensions**
238 Cutting extension hairstyles
239 Styling hair extensions
240 **GH23.5 Maintain and remove hair extensions**
241 Cold fusion systems
241 Hot bonded systems
242 Other systems
243 **GH23.6 Provide aftercare advice**
245 Home-care advice for extensions
246 Typical problems with artificial/synthetic hair extensions
247 Checkerboard
248 Revision questions

Chapter**eleven**

249 **Colouring hair: Unit GH17 Colour hair using a variety of techniques**

249 Creative colouring: quick overview
249 What do I need to do for GH17.1?
250 What do I need to do for GH17.2?
250 What do I need to do for GH17.3?
250 What do I need to do for GH17.4?
250 What do I need to do for GH17.5?
250 What do I need to do for GH17.6?
250 What aspects do I need to cover for GH17.1, GH17.2, GH17.3, GH17.4, GH17.5 and GH17.6?
251 What aspects do I need to know for GH17.1, GH17.2, GH17.3, GH17.4, GH17.5 and GH17.6?
252 Introduction
252 Foreword
252 The principles of colour and colouring
254 Depth and tone
256 Colour types
260 Using hydrogen peroxide
261 **GH17.1 Maintain effective and safe methods of working when colouring and lightening**
261 Safety and preparation
263 Preventing dermatitis
264 **GH17.2 Prepare for colouring and lightening services**
264 Consultation
266 Colour tests
268 Recording the events
269 **GH17.3 Creatively colour and lighten hair**
269 Colour selection principles: 1. Choice, previous processes and current condition
270 Accuracy using measuring flasks and mixing bowls
271 Pre-softening white hair
271 Current condition
272 Pre- and post-colour treatments
272 Timing
273 Temperature
273 Colour selection principles: 2. Harmonising and contrasting effects
275 Step-by-steps
279 **GH17.4 Lighten hair**
279 Lightening hair
280 Types of lightener
282 Step-by-steps
285 **GH17.5 Resolve basic colouring problems**
285 Colouring problems

287 **GH17.6** Provide aftercare advice

288 Explain how routine styling tools can have detrimental effects

288 Show and recommend the products/equipment that you use

289 Demonstrate the techniques that you use

289 Checkerboard

290 Revision questions

Chapter**twelve**

291 **Colour correction: Unit GH18 Provide colour correction services**

291 Colour correction: quick overview

291 What do I need to do for GH18.1?

291 What do I need to do for GH18.2?

292 What do I need to do for GH18.3?

292 What do I need to do for GH18.4?

292 What do I need to do for GH18.5?

292 What aspects do I need to cover for GH18.1, GH18.2, GH18.3, GH18.4 and GH18.5?

293 What aspects do I need to know for GH18.1, GH18.2, GH18.3, GH18.4 and GH18.5?

293 Introduction

294 Foreword

294 **GH18.1** Maintain effective and safe methods of working when colour correcting hair

294 Preparation and safety

297 **GH18.2** Determine the problem

297 Colour correction considerations

298 Consultation for colour correction

300 Colour tests

301 Record the details of your consultation

303 **GH18.3** Plan and agree a course of action to correct colour

303 Colour perfection?

303 Pre-pigmentation

304 Colouring back: Reintroducing colour into bleached hair

304 Decolouring

305 Process preparation

306 Reapplying to natural depth

307 Removal of permanent, synthetic hair dyes

308 Banded hair colour

309 Gradated colour

309 Discoloured highlights/lowlights and partial applications

310 Newly introduced colours

311 Over-porous hair

311 Removing artificial colour

312 **GH18.4** Correct colour

312 Step-by-steps

316 **GH18.5** Provide aftercare advice

316 Lifestyle

318 Checkerboard

319 Revision questions

Chapter**thirteen**

320 **Perming hair: Unit GH22 Create a variety of permed effects**

320 Creative perming: quick overview

320 What do I need to do for GH22.1?

320 What do I need to do for GH22.2?

321 What do I need to do for GH22.3?

321 What do I need to do for GH22.4?

321 What aspects do I need to cover for GH22.1, GH22.2, GH22.3 and GH22.4?

321 What aspects do I need to know for GH22.1, GH22.2, GH22.3 and GH22.4?

322 Introduction

322 Foreword

323 How perms work

324 **GH22.1** Maintain effective and safe methods of working when perming hair

324 Protecting the client and yourself

325 Working effectively

327 Types of perm

327 **GH22.2** Prepare for perming

328 Consultation

329 What should you find out before you start?

330 What contra-indications are you looking for?

331 Hair tests

331 Record the results

331 Pre-perm and post-perm treatments

332 Sensitised hair

334 **GH22.3** Create a variety of permed effects

335 Perming tools and equipment

335 Basic sectioning

335 Basic wind

336 Acid and alkaline perming solutions

339 Alternative/creative winding techniques

341 Other types of perming equipment

342 Straightening hair

344 Neutralising

348 After the perm

349 **GH22.4** Provide aftercare advice

350 Checkerboard
351 Revision questions

Chapter**fourteen**

352 **Develop your creativity: Unit GH21 Develop and enhance your creative hairdressing skills**

352 Developing creativity: quick overview
352 What do I need to do for G21.1?
352 What do I need to do for G21.2?
352 What do I need to do for G21.3?
353 What aspects do I need to cover for G21.1, G21.2 and G21.3?
353 What things do I need to know for G21.1, G21.2 and G21.3?
353 Introduction
353 Foreword
354 **GH21.1 Plan and design a range of images**

354 Hair creativity
354 Pictures and images
355 Thinking about creative design
355 Analysing the essential components
356 Design aspects
359 Other hair aspects
362 **GH21.2 Produce a range of creative images**

362 Photography and photo sessions
364 The photographer
364 The make-up artist
364 Clothes and accessories
365 Storyboard the plan
365 Create your inclusion lists
365 On the day
365 Backdrops and lighting
366 File format
367 Hairdressing competitions
370 **GH21.3 Evaluate your results against the design plan objectives**

370 Checkerboard
371 Revision questions

Part**three**

372 **Supporting management**

Chapter**fifteen**

374 **Health and safety: Unit G22 Monitor procedures to safely control work operations**

374 Health and safety: quick overview
374 What do I need to do for G22.1?
374 What do I need to do for G22.2?
374 What aspects do I need to cover for G22.1 and G22.2?
375 What things do I need to know for G22.1 and G22.2?
375 Introduction
376 **G22.1 Check that health and safety instructions are followed**

376 What health and safety law requires
377 How regulations apply
378 Employees' responsibilities
379 Record keeping
379 Employer's responsibilities
389 **G22.2 Make sure that risks are controlled safely and effectively**

389 Hazard and risk
390 Potential hazards in workplace
391 Process for undertaking COSHH risk assessment
392 Working environment
392 Controlling risks in the workplace
393 Lifting and handling large objects
395 Checkerboard
396 Revision questions

Chapter**sixteen**

397 **Being effective in your work: Unit G11 Contribute to the financial effectiveness of the business**

397 Personal effectiveness: quick overview
397 What do I need to do for G11.1?
397 What do I need to do for G11.2?
398 What aspects do I need to cover for G11.1 and G11.2?
398 What do I need to know for G11.1 and G11.2?
398 Introduction
399 **G11.1 Contribute to the effective use and monitoring of resources**

399 Human resources
399 Working conditions
400 Working hours
402 Staff training
403 Good communication
404 Body language
404 Generally accepted code of conduct at work
404 Dealing with client complaints
405 People's rights and consumer legislation
408 Stock and stock control
413 Time and time management
414 Get organised
415 **G11.2 Meet productivity and development targets**

416 Maintaining productivity
416 Targets
417 SMART productivity
417 Recognise achievement
417 Evaluating results
418 Working together
418 Personal development
418 Measuring effectiveness
420 An example of job description
420 The appraisal process
421 Self-appraisal
421 Checkerboard
422 Revision questions

Chapter**seventeen**

423 **Planning promotional activities:
Unit H32 Contribute to the planning
and implementation of promotional
activities**

423 Promotional activities: quick overview
423 What do I need to do for H32.1?
423 What do I need to do for H32.2?
424 What do I need to do for H32.3?
424 What aspects do I need to cover for H32.1, H32.2 and H32.3?
424 What do I need to know for H32.1, H32.2 and H32.3?
424 Introduction
425 **H32.1 Contribute to the planning and preparation of promotional activities**
425 Initial preparation
426 Working to a budget
426 Decide on the type of promotion
427 Setting your objectives
427 Define your target market
428 Pitch your idea
428 Produce a detailed plan
429 Other things to consider
431 **H32.2 Implement promotional activities**
431 Hairdressing demonstration

431 Select the venue
431 Plan the demonstration
432 Expect the unexpected
432 Make a time schedule
432 Communicating the message
433 Presentation and demonstration skills
434 Advertising, PR and the Press
436 **H32.3 Participate in the evaluation of promotional activities**
437 The purpose of your evaluation
437 Evaluating your promotional response
437 Collect, collate and analyse the information
438 Presenting an evaluation report
438 Checkerboard
439 Revision questions

440 **Appendix 1** Useful addresses and websites
443 **Appendix 2** Accidents, emergencies and manual handling
450 **Appendix 3** End of chapter revision test answers
453 **Appendix 4** People's rights and consumer legislation
456 **Glossary**
459 **Index**

Website

A further two units can be found on
www.cengage.co.uk/prohair

Web Chapter**one**

Facial massage: Unit GB9 Provide face massage services

Web Chapter**two**

Hair patterns and designs: Unit AH35 Design and create patterns in hair

Foreword

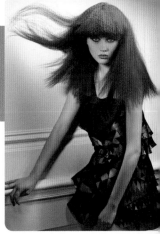

TRACEY DEVINE
@ ANGELS

When we developed the first set of standards for Level 3, we had no idea of the incredible impact they would make on the growing professionalism of the hairdressing industry. Yet without the vision of Martin Green and Leo Palladino, and their seminal book *Professional Hairdressing – The Official Guide to Level 3, Revised 6e*, that impact would not have been as great.

Both Martin and Leo are incredibly passionate and enthusiastic about their industry. But both also have a rare skill: they are able to communicate that passion and enthusiasm to others and translate it into knowledge based on years of experience working in salons and with clients.

Whatever salon issue it is, from dealing with difficult clients to achieving the perfect cut that will leave your customers glowing, Martin and Leo have been there themselves and developed solutions that are tried, tested and effective. Add to that the contribution from Theresa Bullock on hair extensions and *Professional Hairdressing* forms the complete guide for anyone working towards Level 3.

This revised edition also reflects the changes taking place in the Qualifications and Credit Framework (QCF), which means it is completely up to date and flexible, being useful whether you are working towards an NVQ or VRQs.

A testament to the ongoing longevity of *Professional Hairdressing* is that it now forms part of a wider range of learning materials from Habia and Cengage Learning, such as the innovative U2Learn e-learning range, showing just how well it has stood the test of time and why it is the number one choice for Level 3 learners.

I am incredibly proud of the association between Habia and the authors of this book, and hope that this is the starting point to a long and successful career for you.

Alan Goldsbro
Chief Executive Officer
Habia

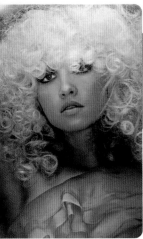

TRACEY DEVINE @ ANGELS

Acknowledgements

The authors and publishers would like to thank the following:

For providing pictures for the book

Adam Harris @ MG Martin Gold, Stanmore
Alamy
Andrew O'Toole (photographer)
Dr Andrew Wright
Anne McGuigan @ Anne McGuigan Hair and Beauty,
    Leighton Buzzard
The Artistic Team @ Jacks of London
The Artistic Team @ TPL Hairdressing
BaByliss Pro
Balmain
Beauty Express
Dr M H Beck
Ben White and the Eleven Hair Art Team
Christopher Appleton @ George's Hair Salon, Leicester
Chubb
Cinderella Hair: www.cinderellahair.co.uk
Clynol
Connect-2-Hair Ltd
Damien Carney for Joico
Daniele Cipriani (photographer)
Denman
Dome Cosmetics
Ellisons
Errol Douglas
Essence PR
Fellowship for British Hairdressing FAME Team 2008
Gloss Communications
Goldwell UK
Gorgeous PR
Great Lengths (www.greatlengths.net)
Habia
Hama Sanders (photographer)
HMSO
i-stock photography

IT&LY
Jemico
Dr John Gray
John Rawson
The John Rawson partnership
Karen Scantlebury @ Ciente, Berkhamsted
Karine Jackson
Ken Picton @ Ken Picton
Kiyoshi Inoue and Tim Hartley for DAVINES
Kyoko Homma (photographer)
L'Oréal Professionnel
Lee Moran @ Sanrizz
Leonardo Rizzo @ Sanrizz
Lewis Moore @ Francesco Group, Streetly
Lynne Welsh @ Mosko, Wishaw
M. Balfre
Mahogany Hairdressing Salons and Academy
    (www.mahoganyhair.co.uk)
Mark Woolley (hair stylist), Pete Webb (photographer)
Matrix
Mediscan
Melanie Tudor@ En Route Hair and Beauty, Wakefield
Michael Barnes for Goldwell
NHF Inspire, Photography: Simon Powell
Paul Falltrick for Matrix
Paul Hawes @ Review, Petersfield and Waterlooville,
Hants
Rae Palmer for Schwarzkopf
REM
Richard Ward
Rush London
Saks Hair and Beauty (www.saks.co.uk)
SANRIZZ Artistic Team
Scott Smurthwaite @ Cream
Sharon Cox @ Sanrizz
Susan Hall @ Reds Hair and Beauty, Sunderland

Terry Calvert and the Clipso Artistic Team
Theresa Bullock
Tim Lawton @ TPL Hairdressing, Nantwich
Tracey Devine @ Angels, Aberdeen
UK Skills
Vicky Turner @ Goldsworthy's
Wahl (UK) Ltd
Wella
Wellcome images
www.gebetterton.co.uk

For their help with the photoshoot

Photoshoot location:
HQ Hair
71 High Street, and 25 Cambray Place, Cheltenham, Gloucestershire

Models:
Alex Bilak
Elisabeth Crabbe
Caroline Palmer
Dale Carney
Dawn Stanley
Es John
Gareth Dazely
Sara Horder
Laura Paoletti
Lucia Parry
Jamie Horder
Holly Batin
Sian Jennings
Sean O'Riley
Teyah Lee
Tom O'Shea
Lucy Dix

Stylists:
HQ Hair Cheltenham
Martin Green
Jodi Green
Becci Fincham

Make up:
Holly Batin

Photography:
Fi Deane

Special Thank You

Goldwell for all their help and support in providing the products and technical assistance within the photo shoot.

Every effort has been made to trace the copyright holders, but if any have been inadvertently overlooked the publisher will be pleased to make the necessary arrangements at the first opportunity. Please contact the publisher directly.

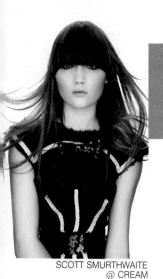

SCOTT SMURTHWAITE
@ CREAM

Introduction

As professional, qualified hairdressers and barbers, you will already be aware of the necessity to do more and to do it better for your clients. Staying the same and offering just enough is never enough; you know what its like, because competition is tough. You have already achieved a lot and travelled a long way down a personal career path, but it wasn't enough; you still wanted more.

You want to be recognized for what you have achieved and now is the time to push that boundary further. You do this so that you can draw a professional distinction between you and the others working in your industry. You have chosen to develop your skills further and want a wider, national acknowledgement, for the services and treatments that you will be providing to your clients in the future.

And that's why you're doing your Level 3 NVQ Diploma.

Good luck

Martin Green

Level 3 NVQ Diploma in Hairdressing or Barbering

SCOTT SMURTHWAITE
@ CREAM

When you previously qualified as a stylist there would have been a wide range of routes and options that you could have taken. Some of you may have followed the NVQ curriculum and that could have been as a full-time college student, or through a salon-based apprenticeship. Some of you may never have had a formal training at all and reached 'qualification' by the 'time-served', experience route.

The National Vocational Qualification has provided the main curriculum route for salon- and college-based training for many years. Historically, the ways in which these qualifications were structured meant that students or trainees would complete a variety of compulsory – or mandatory – units and then could choose from other options, some additional units in order to complete their qualification.

That has now changed. There are now two types of accredited qualification:

1 The VRQ
2 The NVQ

The VRQ or vocationally related qualification is specifically designed for college-based delivery on either a full- or part-time basis. There are a wide variety of qualifications designed to meet VRQ criteria and these can provide students with some practical experience and an insight to what happens 'out in industry'.

The NVQ or NVQ Diploma as it is now called, is the only type of qualification that provides the learner with a 'job ready' qualification. That means that for students who want to be trained up to 'working in a salon' standard, this will be the only option available to them. However, many colleges have chosen the NVQ Diploma as the preferred route and any students enrolled on this type of programme, can expect that at least part of the course will be on work placement out in industry.

The other main changes relate to the 'value' or weighting of the individual units that make up the hairdressing and barbering qualification at all NVQ Diploma levels. Now, both VRQs and NVQs are required to meet the Qualifications and Credit Framework (QCF).

The different units currently have a varying amount of credit values. In order to complete an NVQ Diploma the learner will complete all mandatory units and make up the 'outstanding balance' of credits by choosing from optional units that will make up at least the minimum number of credits that are required to gain full certification.

This may seem confusing but is explained in more detail on the following page.

NVQ Diploma (QCF) – An Introduction

HABIA, The Hair and Beauty Industry Authority, is the representative organization responsible for defining the standards for our hair and beauty industry. The National Occupational Standards (NOS) that they produce are then taken and used by awarding bodies such as City & Guilds (C&G) or VTCT to create the qualifications that you take part in. So in simple terms HABIA produce the standards that you work towards and C&G define the conditions and specifications against which you are assessed.

So all NOS have a common structure and design. That is to say they all follow a particular format for all vocational sectors. Each vocational qualification is structured in the same way and is made up from a number of grouped components.

Level 3 NVQ Diploma in Hairdressing

STRUCTURE OF UNITS:

Candidates must complete **four mandatory units** and gain a **minimum of 37 optional credits** to achieve the qualification.

The mandatory units are:

Unit title	Credit value	Chapter
G22 Monitor procedures to safely control work operations (ENTO HSS3)	4 credits	15
G18 Promote additional services or products to clients (ICS Unit 10)	6 credits	2
G21 Provide hairdressing consultation services	3 credits	1
GH16 Creatively cut hair using a combination of techniques	8 credits	4

(All of these must be completed.)

PLUS a minimum of 37 optional credits from below. Only one unit can be chosen from option group 2 (all optional credits can be chosen from option group 1 if desired)

Option Group 1

Unit title	Credit value	Chapter
GH17 Colour hair using a variety of techniques	12 credits	11
GH18 Provide colour correction services	13 credits	12
GH19 Creatively style and dress hair	4 credits	8
GH20 Creatively dress long hair	5 credits	9
GH21 Develop & enhance your creative hairdressing skills	5 credits	14
GH22 Create a variety of permed effects	8 credits	8
GH23 Provide creative hair extension services	8 credits	10
GH24 Provide specialist consultation services for hair and scalp conditions	5 credits	New for 7th Edition
GH25 Provide specialist hair and scalp treatments (NOTE GH24 and GH25 must be taken together)	7 credits	

Option Group 2

Unit title	Credit value	Chapter
Unit G11 Contribute to the financial effectiveness of the business	4 credits	16
G19 Support client service improvements (ICS Unit 37)	5 credits	3
H32 Contribute to the planning & implementation of promotional activities	5 credits	17

ENTO – Employment National Training Organisation
ICS – Institute of Customer Services

Level 3 NVQ Diploma in Barbering

STRUCTURE OF UNITS:

Candidates must complete **five mandatory units** plus a **minimum of 25 optional credits** to achieve the full qualification.

The mandatory units are:

Unit title	Credit value	Chapter
G22 Monitor procedures to safely control work operations (ENTO HSS3)	4 credits	15
G18 Promote additional services or products to clients (ICS Unit 10)	6 credits	2
G21 Provide hairdressing consultation services	3 credits	1
GB7 Design & create a range of facial hair techniques	4 credits	6
GB8 Creatively cut hair using a combination of barbering techniques	5 credits	5

(All of these must be completed.)

PLUS a minimum of 25 optional credits from below. Only one unit can be chosen from option group 2 (all optional credits can be chosen from option group 1 if desired)

Option Group 1

Unit title	Credit value	Chapter
GB6 Provide shaving services	4 credits	5
Unit GB9 Provide face massage services	4 credits	New
AH35 Design & create patterns in hair	5 credits	New
GH17 Colour hair using a variety of techniques	12 credits	11
GH18 Provide colour correction services	13 credits	12
GH21 Develop & enhance your creative hairdressing skills	5 credits	14
GH22 Create a variety of permed effects	8 credits	8
GH24 Provide specialist consultation services for hair and scalp conditions	5 credits	New for 7th Edition
GH25 Provide specialist hair and scalp treatments (NOTE GH24 and GH25 must be taken together)	7 credits	New for 7th Edition

Option Group 2

Unit title	Credit value	Chapter
Unit G11 Contribute to the financial effectiveness of the business	4 credits	16
G19 Support client service improvements (ICS Unit 37)	5 credits	3
H32 Contribute to the planning & implementation of promotional activities	5 credits	17

ENTO – Employment National Training Organisation
ICS – Institute of Customer Services

Units and main outcomes

The individual units listed above denote the smallest components of the NVQ that can be awarded by certificate. Each unit comprises a unit title and one or more individual learning objectives or **main outcomes** and these are the smallest meaningful components within an NVQ.

Unit title and main outcomes (example Consultation unit)

Unit title	Main outcomes
Unit G21 Provide hairdressing consultation services	G21.1 Identify client's needs and wishes
	G21.2 Analyse the hair, skin and scalp
	G21.3 Make recommendations to clients
	G21.4 Advise clients on hair maintenance and management
	G21.5 Agree services with your client

The main outcomes

Main outcomes are brief statements that outline the tasks that need to be done. Their titles are always expressed in a 'do this' language, e.g. 'Identify the hazards and evaluate the risks in your workplace'. However, while giving you an idea of what **needs** to be done, it doesn't say **how** it's to be done.

The **NOS** cover this in greater detail. They specify how each task is to be performed by listing the **performance criteria**. They also cover the circumstances, conditions or situations in which these actions must be done which is called the **range**.

Performance criteria

The performance criteria are a list of the essential actions. Although these may not be necessarily in the order in which they should be done, they do provide a definitive checklist of what needs doing. During assessment, these performance criteria form the specification of how a task must be done.

Example of performance criteria (G21.1) showing how the task must be done

Main outcome	Performance criteria
G21.1 Identify clients' needs and wishes	**By:** a) encouraging your client to express their wishes and views
	By: b) allowing your client sufficient time to express their wishes and views
	By: c) asking relevant questions in a way your client will understand
	By: d) using visual aids to present clients with suitable ideas to help them reach decision
	By: e) encouraging your client to ask about areas of which they are unsure
	f) confirming your understanding of your client's wishes before making any service recommendations

Range

The range statements provide a number of conditions or applications in which the main outcomes must be performed. Quite simply, they state under what particular circumstances, and on what occasions, or in which special situations, the activity must take place.

Example of range statements – identifying which situations or circumstances need to be included when doing the task

Main outcome	Range
G21.1 Identify clients' needs and wishes	**By means of:** a) questioning
	By means of: b) observation
	By means of: c) testing

Essential Knowledge and understanding (referred to as EKU within this book)

NVQs are not just about doing though; when you do your work properly, you need to know **what** you are doing and **why** you are doing it. The terms 'theory', 'learning' and 'principles' generally refer to essential knowledge and understanding, in other words, **what you must know**.

Typical knowledge statements covering the things you need to know:

Main outcome	What you must know (EKU)
G21.1 Identify clients' needs and wishes	**You should know:** how and when tests are carried out on hair and skin
	You should know: how the following factors limit or affect the services and products that can be offered to clients: - lifestyle - adverse hair, skin and scalp conditions
	You should know: current fashion trends and looks

At the point where a task's performance criteria and range have been covered and knowledge has been learnt and understood, the task is carried out competently and a skill has been acquired.

Shared knowledge

Units and main outcomes often share similar components i.e. some of the performance criteria used within a main outcome from one task is often similar to that used within another.

Example:

GH19.1 Maintain effective and safe methods of working when styling hair and GH16.1 Maintain effective and safe methods of working when cutting.

Similarly, the knowledge that is essential; underpinning one main outcome, will often occur in another. This duplication may at first seem unnecessary, but it happens because of the modular, stand-alone design of NVQ units. (Remember, each individual unit can be awarded on a certificate.)

This can be useful in terms of speeding up the learning process as sometimes knowledge or skills learnt in one activity are then directly applicable to other tasks. This is also useful when it comes to recording these learnt experiences, because the knowledge learnt in one situation can be quickly cross-referenced to other similar activities in your portfolio.

Under assessment

Your competence, your ability to carry out a task to a standard, is measured during **assessment**. Your ability to carry out the task, 'performance evidence', will be observed and checked against the performance criteria. Therefore your assessor will be watching to see how you carry out your work.

Sometimes it is not possible to cover all the situations that might crop up in one performance. So, in that situation, your assessor might ask you questions about what you have done and how you might apply that in different circumstances. To help you get used to this, the activities that appear throughout the book contain lots of the types of questions that you might be asked.

Your understanding and background knowledge of work tasks is also measured through questions asked by your assessor. Sometimes you might be asked to give a personal account of what you have learned. This could take the form of writing a sequence of events that need to be done to complete the task satisfactorily. Other questions may ask you specifically about particular tasks; more often than not, these types of questions take the form of short-answer, or multiple-choice questions. Again, the activities covered within this book give plenty of examples and practice.

About this book

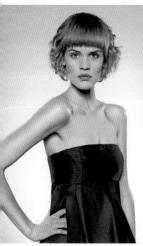

ADAM HARRIS @
MG MARTIN GOLD

The common structure and design that exists within NVQs is mirrored in many ways within this text. For the first time in the hairdressing NVQs official series, revisions and updates have been totally reworked to both 'target' and 'fit' the needs of the learner and the occupational standards. The navigation to standards, access to information, quick referencing and illustration have been redesigned and reorganised in order to help you accelerate through your Level 3 programme. This uniform format or book style incorporates a number of features:

- a common structure and design throughout the text with explanations of the standards and on how to use this book;
- easy referencing systems to include tables, checklists, activities and tips;
- the same format and unit references as NVQs covering both mandatory and the various option groups.

How to use this book

Each chapter addresses specific units from the Level 3 NVQ Diploma. At the beginning of each chapter a referencing system provides a quick signposting to the information you want, providing a variety of starting and finishing points. There is a variety of features and icons used within the text.

What do I need to do? Customised information, telling you about what you need to do to, in order to complete the performance criteria in simple terms.

What aspects do I need to cover? This provides you with a list of things that you need to cover when doing the performance criteria.

What do I need to know? A simple list of things that you need to know in relation to the unit.

Diversion In order to eliminate unnecessary duplication, these references are linked to other relevant information and can be found from the index in the back of this book.

Key words Special or technical terms.

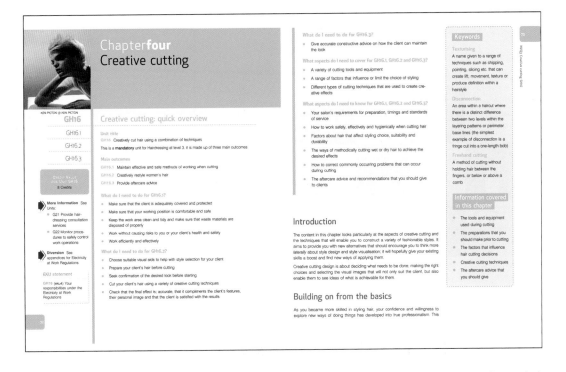

Activity Suggestions for useful learning activities linked with the task.

Remember boxes Tips or hints on points to remember.

Good practice/health and safety Examples of good practice or procedure.

Hair science Scientific principles that relate to hairdressing and barbering.

Learner support signposts Online activities available on the learner side of the eteach hairdressing website.

Tutor support signposts Online activities available on the tutor side of the eteach hairdressing website.

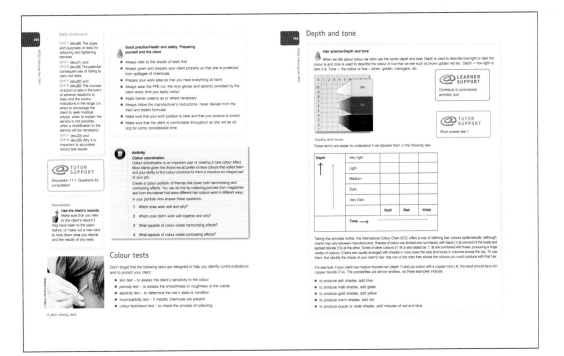

Checkerboard Self-check system and a means of recording progress towards achievement.

Self-test section A variety of self-assessment tests including short answer, multiple choice, true or false, etc.

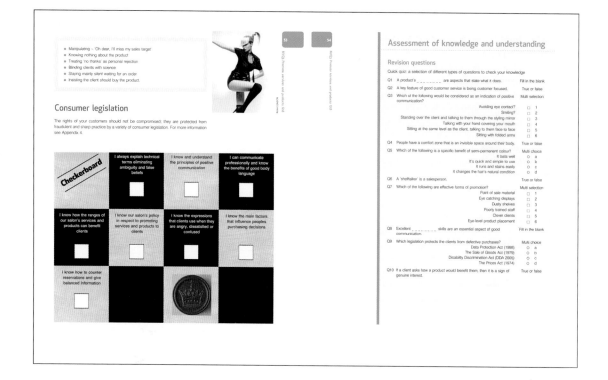

e-teaching website

A **new e-teaching website for trainers** accompanies this textbook. This resource includes **handouts, PowerPoint® slides, interactive assessments,** an **image bank** and **video clips** – all carefully designed to help trainers make classroom delivery more interactive and to provide extra materials for lesson planning.

Please visit **www.eteachhairdressing.co.uk** for more information or contact your Cengage Learning sales representative at **emea.fesales@cengage.com**.

In addition, two further units (*Facial massage: Unit GB9 Provide face massage services* and *Hair patterns and designs: Unit AH35 Design and create patterns in hair*) can be found at **www.cengage.co.uk/prohair**.

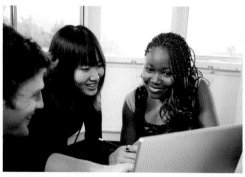

Students! Access your FREE online resources by following the Level 3 student links on www.eteachhairdressing.co.uk and entering your password 'perming'.

Essential knowledge mapping

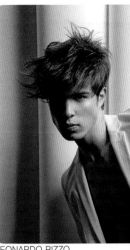

LEONARDO RIZZO
@ SANRIZZ

To use this essential knowledge mapping grid simply find the EKU statement in the standards that you want to learn more about. Then using this grid match the number to its corresponding page.

For example, say that you want to look up the information about **G18.6 How to give appropriate balanced information to clients about services or products** from within **Unit G18 Promote additional products or services to clients**, just look in the table G18 below and look at the corresponding page for EKU number 6.

Green units are applicable to both Barbering and Hairdressing		Blue units are applicable to Barbering at Level 3		Orange units are applicable to Hairdressing at Level 3	

G21 Provide hairdressing consultation services

EKU	1	2	3	4	5	6	7	8	9	10	11	12	13	14	15	16	17	18	19
Page	4	4	20	40	36	35	39	40	35	20	35	35	15	15	15	15	10	21	15
EKU	20	21	22	23	24	25	26	27	28	29	30	31	32	33	34	35			
Page	23	23	23	20	20	8	40	7	11	37	38	38	37	38	38				

G18 Promote additional products or services to clients

EKU	1	2	3	4	5	6
Page	46	46	46	46	36	50

G19 Support client service improvements

EKU	1	2	3	4
Page	56	57	60	65

GH16 Creatively cut hair using a combination of techniques

EKU	1	2	3	4	5	6	7	8	9	10	11	12	13	14	15	16	17	18	19
Page	74	78	76	72	78	74	74	78	74	77	77	77	77	84	77	75	79	79	81
EKU	20	21	22	23	24	25	26	27	28	29	30	31	32	33	34	35	36	37	38
Page	83	85	85	74	101	94	94	79	90	84	88	87	91	94	89	89	75	88	75

EKU	39	40	41	42															
Page	89	100	101	101															

GB8 Creatively cut hair using a combination of barbering techniques

EKU	1	2	3	4	5	6	7	8	9	10	11	12	13	14	15	16	17	18	19
Page	107	108	109	104	109	108	107	107	107	107	109	107	109	107	116	107	107	125	111
EKU	20	21	22	23	24	25	26	27	28	29	30	31	32	33	34	35	36	37	38
Page	113	113	111	111	108	123	114	122	118	116	123	123	121	120	118	118	123	123	116
EKU	39	40	41	42	43	44	45	46	47	48									
Page	123	120	122	126	126	126	109	109	109	126									

GB7 Design and create a range of facial hair shapes

EKU	1	2	3	4	5	6	7	8	9	10	11	12	13	14	15	16	17	18	19
Page	131	132	133	129	131	140	131	131	131	133	132	132	133	132	132	137	137	138	137
EKU	20	21	22	23	24	25	26	27	28	29	30	31	32	33	34	35	36	37	38
Page	134	143	143	133	134	134	141	139	139	139	139	139	139	135	142	143	142	143	143
EKU	39	40	41	42	43														
Page	133	129	134	134	133														

GB6 Provide shaving services

EKU	1	2	3	4	5	6	7	8	9	10	11	12	13	14	15	16	17	18	19
Page	148	148	156	146	156	148	152	149	152	148	151	148	148	149	149	151	149	148	153
EKU	20	21	22	23	24	25	26	27	28	29	30	31	32	33	34	35	36	37	38
Page	154	154	154	154	153	154	154	154	157	150	151	154	157	153	149	154	154	155	154
EKU	39	40	41	42	43	44	45	46	47	48									
Page	156	156	156	156	156	157	157	157	157	156									

GB9 Provide face massage services (on website www.cengage.co.uk/prohair)

EKU	1	2	3	4	5	6	7	8	9	10	11	12	13	14	15	16	17	18	19
Page	9	9	9	15	1	1	1	9	9	9	9	9	10	10	10	10	10	11	11
EKU	20	21	22	23	24	25	26	27	28	29	30	31	32	33	34	35	36	37	38
Page	11	11	11	11	12	12	12	12	12	12	12	12	3	6	6	6	3	3	3
EKU	39	40	41	42	43	44	45												
Page	3	3	15	15	15	15	15												

AH35 Design and create patterns in hair (on website www.cengage.co.uk/prohair)

EKU	1	2	3	4	5	6	7	8	9	10	11	12	13	14	15	16	17	18	19
Page	3	4	3	1	4	3	3	4	3	3	3	3	3	4	4	3	10	10	10
EKU	20	21	22	23	24	25	26	27	28	29	30	31	32	33	34	35	36	37	38
Page	10	5	11	6	6	6	6	9	10	16	16	16	11	11	11	6	6	11	11
EKU	39	40	41	42	43	44	45	46	47										
Page	10	11	13	16	13	10	9	13	14										

GH19 Creatively style and dress hair

EKU	1	2	3	4	5	6	7	8	9	10	11	12	13	14	15	16	17	18	19
Page	162	163	160	160	163	163	162	162	162	162	163	162	162	163	160	160	163	169	164
EKU	20	21	22	23	24	25	26	27	28	29	30	31	32	33	34	35	36	37	38
Page	179	169	169	169	172	172	181	181	163	164	164	168	175	181	175	175	175	181	175
EKU	39	40	41	42	43	44													
Page	175	182	184	184	181	184													

GH20 Creatively dress long hair

EKU	1	2	3	4	5	6	7	8	9	10	11	12	13	14	15	16	17	18	19
Page	189	197	187	190	190	189	189	189	189	189	189	189	189	189	195	211	191	197	200
EKU	20	21	22	23	24	25	26	27	28	29	30	31	32	33	34	35	36	37	38
Page	200	199	195	193	195	195	190	191	191	194	198	200	204	203	204	198	204	204	197
EKU	39	40	41	42	43	44	45												
Page	198	211	211	211	211														

GH23 Provide creative hair extension services

EKU	1	2	3	4	5	6	7	8	9	10	11	12	13	14	15	16	17	18	19
Page	216	226	217	214	214	216	214	216	216	216	217	216	218	216	217	217	216	218	216
EKU	20	21	22	23	24	25	26	27	28	29	30	31	32	33	34	35	36	37	38
Page	226	226	226	224	224	224	224	224	224	224	224	222	226	217	217	226	223	218	227
EKU	39	40	41	42	43	44	45	46	47	48	49	50	51	52	53	54	55	56	57
Page	228	227	224	227	222	218	218	226	234	237	237	229	217	218	229	229	229	242	240
EKU	58	59	60	61	62	63	64	65	66	67	68	69	70	71	72	73	74	75	76
Page	242	245	222	237	237	237	237	237	242	242	240	245	245	245	245	245	245	245	245
EKU	77	78	79	80	81	82													
Page	245	245	245	242	242	242													

GH17 Colour hair using a variety of techniques

EKU	1	2	3	4	5	6	7	8	9	10	11	12	13	14	15	16	17	18	19
Page	252	252	252	252	252	252	249	263	260	260	260	260	260	263	283	279	281	260	260
EKU	20	21	22	23	24	25	26	27	28	29	30	31	32	33	34	35	36	37	38
Page	260	280	260	268	268	268	266	268	268	269	280	256	266	266	256	258	253	265	253
EKU	39	40	41	42	43	44	45	46	47	48	49	50	51	52	53	54	55	56	57
Page	279	256	259	272	260	279	272	281	271	256	264	269	256	264	270	270	270	272	270
EKU	58	59	60	61	62	63	64	65	66	67	68	69	70	71	72	73	74	75	76
Page	264	269	269	280	275	273	281	269	280	285	272	269	279	272	285	288	286	286	286
EKU	77	78	79																
Page	286	286	286																

GH18 Provide colour correction services

EKU	1	2	3	4	5	6	7	8	9	10	11	12	13	14	15	16	17	18	19
Page	295	295	291	291	291	296	296	296	296	296	296	296	296	296	296	296	296	296	296
EKU	20	21	22	23	24	25	26	27	28	29	30	31	32	33	34	35	36	37	38
Page	296	296	296	296	300	300	300	300	300	300	300	302	303	302	302	302	302	303	302
EKU	39	40	41	42	43	44	45	46	47	48	49	50	51	52	53	54	55	56	57
Page	302	302	302	302	302	311	302	302	303	303	303	303	303	303	303	305	303	303	311
EKU	58	59	60	61	62	63	64	65	66	67	68	69	70	71					
Page	308	303	306	309	304	304	304	316	316	316	316	316	316	316					

GH22 Create a variety of permed effects

EKU	1	2	3	4	5	6	7	8	9	10	11	12	13	14	15	16	17	18	19
Page	324	324	331	326	320	325	320	324	326	324	324	324	324	324	324	324	325	325	325
EKU	20	21	22	23	24	25	26	27	28	29	30	31	32	33	34	35	36	37	38
Page	325	325	325	328	331	331	330	330	330	330	330	330	323	332	332	332	332	338	332
EKU	39	40	41	42	43	44	45	46	47	48	49	50	51	52	53	54	55	56	57
Page	323	337	327	332	344	327	329	339	333	341	332	332	344	338	343	347	347	347	347
EKU	58	59	60	61	62	63													
Page	347	347	347	347	347	347													

GH21 Develop and enhance your creative hairdressing skills

EKU	1	2	3	4	5	6	7	8	9	10	11	12	13	14	15	16	17	18	19
Page	363	363	363	363	363	356	356	356	356	356	370	370	370	370	363	363	363	363	363
EKU	20	21	22	23	24	25	26	27	28	29	30	31	32	33	34	35			
Page	363	354	354	354	354	354	354	354	354	363	359	359	359	359	359	359			

G22 monitor procedures to safely control work operations

EKU	1	2	3	4	5	6	7	8	9	10	11	12	13	14	15	16			
Page	378	378	378	378	389	390	389	375	378	386	380	390	390	380	380	378			

G11 Contribute to the financial effectiveness of the business

EKU	1	2	3	4	5	6	7	8	9	10	11	12	13	14	15	16	17	18	19
Page	399	405	406	399	415	407	399	407	409	407	407	407	399	403	403	420	403	403	420
EKU	20	21	22	23	24	25	26	27											
Page	413	417	415	415	415	415	420	420											

H32 Contribute to the planning and implementation of promotional activities

EKU	1	2	3	4	5	6	7	8	9	10	11	12	13	14	15	16	17	18	19
Page	430	430	430	430	430	430	425	425	425	425	425	425	425	425	425	425	430	430	431
EKU	20	21	22	23	24	25	26	27	28	29	30	31	32	33	34				
Page	426	423	423	423	436	436	436	436	433	433	436	436	436	436	436				

PROFESSIONAL HAIRDRESSING
VRQ mapping grid

Unit Ref	Unit credit (QCF)	VRQ Unit Title	Unit Level	Ch1 G21	Ch2 G18	Ch3 G19	Ch4 GH16	Ch5 GB8	Ch6 GB7	Ch7 GB6	Ch8 GH19	Ch9 GH20	Ch10 GH23	Ch11 GH17	Ch12 GH18	Ch13 GH22	Ch14 GH21	Ch15 G22	Ch16 G11	Ch17 H32	Web Ch1 GB9	Web Ch2 AH35
R/600/8780	4	Monitor and maintain health and safety practice in the salon	3															X				
T/600/8769	2	Promote products and services to clients in a salon	3		X																	
D/600/8779	7	Maintaining personal health and wellbeing	3				X															
Y/600/8635	8	Cut women's hair to create a variety of looks	3				X															
R/600/8634	7	Style and dress hair using a variety of techniques	3								X	X										
D/6008636	11	Colour hair to create a variety of looks	3											X								
H/600/8637	8	Creative Hairdressing design skills	3														X					

PROFESSIONAL HAIRDRESSING
VRQ mapping grid

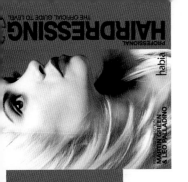

Unit Ref	Unit credit (QCF)	VRQ Unit Title	Unit Level	Ch1 G21	Ch2 G18	Ch3 G19	Ch4 GH16	Ch5 GB8	Ch6 GB7	Ch7 GB6	Ch8 GH19	Ch9 GH20	Ch10 GH23	Ch11 GH17	Ch12 GH18	Ch13 GH22	Ch14 GH21	Ch15 G22	Ch16 G11	Ch17 H32	Web Ch1 GB9	Web Ch2 AH35
J/600/8632	6	Create an Image based on a theme within the hair and beauty Sector	3	X																		
H/600/9061	3	Hairdressing consultation support for colleagues	3														X					
D/600/9060	4	Cut facial hair to create a variety of looks	3						X													
K/600/9062	5	Cut men's hair to create a variety of looks	3					X														
K/600/9059	4	Bridal hairstyling	3																			
A/600/9034	5	Hair Extension services	3										X									
M/601/2481	7	Human Resource Management within the hair and beauty sector	3																X			

PROFESSIONAL HAIRDRESSING
VRQ mapping grid

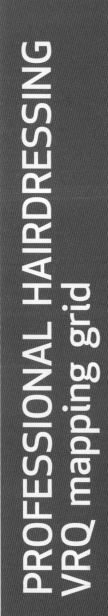

Unit Ref	Unit credit (QCF)	VRQ Unit Title	Unit Level	Ch1 G21	Ch2 G18	Ch3 G19	Ch4 GH16	Ch5 GB8	Ch6 GB7	Ch7 GB6	Ch8 GH19	Ch9 GH20	Ch10 GH23	Ch11 GH17	Ch12 GH18	Ch13 GH22	Ch14 GH21	Ch15 G22	Ch16 G11	Ch17 H32	Web Ch1 GB9	Web Ch2 AH35
A/600/8532	5	Style and finish African Type women's hair using a variety of techniques - VR184 (VTCT)	3																			
D/600/8538	5	Relaxing services for African Type Hair	3																			
F/600/8533	7	Perm hair to create a variety of looks	3													X						
M/601/5378	5	Cultural, social and technological influences on the hair industry	3																			
F/601/4459	5	Cultural, social and technological influences on the hair industry	3																			
A/601/5366	5	Wig Services	3																			
K/600/8638	6	Make and style a hair addition	3																			

Hairdressing
E-Teaching Website

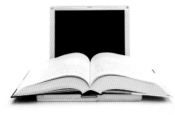

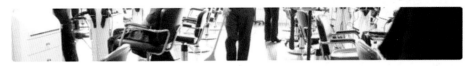

e-teaching website

A **new e-teaching website** for trainers accompanies this text book.

This resource includes **handouts, PowerPoint™ slides, interactive quizzes,** an **image bank** and **videoclips** – all carefully designed to help trainers make classroom delivery more interactive and to provide extra materials for lesson planning.

Please visit www.eteachhairdressing.co.uk for more information or contact your Cengage Learning sales representative at emea.fesales@cengage.com.

Students! Access your FREE online resources by following the Level 3 student links on www.eteachhairdressing.co.uk and entering your password 'perming'.

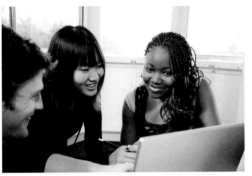

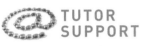

Hairdressing
E-Teaching Website

Leveltwo – Hairdressing the Foundations

| Unit G7 | Advise and consult with clients |

Activity 1

Purpose of consultation

Consultation is a meeting where advice is given and taken. It consists of talking to the client, listening to them so you can establish their needs and jointly negotiating a suitable course of action.

To carry out a good consultation there are 8 steps that you should include. In the table below write down the 8 steps. Use your textbook to help you.

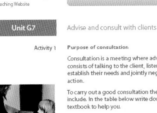

Steps	Good consultation includes:
1	
2	
3	
4	
5	
6	
7	
8	

TUTOR SUPPORT

Links to the e-teach resources are flagged throughout the text. If your trainer subscribes to the e-teaching website, they will be able to download these and use them in class.

LEARNER SUPPORT

Free online student resources are available wherever you see this red symbol.

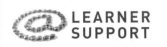

Hairdressing
E-Teaching Website

Leveltwo - Hairdressing the Foundations
Logged in as lucy mills (logout)

Change level:

Level 2 contents

Units

G8	G4	G7
GH12	AH21	GH9/GB2
Gen 1	Gen 2	Gen 3
Gen 4		

Key Teaching Strategies

Glossary

Feedback

Useful weblinks

Fun weblinks

Video

Coming soon, a selection of videos demonstrating professional cutting techniques.

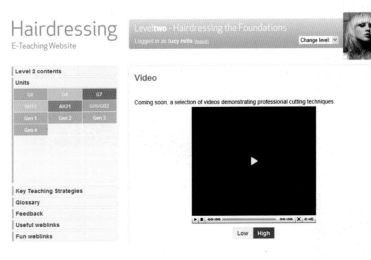

Low High

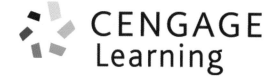 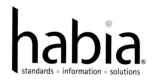

CENGAGE Learning

habia
standards • information • solutions

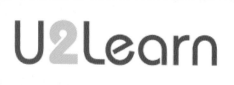

ONLINE LEARNING RESOURCES
FOR HAIRDRESSERS AND BEAUTY THERAPISTS

Produced in partnership by Cengage Learning and Habia, U2Learn is a ground-breaking e-learning solution for Beauty Therapy and Hairdressing students. Available online to provide qualification coverage in class, in the salon or at home. U2Learn is interactive and fun for you and your learners and offers a wealth of video clips, animations and activities to bring learning to life! Each U2Learn product offers you flexibility in your purchasing and can be bought as a complete package or per module.

For more information about our U2Learn solutions, contact our sales team at emea_fesales@cengage.com

U2Learn Hairdressing

U2Learn Hairdressing offers a one-stop-shop e-learning solution for Hairdressing at Level 2.

U2Learn Hairdressing can be purchased **per module** or as a **whole package**:

The modules within U2Learn Hairdressing are:

- Salon legislation
- Salon reception
- Selling skills
- Consultation
- Positive effectiveness
- Cut hair

- Shampoo, condition and treat the hair and scalp
- Style and set hair
- Perm and neutralise hair
- Colour hair
- Plait and twist hair – Coming soon!
- Attach hair to enhance a style – Coming soon!

U2Learn Hairdressing is the perfect partner to *Palladino's Hairdressing: The Foundations - The Official Guide to Hairdressing Level 2* textbook, but can also be used as a stand-alone teaching and learning resource.

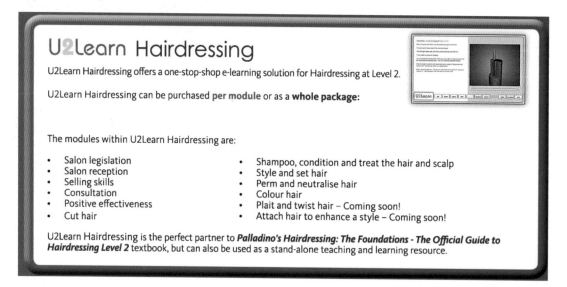

Professional

Hairdressing

Revised 6th Edition

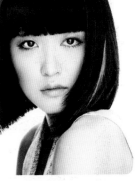

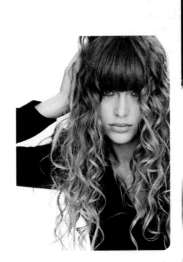

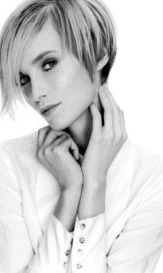

SCOTT SMURTHWAITE @ CREAM

Part**one**
Customer-centred services

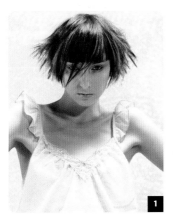

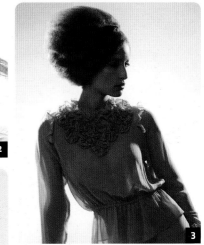

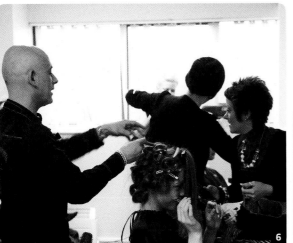

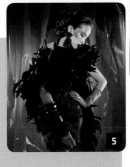

1 Vicky Turner @ Goldsworthy's 2 Paul Hawes @ Review,
Petersfield * Waterlooville, Hants 3 Ken Picton @ Ken Picton
4 Vicky Turner @ Goldsworthy's 5 Hair: Richard Ward,
Photography: Daniele Cipriani 6 Hair: NHF Inspire, Photography:
Simon Powell Left Hair by Lewis Moore @ Francesco Group,
Streetly, Photography by John Rawson@TRP

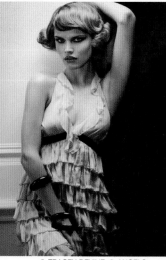

Chapter**one**
Consultation and advice

G21

| G21.1 |
| G21.2 |
| G21.3 |
| G21.4 |
| G21.5 |

**CREDIT VALUE
FOR UNIT G21**
3 Credits

More Information See
Appendices for relevant
legislation:

- Data protection Act
  (1998) G21 (eku1)
- Equal opportunities
- Consumer rights
  G21 (eku2)

Consultation: quick overview

Unit title

G21 Provide hairdressing consultation services

This is a **mandatory** unit and is made up of five main outcomes

Main outcomes

G21.1 Identify clients' needs and wishes

G21.2 Analyse the hair, skin and scalp

G21.3 Make recommendations to clients

G21.4 Advise clients on hair maintenance and management

G21.5 Agree services with your client

What do I need to do for G21.1?

- Encourage and allow clients to express their ideas
- Find out what clients want with simple questioning
- Use a variety of visual aids to get different ideas
- Ask about uncertainties and confirm your plan of action with the client

What do I need to do for G21.2?

- Look for signs that will influence, limit or change your plan of action
- Carry out any necessary tests beforehand
- Check previous records for any indications that might affect your plan
- Help others with their consultations when needed

What do I need to do for G21.3?

- Make recommendations based upon your findings
- If necessary, provide alternatives for services and products

- Provide the client with advise and courses of action
- Maintain a professional level of contact with the client

What do I need to do for G21.4?

- Select a suitable care regimen for the client
- Explain the benefits of following the care regimen and the possible outcomes if that advice is ignored
- Explain how they can manage their hair themselves

What do I need to do for G21.5?

- Make the client aware of service duration and involvements
- Agree services and products to be carried out
- Agree costs for services and products
- Update client records accurately

What aspects do I need to cover for G21.1, G21.2, G21.3, G21.4 and G21.5?

- The different ways of getting an accurate understanding of your clients hair
- Any factors that might have an impact or limit the hairdressing options
- Referrals to other professionals when needed
- Factors of costs, hair maintenance and any future style limitations

What do I need to know for G21.1, G21.2, G21.3, G21.4 and G21.5?

- The legal and salon requirements affecting your consultation and advice
- The ranges of products and services available; their costs, timings and applications
- How hair grows and the effects of different types and textures
- A range of adverse hair and skin conditions their possible causes and the ways in which they affect styling options
- Which adverse hair and skin conditions require professional referral
- The importance of a confidential and professional communication with clients
- How to provide professional advice for home care regimens

Keywords

Trichology
The scientific study of the hair and scalp

Referral
the situations where you need to redirect clients to other sources of treatment or service; i.e. adverse hair and skin conditions, or because of other services that your salon doesn't provide

Incompatibility
As a hairdressing term this refers to your planned service, being incompatible/unsuitable with what has previously been carried out on the hair. When incompatibles are present within the hair – e.g. metallic salts found in colour restorers or compound henna – no professional salon colour service can be provided

Adverse hair and scalp condition
is something that will affect the way in which a service is or can be carried out; for example, a double crown – this will influence the way in which the hair can be cut in order to camouflage the growth pattern

Information covered in this chapter

- Hair tests
- Hair and scalp disorders
- Using visual aids
- Limiting and influencing factors affecting styling choices
- Product advice and home care maintenance

Introduction

Consultation is arguably the most important service provided in a hairdressing salon, although the professional advice it produces for its clients often seems undervalued in relation to other professional sectors. But make no mistake: the service of consultation is fundamental to all other services and treatments that take place within the salon and without it salon–based hairdressing would not survive.

But in many salons consultation is a service that is often 'squeezed into or bolted on to' other booked services, when this is rushed, you run the risk of unexpected outcomes or potential disasters. Conversely, when too much time is taken, it often erodes into the service time; causing a 'knock-on' effect that will either make the stylist and client run late or not allow enough time to do the job properly.

So, taking that on board, it is essential that you get the balance right. Enough time must be given to:

- gain the client's trust and professional respect
- use visual aids either brought by the client or available from the salon
- conduct an analysis of the starting situation
- discuss the client's expectations in line with your analysis
- negotiate and then agree the best course of action
- provide home care maintenance and management advice.

During consultation a client begins to learn about your 'professional wizardry', the breadth and depth of technical knowledge and subject expertise, whereas the communication that takes place during routine services takes on a very different relationship. The bond that develops during consultation sets the tone for an ongoing business relationship.

About you – the senior stylist

As a true professional you lead by example; you are responsible for the quality of service that you provide to your clients and as a senior operator you are also a focal point to the other staff for back-up, support, advice and reassurance. Your experience is respected

Remember

A professional *distance* is created during consultation that does not happen at any other time. From the clients' perspective they are on the outside, observing; they are able to sample the salon's ability to deliver without any commitment. It is therefore the one chance to maximise this commitment and creating a strong mutual respect and a first impression that lasts.

Remember

Even if your regular customers are totally happy with what you provide, take the opportunity to enhance the professional balance by treating them to the occasional consultation review. (Otherwise they might go somewhere else.)

Remember

Effective communication relies upon listening to the client, hearing what they have to say, responding to them positively in what you say and backing that up with the right body language.

Activity

Putting consultation into practice

Client consultation can be practised within the salon/barber's shop with your work colleagues; the service lends itself well to role plays.

So, to develop these skills further, simulate your consultation skills by conducting a consultation for the following services upon each other.

Hairdressers	Colour correction
	Bridal hairstyle
	Perming
	Hair extensions
Barbers	Colour correction
	Shaving
	Perming
	Hair patterns/design

and your opinions are valued, the directions taken by other less senior staff maybe dependant on your actions. The trust invested in you by your colleagues marks you as different; a career professional, a valuable salon asset, the *backbone* of the salon team.

'Does that sound like something to aim for?'

A professional

So what are the true attributes of the professional hairdresser? One way of looking at it would be from the employer's point of view, that is, in the profile they draw up in the form of a person specification. When recruiting staff, in the early stages long before selection takes place, employers will create a basic profile for the person they are looking for. Obviously within this specification there will be references to the skills that are deemed essential and those that are preferred. However, technical skills are not the only attributes that employers are looking for. There will also be certain personality features too.

We could now look at hairdressing from the young, aspiring professional's point of view. Why do they go into hairdressing? What are their expectations? Do they really know from the outset what is required of them? We know what the 'industry drivers' are in hairdressing and we can accept that they will already have been stimulated by fashions, celebrities and the music industry. They may also have friends or relatives employed within the industry. For the young people joining the craft after leaving school, it is unlikely that they know what is really needed. This key factor is one of the main reasons for why the industry has a high fallout rate. In other words, many people join the craft with an uninformed, unrealistic view of what it is all about.

People joining the craft later in life, perhaps wanting a career change, probably have more idea. Why would that be? Well for one thing this group of people has experienced something over a long period of time that the others have not. They have all been clients. So what difference does that make? A huge one – these people have spent more time on the outside looking in than on the inside looking out – so their perspective is very different. They have had the opportunity to observe and receive at first hand all that the industry has to offer.

Remember

You have to earn respect; your client is already paying for it.

G21.1 Identify clients' needs and wishes

Hairdressing is about relationships – the relationships that are created through good communication. Many people find it difficult to convey what they really mean; they try to use technical terms inaccurately, they don't necessarily say what they really want to, they see aspects and parts of styles in pictures that they like, but cannot easily express or convey these aspects to you.

EKU *statement*

G21 (eku27) Make openings in conversations to encourage clients to speak

Remember

Visualisation is a rare skill: being able to see what something will be like before actually doing it is often very difficult for stylists let alone clients.

Remember

Advising clients means listening to what they have to say about their hair, asking appropriate questions and coming up with suitable suggestions for styles and treatments.

Always: Check that you have the right information by summarising their points and repeating back to them your understanding.

Always: Gain agreement before you start anything.

EKU *statement*

G21 (eku25) The importance of effective communication

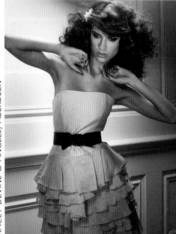

So your communication skills need to be well developed to get through this smoke screen and get to the real person underneath. It's not that clients want to mislead us; its more to do with the fact that people find discussing personal matters or things to do with their appearance a difficult issue to address.

Most people have no self-visualisation; they have an inability to imagine what a style would look like on them. Many others would not want to disclose physical features or aspects about themselves that they aren't happy with. So you are tasked with the challenge of sympathetically discovering these features and, more importantly, finding ways of optimising your clients appearance in light of the real limiting factors that you see professionally.

Activity
Communication
In client consultation, what are the key features of positive communication and conversely poor communication? Give some examples of each and record your findings within your portfolio.

Good, effective communication

Good communicators use a mixture of skills in their daily routines. This 'toolbox' of skills is made up from the following essential components.

1 *Excellent listening skills*. This is the ability to hear and understand what the client is saying. This is particularly useful when the one requiring/initiating a change is not the client in the chair.

2 *A good speaker*. Long pauses during conversations can often be uncomfortable. Knowing when it is right to speak or keep quiet is an invaluable interpersonal skill. During normal consultation you, the hairdresser, will be taking the lead. You will be asking questions; i.e. trying to elicit enough information in the time span available to make the right judgements. You will be weighing up what the client wants against the limitations arising from the analysis. You will be getting the client to agree on the various possible options and planning the necessary course of action.

3 *'Reading' skills*. The ability to read situations, to understand what has been said or not said, is exceptionally useful. There are times when your client will look a certain way or say something that makes you think. In these situations, your ability to read the situation, i.e. your perceptiveness in picking this up and responding appropriately may have a crucial impact on your long-term relationship.

Body language

We have always relied upon our ability to speak and hear as the natural way of communicating. In fact we use all of our senses to communicate. But do we use all of our senses equally? The way we use our sight is probably at the top of the list. This is the fastest but very often unreliable way of drawing conclusions. As well as using words we show our interest, attitude and feelings by bodily expressions. Non-verbal communication (NVC) or body language to put it more simply, is especially important. It can truly show what we are feeling, even if our mouths are saying something quite different!

In the animal world the main form of communication and interaction from one creature to another is through body language. The cat that is alarmed at being confronted by a dog on the street turns sideways on and hunches up. This makes him look larger than he actually is. Size means everything. You pull the dog away sharply and when you get home he sulks; he gets right in your view and turns his back to you. The positioning, posturing and mannerisms of animals all mean something, conveying very clear and strong messages.

We too express our interest and attitudes with NVC through eye contact, posture and general body positioning. So it is very important that we send the right message, particularly when dealing with clients and potential customers.

Eye contact

Eye level Always maintain eye contact when in conversation with your client. Where possible, maintain the same eye level. For example, when you carry out a consultation with the client and they are seated, sit beside the client or opposite them. Standing over or above them and looking down will convey a feeling of authority, and might appear as if you are trying to assert yourself and take control. This is threatening, intimidating and definitely the wrong signal to send to a potential client.

I love you The eyes give away our innermost feelings too, this is particularly obvious when we show attraction to someone. When we are attracted to someone, the dark centres of the eye, i.e. the pupils, grow wider and dilate. Look into them and you'll soon know if attraction is mutual, eye contact lasts longer with attraction and the eyes form a more intense gaze. The reason people's pupils dilate is adrenaline which is released when you are excited or afraid. So, whether you fancy someone, think you're about to win a poker hand, or are telling lies then they will dilate.

Physical contact

Most people are embarrassed by physical contact from someone they do not know well.

Posture, body position and gestures

Much has been written on the subject of body language and the psychological effects that it has on those reading it. It is far too complex a subject to address in a few simple paragraphs. Posture, or composure of the body, is a form of body language in this context. Reading the message of this form of communication is a skill that develops over time and once learnt is never forgotten. However, there are few obvious rules that can help to convey the right message and create a right impression.

- Folded arms and the crossing of arms on the chest is a protective gesture that portrays a closed mind or shows defensiveness.
- Open palms, as a gesture supporting explanation or information, with hands at waist height and palms upward, indicates that the person has nothing to hide. This is interpreted as openness or honesty.
- Scratching behind the ear or the back of the neck whilst listening indicates that the listener is uncertain or doesn't understand. Rubbing the nose whilst listening can indicate that you don't believe what you are hearing.

Remember

 Your body may be saying things that your mouth is not!

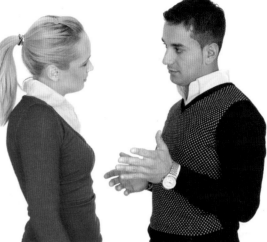

ISTOCKPHOTO.COM/SANDRA GLIGORIJEVIC

Remember

Body zones – Proxemics
Do not crowd or appear over-familiar with your client. Imagine how you would feel if someone came up to you and got a little too close. What do you do? Immediately back off and go onto the defensive.

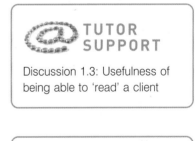 **TUTOR SUPPORT**

Discussion 1.3: Usefulness of being able to 'read' a client

 **TUTOR SUPPORT**

Discussion 1.4: Recognising client signs

- Inspecting fingernails or looking at a watch is a plain and simple indication of boredom or vanity.

- Talking with your hand in front your mouth may lead the listener to believe you are not being honest. You're hiding yourself by your gestures.

- Shifting from foot to foot: This shows that you're worrying about getting found out! It also says that you would rather be somewhere else, to get away so that no guilty expressions are spotted.

These forms of communication are only an indication of feelings and emotions. In isolation they may not mean anything at all. However, taken together they can convey a very clear message. Make sure that you send the appropriate signals and look interested, keen, ready to help and positive. And above all show that you can listen.

Mirroring posture If you're in tune with the person you're speaking to you will often find you unconsciously mirror each other's body postures. So, if you rest your hand on your chin, the other person will follow you. If he or she leans forwards you'll find yourself making the same move and so on.

This technique is often used in interviews by helping to make the candidates feel at ease. Conversely, the technique is used as a subconscious sales tool, when sales representatives want us to part with our money.

You're a liar!

- Sweating.
- Excessive hand movements.
- Biting of fingernails.

- Chewing of the inside of the mouth.
- Drying up of the mouth.
- Lack of eye contact.

Effective body language during consultation Remember as a professional you should be attentive, positive and actively participating in the consultation process. You can show this in the way that you:

- sit to the front edge of your chair or stool, facing the client (not through the mirror)
- maintain eye contact and eye level, do not look down on them
- acknowledge what has been said by nodding or confirming with a 'yes' at the appropriate moments.

EKU statement

G21 (eku25) The importance of effective communication

EKU statement

G21 (eku27) Make openings in conversations to encourage clients to speak

G21 (eku17) Why it is important to identify factors that may limit or affect services and products which can be used

Activity

The illustration below shows the differences between question styles. Use this as a discussion point that you could use with your colleagues in role play. Try out different question techniques to see how they prompt for additional information then answer the following questions.

1 Which questioning style created the most response?

2 Which questioning style created the least response?

3 Which style do you think you would try to use in your consultations with clients?

Questioning techniques

There are three main types of question that you could use during your consultation.

Open questions – these are good to use if you want to gain more in-depth information from the client. They start with 'who,' 'what,' 'when,' 'why,' 'where' and 'how'. Examples:

- What products do you use on your hair?
- When did you last wash your hair?
- How often do you use the straightening irons on your hair?

Closed questions – these are useful for a quick 'yes' or 'no' elimination response. Examples:

- Have you had permanent colour on your hair before?
- Would you like me to do it in your lunch hour today for you?
- Are you against moving the parting from the centre?

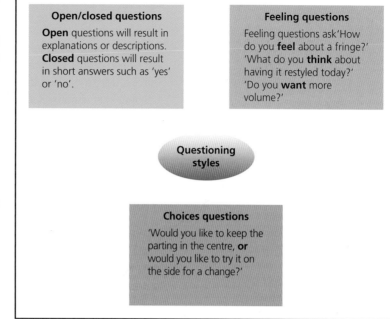

Open/closed questions
Open questions will result in explanations or descriptions. **Closed** questions will result in short answers such as 'yes' or 'no'.

Feeling questions
Feeling questions ask 'How do you **feel** about a fringe?' 'What do you **think** about having it restyled today?' 'Do you **want** more volume?'

Questioning styles

Choices questions
'Would you like to keep the parting in the centre, **or** would you like to try it on the side for a change?'

Different question styles

Feeling questions – these types of questions focus upon the client and are good to use when you are trying to gauge a personal opinion or feeling. Examples:

- How do you feel about taking the length back up to the shoulders?
- Do you want me to talk you through the home care for this style now?
- What do you think about a complete colour change today?

Choices questions – they could be considered to be leading and are a good sales tactic when trying to pinpoint a few possible options. Examples:

- Would you prefer the smaller intense leave-in treatment or the normal after–shampoo conditioner?
- Shall we see if there is time today to do it all, or would you rather make a separate appointment for the highlights after the cut?
- Where would you like to wear the bulk of the hair? Piled on top, at the side or smooth on the sides and fixed at the back?

Whatever style of question you choose to use, you must make sure that you:

- Identify the limitations or influencing factors – some of these will crop up in your conversation, but the main influencing factors are going to arise during your visual inspection of the hair and scalp. So whether you do your inspection first or later will depend on the service that you are going to do, or how comfortable the client is with the consultation process.
- Avoid misunderstandings – you need to adapt your consultation style to suit the level of understanding of the client. Don't expect the clients to know what a reverse graduated bob is with sliced and shattered edges. It's showing off! It's not clever and may (to them) sound conceited.

Remember

If you find that your line of questions isn't getting the information that you need, try asking again but in a different way. For example: 'Well, how do you feel about changing the colour?' or, 'What other things do you find that also work well on your hair?'

EKU *statement*

G21 (eku28) The importance of confirming your understanding of what the client has said to you

Remember

 It's easy to confuse clients if you start using technical terms. Keep it simple.

@ **TUTOR SUPPORT**

Project 1.1: Consultation plan

Remember

Being highly self-motivated affects others too. The way in which we conduct ourselves at work has a direct, positive impact on those around us. Conversely, poor motivation spreads like a disease!

• Avoid *our* technical jargon; keep it for the training salon. Inevitably, you want the client to be happy with the final effect, so keep it simple. If a client uses our technical jargon with you, find out exactly what she means; it might not be what we mean by it.

• Allow time for the client to consider your advice. Don't rush them into making swift decisions; you need to take them with you every step along the journey. If they do feel rushed or that you are 'pushy' you will be alienating them from the outset. That's a difficult position to be in as you will *feel* the tension during the service and then that's an uncomfortable position for a stylist to be in.

• Urge the clients to provide their input – you need all the facts before you start. 'If the engine seems a little cold', you might find that you need to just sit and ask a few questions before you make any examinations. Many people can be intimidated by having to walk into salon in front of others. Be sensitive to their needs and watch their body language for the signs of defence and remember to be patient throughout the service.

• Listen to their responses – hear what the client is saying, if there seems to be hesitation or reluctance, be positive, give reasons for your plan of action. If you can't dispel the concerns, you had better find another plan as your first is going to crash!

• Confirm and agree – at any point where some decision is being made. Make sure that you confirm and summarise at all the points along the way. Only after you have both agreed a course of action can you take things to the next stage.

Activity

Dealing with customer resistance

Most of the resistance from clients about services or products that you recommend is more to do with a lack of understanding rather than disinterest. Your professionalism enables you to explain what would be right for them and the benefits that they can provide.

Complete this activity by filling in the missing information in the table below. We have started you off with the first one.

Consultation aspect	What might a client say in a defensive way?	What can you say to dispel resistance, uncertainty, hesitation or general confusion?
Recommending a retail product	No thanks I have bought mousse before at the supermarket and it didn't work	Well, that was an unfortunate waste of money. What was it that you found a disappointment?
Recommending a new hairstyle		
Recommending a conditioning treatment		
Recommending further (unplanned) salon services		

Activity

Hair fashions are strongly linked to the trends in the general fashion industry.

So how would you keep abreast of the current fashions? Use the internet, hair magazines, and professional trade press to:

(a) Create a collection of work, comprising of the latest looks for reference in your portfolio.

(b) Then, after creating the collection, complete the information in the table below.

Keep your completed information within your portfolio.

	Describe the looks	How does it differ from previous looks?	Where did you find your source data/information?
Current hair fashions			
New trends i.e. emerging looks			

Avoid misunderstandings

Have empathy

Clients don't come to the salon just when there is a celebration. Because hair grows at an even rate, they are likely to arrive when all sorts of things are going on in their lives and in yours too. It's easy to have sympathy. As hairdressers we do it every day. We can all relate to the stories told by our fellow staff over lunch or during breaks – the stories about our clients in certain situations and circumstances. That's life. However, having the ability to put yourself in somebody else's shoes is quite difficult. It's easy to say 'how sad', or 'you poor thing', but beware because sincerity is an emotion that is easily *read* through your body language and thus people can usually tell if you are being *in*sincere.

The close bond that forms between client and hairdresser is often tested at times like these. Not all clients can be upbeat all of the time. Due to modern living, people's lives have become more stressful. As a result there is an increase in general unhappiness. From the client's point of view, the visit to the salon is not just about having their hair done; it's a lot to do with the feel-good factor too. As hairdressers we must recognise this. The hairdresser's role seems to involve a number of occupations – a little bit of social worker, a touch of psychologist, a bit of entertainer and a huge companion. In order to be this well-rounded individual, we need to *have and show* empathy. It is an extremely useful personal attribute for supporting and understanding others.

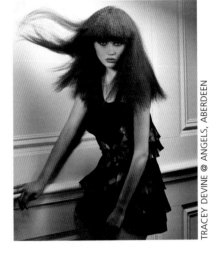

TRACEY DEVINE @ ANGELS, ABERDEEN

Remember

Customer Expectations

During consultation with your client, take a little extra time to find out what specific service expectations are required.

1 What aspects of customer service are already delivered?

2 What aspects are omitted? Of these, which would it be feasible to introduce?

Would they be happy to pay for these additions?

Remember

Motivation

Discuss with your fellow staff members the benefits of self-motivation and the impact that it has on the whole team. Then discuss the disadvantages of demotivation and the impact it will have. Summarise and record your findings.

Remember

Visual aids are an extremely useful way of conveying information.

What types of visual aid do you use during client consultation?

Remember

Trust is hard earned. Gaining a customer's trust and loyalty takes time. Once you have earned this, the bond remains fragile, so handle with care.

Remember

You have to have the confidence to lead during consultation. It is your positive approach and outlook that will draw your client in to the conversation and draw the vital information out.

Who are we dealing with?

The analytical skills used during client consultation will at a higher professional level draw down on the objective and the subjective. These aspects are not examined at level 2 as we take a more *prescriptive* view of the client before us. At level 2 the stylist makes a number of observations, looking for influencing factors that control their thinking and arriving at a technically sound course of action. Fine.

At NVQ level 3, through the very experience of working with people we modify the way that we approach the work in hand. We start to work *intuitively*; in fact we subconsciously draw information from the client that shapes the way in which we arrive at a conclusion. It is a natural thought process that makes us look for patterns. In finding those patterns we then sort them into order and compartmentalise them. Obviously, different people will do this to a different extent. The individual who tries to approach things in a logical, systematic way will do this more than someone who does not. Unfortunately, we need to do this, albeit subconsciously, as this gives us the professional edge. The artistic stylist who just visualises the perfect style for their new client without any previous analysis, saying 'leave it to me', is playing Russian roulette. When it works it is fantastic, but the law of percentages is against it. So what information do you need in order to get it right?

Activity

Standardising a consultation within the salon

It is very easy to overlook small details during consultation and this may have an impact on the final results. One simple way of combating this issue would be to devise a standardised consultation process for all salon staff.

1   What sorts of things would you need to include within your consultation system?

2   What other aids or information would you need for the system?

3   What sorts of things do you need to record?

4   How would you keep records of the consultations?

Create a copy of this system and keep it within your portfolio.

Leading the consultation

The biggest difference between consultation at level 3 and level 2 is that the level 3 stylist will need to have a broader understanding of people. Experience enables you to combine improved communication skills with a wider range of technical skills and this is directly proportional to the ability to reach the desired result. So from this we can conclude that the level 3 stylist (or someone with the same experience) is more likely to be able to handle a far greater range of people, personalities and their styling requirements. There are two specific attributes that relate to this type of communication at level 3 which you must take on board:

- control
- responsibility.

Taking control of the whole situation is essential. This will occur at the moment when the new potential client realises that it is you who is going to conduct the consultation.

However, in taking charge and leading the client through this process you have to give something in return. The cost for being allowed to lead is responsibility. In assuming control, you have to gain the trust of the client. This can only happen if you are prepared to shoulder the responsibility for the eventual outcome. So this is it, the big chance to get it right and win over another client into your following.

G21.2   Analyse the hair, skin and scalp

You need a thorough understanding of all the hair and skin problems that could affect your choices in selecting a suitable course of action for your client. This section addresses the following hair analysis aspects:

Structure of hair and skin pg 5	Cortex, cuticle, medulla, physical properties of hair and skin, hair follicle
Growth cycle of hair pg 19	Anagen, catagen, telogen
Hair texture pg 20	Coarse, medium, fine
Hair tests pg 20	Sensitivity test, strand test, colour test, test cutting, test curl, curl check, peroxide test, incompatibility test, elasticity test, porosity test
Infectious skin and scalp pg 24	Impetigo, scalp ringworm (tinea conditions capitis), head lice (pediculosis capitis)
Non-infectious skin and scalp pg 26	Folliculitis, dandruff (pityriasis conditions capitis), alopecia, seborrhoea, psoriasis, eczema
Hair defects pg 28	Split ends (fragilitis crinium), damaged cuticle, trichorrexis nodosa, monilethrix
Head and face shapes pg 30	Oval, round, rectangular, square, heart-shaped
Other important physical features pg 31	Hair growth patterns, ears, nose, eyes, etc.

EKU statement

G21 (eku13) The basic structure of hair and skin

EKU statement

G21 (eku14) The growth cycle of hair

EKU statement

G21 (eku15) The characteristics of different hair types and textures

EKU statement

G21 (eku19) How to visually recognise indications of ringworm, impetigo, scabies, eczema, alopecia, psoriasis, folliculitis, dandruff, ingrowing hair and head lice

EKU statement

G21 (eku16) The general factors that contribute to healthy hair (e.g. health, environment, chemicals)

Structure of hair and skin

Hair

The cross-section taken through the hair lengthways shown in the diagram provides us with a microscopic view of the three specific layers.

The *cuticle* is the outer layer of colourless cells which forms a protective surface to the hair. It regulates the chemicals entering and damaging the hair and protects the hair from excessive heat and drying. The cells overlap like tiles on a roof with the free edges pointing towards the tips of the hair. The amount of layers is proportional to hair texture. Hair with fewer layers of cuticle is finer than coarser hair types which have several layers. Hair in good condition has a cuticle that is tightly closed, limiting the penetration of moisture and chemicals. Conversely, hair that is in a dry or porous condition has damaged or partially missing cuticle layers. One simple indicator of cuticle condition relates to the time taken to blow-dry hair. Hair in good condition will dry quickly in proportion to the amount of hair on the head (*density*). The closely packed cuticle allows the drier to chase the water from the hairshaft. Porous hair absorbs moisture and therefore takes far longer to dry and is unfortunately subjected to more heat, which exacerbates the problem.

Remember

A closed smooth cuticle is the most important sign of healthy hair. Healthy hair imparts shine, dries more quickly, is resistant to chemical treatments and holds styles and colours better than hair with a raised/damaged cuticle.

The *cortex* is the middle and largest layer. It is made up of a long fibrous material which has the appearance of rope. If looked at more closely, each of the fibres is made up of even smaller chains of fibres. The quality and condition of these bundles of fibres will determine the hair's strength. The way in which they are *bonded* together has a direct effect upon curl and ability to stretch (*hair elasticity*). It is within this part of the hair that the natural hair colour is distributed. These pigments are diffused throughout the cortex and their colour(s) and rate of distribution determine the colour that we can see. It is also in this layer that both synthetic colours and permanent waves make the permanent chemical changes.

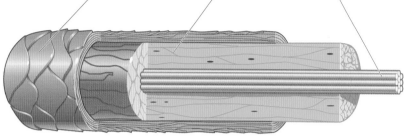

Hair cuticle   Cortex   Medulla

Cross section of hair

The *medulla* is the central, most inner part of the hair. It only exists in medium to coarser hair types and is often intermittent throughout the length. The medulla does not play any useful part in hairdressing processes and treatments.

Chemical properties of hair

The bundles of fibres found in the cortex are made from molecules of *amino acids*. There are about 22 amino acids in hair and the molecules of each contain atoms of elements in different proportions. Overall, the elements in hair are in approximately these proportions:

carbon: 50%

hydrogen: 7%

nitrogen: 18%

oxygen: 21%

sulphur: 4%

The amino acids combine to form larger molecules, in the form of long chains called polypeptides, or, if they are long enough, *proteins*. One of the most important of these is keratin. Keratin is an important component of nails, skin and hair. It is this protein which makes them flexible and elastic. Because of the keratin it contains, hair can be elastic, and allows the hair to be stretched, curled and waved.

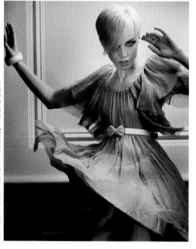

In hair, keratin forms long chains which coil up like springs. They are held in this shape by cross-links between chains. The three kinds of link are *disulphide bridges* (*sulphur bonds*), *salt bonds* and *hydrogen bonds*. Salt bonds and hydrogen bonds are relatively weak and easily broken, allowing the springs to be stretched out. This is what happens in curling. The normal, coiled form of keratin is called **alpha keratin**. When it has been stretched, set and dried it is called **beta keratin**. The change is only temporary. Once the hair has been made wet or has gradually absorbed moisture from the air, it relaxes back to the alpha state. Disulphide bridges are much stronger but these too can be altered, as in perming.

Physical properties of hair

EKU statement

G21 (eku16) The general factors that contribute to healthy hair (e.g. health, environment, chemicals)

Hair *naturally* contains a certain amount of natural moisture that lubricates it, allowing it to stretch and recoil. Hair that is dry and in poor condition is less elastic. Hair is *hygroscopic*; it absorbs water from the surrounding air. How much water is taken up depends on the dryness of the hair and the moistness of the atmosphere. Hair is also *porous*. There are tiny tube-like spaces within the hair structure and the water flows into these by *capillary* action, rather like blotting paper absorbing ink. Drying hair in the ordinary way evaporates only the surface moisture, but drying over long periods or at too high a temperature removes water from within the hair, leaving it brittle and in poor condition. Damaged hair is more porous than healthy hair and easily loses any water, which makes it hard to stretch and mould. Curled hair returns to its former shape as it takes up water, so the drier the atmosphere, the longer the curl or set lasts.

Hair health and condition

Moisture levels within the hair are essential for maintaining good condition. We can see the evidence of this moisture from the shine that we associate with great-looking hair. 'Bad hair' denotes poor condition and the lack of shine is due to the unevenness of the hair's surface, i.e. the cuticle. A roughened cuticle surface is an indicator of either physical or chemical damage. Each of these states is difficult to correct. In mild cases of dryness, treatments can be applied to improve the hair's manageability and handling. In more serious situations of porous hair, the hair's ability to resist the ingress of chemicals and moisture is severely impaired. There are no long-lasting remedies for this so regular reconditioning treatments must be used.

So the health and the condition of the hair is your starting point. Whatever happens next should be a process of improving what went on before. A client will expect the service or treatment that you advise to be a step in the right direction. You will need to look for each of the following properties and aspects:

Features of hair in good condition

- Shine and lustre.
- Good elasticity.
- Smooth outer cuticle surface.
- Good natural moisture levels.
- Strength and resistance.

Features of hair in poor condition

- Raised or open cuticle.
- Low strength and resistance.
- Damaged torn hair shaft.
- Over-elastic/stretchy.
- Split ends.
- Dry, porous lengths or ends.

Physical hair damage is caused by

- harsh, or incorrect usage of brushes and/or combs
- excessive heat from styling equipment.

Chemical hair damage is caused by

- incorrect over-timing of all colouring and perming treatments
- strengths of hydrogen peroxide
- over-bleaching and highlighting services
- excessive overuse of colouring products
- perm products that are too strong or over-processing
- chlorine from swimming pools.

Weathering

- Hair is also damaged by excesses of sunlight.

And generally speaking

- The normal and abnormal working of the body has a direct effect on the hair and scalp. Good health is reflected in good hair and skin. A balanced diet with plenty of fresh foods contributes to good health.

Remember

Hair in good condition has natural moisture levels that help to give it elasticity and shine.

Remember

Curling dry hair is most effective just after the hair has been washed because, although the surface is dry, the hair will have absorbed water internally. Blow-styling and curling with hot irons, heated rollers, hot combs and hot brushes all have similar temporary effects.

Remember

It is far easier to keep good conditioned hair in good condition than it is to try to correct hair in bad condition.

- Disease and drugs used in the treatment of disease take their toll on the hair and skin.
- Genetic factors affecting hair growth determine hair strength and texture.
- The hair of women is usually at its best during pregnancy.
- Deterioration of the hair and skin after giving birth is usually due to stress and tiredness.

The skin

The epidermis The epidermis is the front line of defence. This outer protective layer of the skin is called the *stratum corneum* and is a hard, cornified layer, consisting of 15 to 40 layers of flattened skin cells or corneocytes, which constantly migrate up from deeper regions and fully replace themselves about once a month. The *corneocytes* are filled with keratin and a fatty *lipid* that make a barrier to prevent loss of water through the skin.

Beneath the stratum corneum lie *keratinocytes* which produce keratin and form the building blocks of the epidermis. In the same area, *langerhans cells* scout for invading pathogens while *melanocytes* produce the pigment melanin that protects the skin from UV radiation. *Merkel* or nerve cells send messages via the nerve receptors to the brain to register sensation.

The dermis The dermis is the thickest layer of the skin. It is here that the hair follicle is formed. The dermis is made up of elastic and connective tissue and is well supplied with blood and lymph vessels. The skin receives its nutrient supply from this area. The upper part of the dermis, the *papillary layer*, contains the organs of touch, heat and cold, and pain. The lower part of the dermis, the *reticular layer*, forms a looser network of cells.

The subcutaneous fat lies below the dermis. It is also known as the *subcutis*, or occasionally as the *hypodermis*. It is composed of loose cell tissue and contains stores of fat. The base of the hair follicle is situated just above this area, or sometimes in it.

Subcutaneous tissue gives roundness to the body and fills the space between the dermis and muscle tissue that may lie below.

The hair follicle Hair grows from a thin, tube-like space in the skin called a *hair follicle*.

- At the bottom of the follicles are areas well supplied with nerves and blood vessels, which nourish the cellular activity. These are called *hair papillae*.
- Immediately surrounding each papilla is the *germinal matrix* which consists of actively forming *hair cells*.
- As the new hair cells develop, the lowest part of the hair is shaped into the *hair bulb*.

Remember

The skin is the largest organ of the body and if laid flat would cover an area of about 21 square feet. It forms the barrier to a multitude of external forces and is made up of many layers.

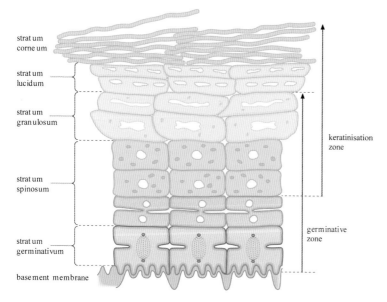

strat um
corne um

strat um
lucidum

strat um
gran ulosum

keratinisation
zone

strat um
spinosum

germinative
zone

strat um
germinativum

base ment membrane

Layers of the epidermis

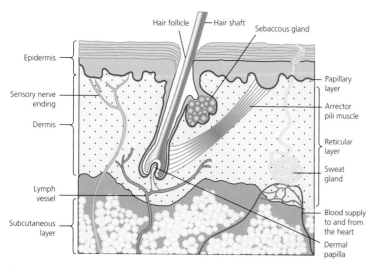

Hair follicle — Hair shaft
Sebaccous gland

Epidermis

Sensory nerve
ending

Dermis

Papillary
layer

Arrector
pili muscle

Reticular
layer

Sweat
gland

Lymph
vessel

Subcutaneous
layer

Blood supply
to and from
the heart

Dermal
papilla

The hair in skin

- The cells continue to take shape and form as they push along the follicle until they appear at the skin surface as *hair fibres*.
- The cells gradually harden and die. The hair is formed of dead tissue. It retains its elasticity due to its chemical structure and keratin content.

Sebaceous gland   The oil gland, or *sebaceous gland*, is situated in the skin and opens out into the upper third of the follicle. Oil or *sebum* is secreted into the follicle and onto the hair and skin surface.

Sebum helps to prevent the skin and hair from drying. By retaining moisture it helps the hair and skin to stay pliable. Sebum is slightly acid – about pH 5.6 – and forms a protective antibacterial covering for the skin.

Sweat glands   The sweat gland lies beside each hair follicle. These are appendages of the skin. They secrete sweat which passes out through the sweat ducts. The ends of these ducts can be seen at the surface of the skin as sweat *pores*. There are two types of sweat gland: the larger, associated closely with the hair follicles, are the apocrine glands; the smaller, found over most of the skin's surface, are the *eccrine glands*.

Sweat is mainly water with salt and other minerals. In abnormal conditions sweat contains larger amounts of waste material. Evaporation of sweat cools the skin. The function of sweat, and thus the sweat glands, is to protect the body by helping to maintain the normal temperature.

The arrector pili muscle   The hair muscle, or *arrector pili*, is attached at one end to the hair follicle and at the other to the underlying tissue of the epidermis. When it contracts it pulls the hair and follicle upright. Upright hairs trap a warm layer of air around the skin. The hairs also act as a warning system; for example, you soon notice if an insect crawls over your skin.

Hair growth

Hair is constantly growing. Over a period of between one and six years an individual hair actively grows, then stops, the follicle rests, degenerates and the hair finally falls out. Before the hair leaves the follicle, the new hair is normally ready to replace it. If a hair is not replaced then a tiny area of baldness results. The lives of individual hairs vary and are subject to variations in the body. Some are actively growing while others are resting. Hairs on the head are at different stages of growth.

Stages of growth   The life cycle of hair is as follows:

- **Anagen** (growing stage) is the active growing stage of the hair, a period of activity of the papilla and germinal matrix. This stage may last from a few months to several years. It is at this stage of formation at the base of the follicle that the hair's thickness is determined. Hair colour too is formed in the early part of anagen.
- **Catagen** (preparing to rest) is a period when the hair stops growing but cellular activity continues at the papilla. The hair bulb gradually separates from the papilla and moves further up the follicle.
- **Telogen** (resting stage) is the final stage, when there is no further growth or activity at the papilla. The follicle begins to shrink and completely separates from the papilla area. This resting stage does not last long. Towards the end of the telogen stage, cells begin to activate in preparation for the new anagen stage of regrowth.

The new anagen period involves the hair follicle beginning to grow down again. Vigorous papilla activity generates a new hair at the germinal matrix. At the same time the old hair

Remember

Hair texture
The more layers of cuticle that the hair has, the greater its resistance to absorbing moisture and chemicals. Therefore coarse hair in good condition can often take longer to perm than finer hair types.

EKU *statement*

G21 (eku23) The importance of carrying out tests and the potential consequences of failing to do so

G21 (eku24) How and when tests are carried out on hair and skin

G21 (eku10) The services for which you would need to give clients special advice prior to their visit and the type of advice to give (i.e., whether the service could affect their comfort, any special clothing requirements, the need for any tests, any special preparation activities)

G21 (eku3) Salon procedures and manufacturers' instructions in relation to conducting tests

Remember

Tests are a vital part of general hairdressing services. If they are missed or ignored you and the salon run the risk of a potential disaster.

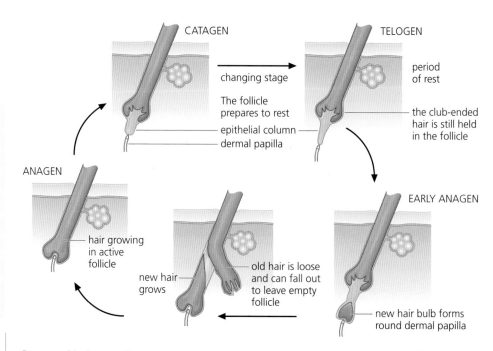

Stages of hair growth

is slowly making its way up and out of the follicle. Often the old and new hair can be seen at the same time in the follicle.

In some animals most of the hairs follow their life cycle in step, passing through anagen, catagen and telogen together. This results in moulting. Human hair, however, develops at an uneven rate and few follicles shed their hair at the same time. (If all hairs fell at the same time we would have bald periods.)

Hair texture

Individual hair thickness is referred to as hair texture and the main types are:

- very fine hair
- medium hair
- fine hair
- coarse hair.

The main differences between the hair textures relate to the number of layers of cuticle.

Hair and skin tests

To minimise the likelihood of problems arising, there are a number of tests that you can carry out to help diagnose the condition and likely reaction of your client's skin and hair. These tests will assist you to decide what action to take before, during and after the application of hairdressing processes. You will need to record all these results onto the client's record file.

Development strand test

A strand test or hair strand colour test is used to assess the development of a colour, whilst the hair is processing. It is carried out as follows:

1 Most colouring products just require the time recommended by the manufacturer – check their instructions.

2 Rub a strand of hair lightly with the back of a comb to remove the surplus colour.

3 Check whether the colour remaining is evenly distributed throughout the hair's length. If it is even, remove the rest of the colour. If it is uneven, allow processing to continue, if necessary applying more colour. If any of the hair on the head is not being treated, you can compare the evenness of colour in the coloured hair with that in the uncoloured hair.

Colour test

This test is used to assess the suitability of a chosen colour, the amount of processing time required and the final colour result. Apply the colour or bleaching products you propose to use to a cutting of the client's hair and process as recommended.

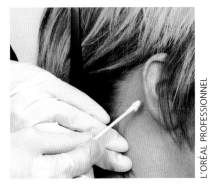

Skin test

Good practice/health and safety: sensitivity test

(Also known as patch test or skin test)
The sensitivity test is used to assess the reaction of the skin to chemicals or chemical products. In the salon it is mainly used before colouring. Some people are allergic to external contact of chemicals such as PPD (found in permanent colour). This can cause dermatitis or, in more severe cases, permanent scarring of skin tissue and hair loss. Some people are allergic to irritants reacting internally, causing asthma and hay fever. Others may be allergic to both internal and external irritants. To find out whether a client's skin reacts to chemicals in permanent colours, the following test should be carried out at least 24 hours prior to the chemical process.

Note: Skin testing is not just for new clients, it has now been found that clients can develop sensitivity to chemicals through prolonged use of the same or similar products. Therefore periodic testing for adverse reactions is essential and should be carried out routinely from time to time.

1 Mix a little of the colour to be used with the correct amount of hydrogen peroxide – as recommended by the manufacturer.

2 Clean an area of skin about 8 mm square behind the ear or in the fold of the arm. Use a little spirit on cotton wool to remove the grease from the skin.

3 Apply a little of the colour mixture to skin.

4 Cover the colour patch with a simple dressing to protect it. Ask your client to report any discomfort or irritation that occurs over the next 24 hours. Arrange to see your client at the end of this time so that you can check for signs of reaction.

5 If there is a *positive response*, i.e. a skin reaction such as inflammation, soreness, swelling, irritation or discomfort, do not carry out the intended service. Never ignore the result of a skin test. If a skin test showed a reaction and you carried on anyway, there might be a more serious reaction which could affect the whole body.

6 If there is a *negative response*, i.e. no reaction to the chemicals, then carry out the treatment as proposed.

Warning: In recent years there have been a growing number of successful personal injury claims made against salons where the necessary precautions have not been taken.

Remember

Always follow the manufacturer's instructions when conducting/carrying out tests.

Remember

Contra-indications
A contra-indication is something that signifies that a service CANNOT be carried out.

EKU *statement*

G21 (eku18) How the following factors limit or affect the services and products that can be offered to clients

Test cutting

In this test a piece of hair cut from the head is processed to check its suitability, the amount of processing required and the timing, before the process is carried out. The test is used for colouring, straightening, relaxing, reducing synthetic colouring, i.e. decolouring, bleaching and incompatibility.

Test curl

This test is made on the hair to determine the lotion suitability, the strength, the curler size, the timing of processing and the development. It is used before perming. This is done by winding test roller(s) up at the back of the head and then applying the perm solution, allowing it to develop and finally neutralising.

Curl check or development test curl

This test is used to assess the development of curl in the perming process. The test is used periodically throughout a perm by looking for the optimal 'S' development of the wound hair.

Incompatibility test

Perm lotions and other chemicals applied to the hair may react with chemicals that have already been used such as home-use products. The incompatibility test is therefore used to detect chemicals/elements which could react with hairdressing processes such as colouring and perming. The test is carried out as follows:

1 Protect your hands by wearing gloves.
2 Place a small cutting of hair in a small dish.
3 Pour into the dish a mixture of 20 parts of 6 per cent hydrogen peroxide and one part ammonium thioglycolate (general purpose perm solution). Make sure that you are not bending over the dish to avoid splashing the chemicals on to your face or inhaling any resultant released fumes.
4 Watch for signs of bubbling, heating or discolouration. These indicate that the hair already contains incompatible chemicals. The hair should not be permed, coloured or bleached if there are any signs of reaction. Perming treatment might discolour or break the hair and could burn the skin.

Elasticity test

This test is carried out on a dry single hair and used to determine how much the hair will stretch and then return to its original position. It is an indicator of the internal condition of the hair's bonded structure and ability to retain moisture. By taking a hair between the fingers and stretching it you can assess the amount of spring it has. If the hair breaks easily, care needs to be taken before applying any hairdressing process and further tests are indicated – a test curl or a test cutting, for example. Natural healthy hair in good condition will be elastic and more likely to retain the effects of physical curling, setting or blow shaping longer. It will also take chemical processes more readily. Hair with little elasticity will not hold physical shaping or chemical processes satisfactorily.

Remember

Incompatible chemistry
Henna is still widely used throughout the world as a hair and skin dyeing compound. In the UK people using natural henna will often add other ingredients such as coffee, wine, lemon juice, etc. to intensify the final colour. However, people in other countries also add compounds to henna; for example, in India and Turkey people sometimes add iron ore deposits which are crushed into the powder to increase the 'reddening' effect. If this mix subsequently comes into contact with hydrogen peroxide (either through colouring or perming), a chemical reaction will take place. In the exchange that takes place permanent damage and breakage will occur.

Remember

Sensitivity and PPD
This test is used to assess the client's tolerance of chemicals introduced to the skin – PPD. The abbreviation stands for paraphenylenediamine (para-dyes), the main ingredient within permanent colour that is a known irritant to skin and eyes and can cause an allergic reaction.

Remember

Always wear vinyl disposable gloves when conducting a chemical process.

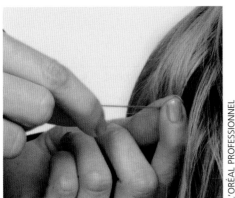

L'ORÉAL PROFESSIONNEL

Porosity Test

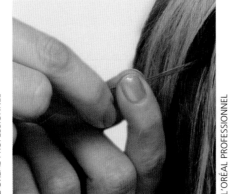

L'ORÉAL PROFESSIONNEL

Porosity Test

Porosity test

The porosity test is will assess the amount of damage to the cuticle layer and therefore the hair's ability to absorb moisture or liquids – another indicator of poor condition. If the cuticle is torn or broken, it will soon lose its moisture and become dry. It may be able to absorb liquids quicker, but its ability to retain them is reduced. If the cuticle is smooth, unbroken and tightly packed, it may resist the passage of moisture or liquids. By running the fingertips through the hair, from points to roots, you can assess the degree of roughness. The rougher the hair, the more porous it will be and the faster it will absorb chemicals.

Remember

Natural moisture levels

The natural moisture levels in hair play a significant part in the way that hair responds to treatments and styling. If the natural levels can be retained following perming, colouring and bleaching the client's hair will remain manageable, easier to detangle and able to hold thermal styling effects for far longer.

Deplete those natural levels and the hair becomes porous and will tangle easily, is less manageable and not able to hold a set for long. Pre-chemical treatments help to reduce the hair's moisture reduction.

EKU statement

G21 (eku20) The likely causes of various adverse hair, skin and scalp conditions (i.e. ringworm, impetigo, scabies, eczema, alopecia, psoriasis, folliculitis, dandruff, ingrowing hair and head lice)

G21 (eku21) Which hair, scalp conditions and disorders should be referred to a pharmacist, general practitioner or registered trichologist and why

G21 (eku22) The importance of, and reasons for, not naming specific conditions when referring clients to a general practitioner or trichologist

Hair and scalp diseases, conditions and defects

Diseases of the hair and scalp may be caused by a variety of infectious organisms and particular *tell-tale* signs or symptoms enable us to identify them. An initial examination should be carried out before any hairdressing process occurs, so that any adverse conditions can be identified. If this is not done a variety of serious outcomes can occur. However, not all hair and scalp conditions are dangerous; some non-infectious conditions can easily be addressed within the salon.

You have to differentiate between them.

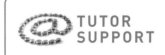

TUTOR SUPPORT

Discussion 1.6: Situations necessary to refuse to carry out a service

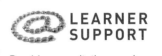

LEARNER SUPPORT

Provide consultation services crossword

Infectious diseases

Bacterial diseases

Condition	Symptoms	Cause	Treatment	Infectious
Folliculitis Inflammation of the hair follicles	Inflamed follicles, a common symptom of certain skin diseases	A contact bacterial infection, or due to chemical or physical action	Medical referral to GP	Yes
Impetigo A bacterial infection of the upper skin layers	At first a burning sensation, followed by spots becoming dry; honey-coloured, crusts form and spread	A staphylococcal or streptococcal infection	Medical referral to GP	Yes
Sycosis A bacterial infection of the hairy parts of the face	Small, yellow spots around the follicle mouth, burning, irritation and general inflammation	Bacteria attack the upper part of the hair follicle, spreading to the lower follicle	Medical referral to GP	Yes
Furunculosis Boils or abscesses	Raised, inflamed, pus-filled spots, irritation, swelling and pain	An infection of the hair follicles by staphylococcal bacteria	Medical referral to GP	Yes

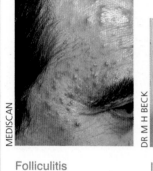

MEDISCAN

Folliculitis

DR M H BECK

Impetigo

DR ANDREW WRIGHT

Sycosis

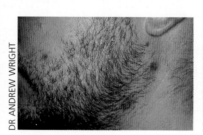

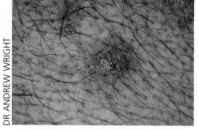

DR ANDREW WRIGHT

Furunculosis

Viral diseases

Condition	Symptoms	Cause	Treatment	Infectious
Herpes simplex (cold sore) A viral infection of the skin	Burning, irritation, swelling and inflammation precede the appearance of fluid-filled blisters, usually on the lips and surrounding areas	Possibly exposure to extreme heat or cold, or a reaction to food or drugs; the skin may carry the virus for years without exhibiting any symptoms	Medical referral to pharmacist	Yes
Warts A viral infection of the skin	Raised, roughened skin, often brown or discoloured. There may be irritation and soreness. Warts are common on the hands and face	The lower epidermis is attacked by the virus, which causes the skin to harden and skin cells to multiply	Medical referral to pharmacist	Yes

DR M H BECK

Herpes simplex

COURTESY OF MEDISCAN

Warts

Animal (parasitic) infestations

Condition	Symptoms	Cause	Treatment	Infectious
Head lice (Pediculosis capitis) Infestation of the hair and scalp by head lice	An itchy reaction to the biting head louse, 'peppering' on pillowcases and minute egg cases (nits) attached to the upper hair shaft close to the scalp	The head louse bites the scalp feeding on the victim's blood. Breeding produces eggs, which are laid and cemented onto the hair shaft for incubation until the immature louse emerges	Referral to a pharmacist	Yes
Scabies An allergic reaction to the itch mite	A rash in the skin folds around the midriff and on the inside of the thighs, extremely itchy at night	The itch mite burrows under the skin where it lays eggs	Medical referral to GP	Yes

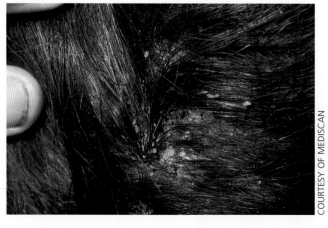

Head lice

COURTESY OF MEDISCAN

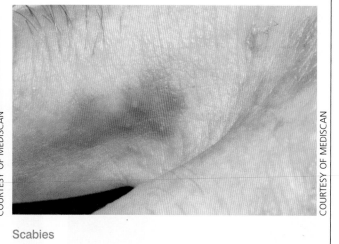

Scabies

COURTESY OF MEDISCAN

Fungal diseases

Condition	Symptoms	Cause	Treatment	Infectious
Tinea capitis Ringworm of the head	Circular bald patch of grey or whitish skin surrounded by red, active rings; hairs broken close to the skin, which looks dull and rough. The fungus lives off the keratin in the skin and hair. This disease is common in children	Fungal infection of the skin or hair	Medical referral to GP	Yes

Tinea capitis

DR JOHN GRAY

Non-infectious diseases

Conditions of the hair and skin

Condition	Symptoms	Cause	Treatment	Infectious
Acne Disorder affecting the hair follicles and sebaceous glands	Raised spots and bumps within the skin, commonly upon the face in adolescents	Increased sebum and other secretions block the follicle and a skin reaction occurs	Medical referral to GP	No
Eczema and dermatitis In its simplest form a reddening of the skin	Ranging from slightly inflamed areas of the skin to severe splitting and weeping areas with irritation and soreness	Many possible causes, eczema often associated with internal factors, i.e. allergies or stress Dermatitis a reaction or allergy to external factors.	Medical referral to GP	No
Psoriasis An inflamed, abnormal thickening of the skin	Areas of thickened skin, often raised and patchy. Often on the scalp and also at the joints (arms and legs)	Unknown	Medical referral to GP	No

COURTESY OF MEDISCAN

Acne

HMSO

Dermititis

ISTOCKPHOTO.COM\KEN ROBERTS

Psoriasis

Conditions of the hair and skin

Condition	Symptoms	Cause	Treatment	Infectious
Dandruff (Pityriasis capitis)	Dry, small, irritating flakes	Fungal (yeast-like) infection, or physical or chemical irritants	Anti-dandruff treatments	No
Seborrhea Excessive	Very greasy, lank hair and greasy skin, making styling difficult	Over-production of sebum	Astringent shampoos	No
Alopecia (hair loss) Alopecia **areata**	The name given to balding patches over the scalp. Often starts around or above the ears, circular in pattern ranging from 1–2.5 cm in diameter		Trichological referral	
Traction **alopecia**	Hair loss as a result of excessive pulling at the roots from brushing, curling and straightening. Very often seen with younger girls tying, plaiting or braiding long hair		None	
Alopecia totalis	Complete hair loss sometimes as a result of alopecia areata spreading and joining up across the scalp		Trichological referral	

Alopecia (hair loss)

Cicatrical alopecia   Baldness due to scarring of the skin arising from chemical or physical injury.
The hair follicle is damaged and permanent baldness results

Male pattern   Male baldness or thinning of hair occurring in teens or early twenties. Hair
recedes at the hairline or loss at the crown area. Condition is hereditary
(passed on in families)

Remedies currently
being developed

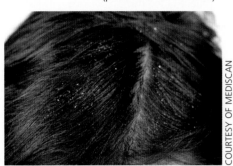

Dandruff

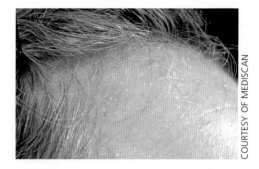

Seborrhea

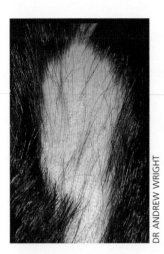

Alopecia areata

Traction alopecia

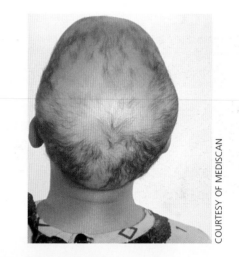

Alopecia totalis

Cicatrical alopecia

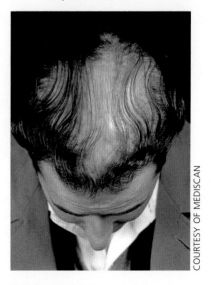

Male pattern baldness

Condition	Symptom	Cause	Treatment
Split ends (Fragilitis crinium) Fragile, poorly conditioned hair	Dry, splitting hair ends	Harsh physical or chemical treatments	Cutting off or special treatment conditioners
Monilethrix Beaded hair	Beadlike swellings along the hair shaft, hair often breaks at weaker points	Irregular development of the hair forming during cellular production	None
Trichorrexis nodosa Nodules forming on the hair shaft	Areas of swelling at locations along the hair shaft, splitting and rupturing the cuticle layer	Harsh physical or chemical processing	None, although cutting and conditioning may help
Sebaceous cyst Swelling of the oil gland	Bumps, lumps and swellings on the scalp containing fluid, soft to the touch	Sebaceous gland becomes blocked allowing a build-up of fluid to take place	Medical referral
Damaged cuticle Broken, split, torn hair	Rough, raised, missing areas of cuticle; hair loses its moisture and becomes dry and porous	Harsh physical or chemical processes	None, although cutting and conditioning may help

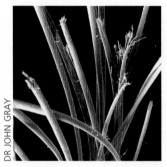

Split ends

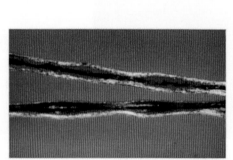

Monilethrix

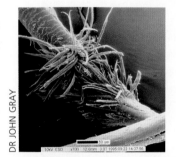

Trichorrexis nodosa

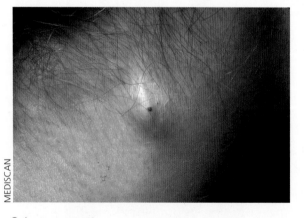

Sebaceous cyst

Damaged cuticle

Influencing factors and features

The purpose of consultation is to arrive at a suitable hairdressing outcome through the process of analysis and evaluation. It should be done in a way that gives the client confidence in both the salon and in you.

It is necessary to study the 'complete picture' when you first meet the client. This is to make sure that you have enough information to advise the client properly. Your aim is not to alter what the client wears or their self-image, but to work with these aspects to achieve satisfaction.

During consultation you will be considering all the aspects of the client's physical features. Is there anything that doesn't work? Is the client happy with the existing style? They may point to areas which you feel are wrong or unnecessary, so you need to be able to express your technical appraisal in a clear, simple way without confusion. Avoid using any technical jargon or trade terms.

Consultation is *customised* for the client. It is personal and individual on each and every occasion. We therefore have to consider technical and personal image aspects:

- cutting and final shape of the hair
- volume or colour which will enhance the style
- finishing options of blow-drying or dressing the hair
- their type, hair growth, natural colour and face shape
- their personal image, lifestyle and personality
- amount of time they can give to their hair.

Expression

Look for responses to your suggestions. Facial expression reflects the client's mood or how they are feeling. You need to pick up on these expressions and react to them appropriately. This will help to understand the client's wants and needs more easily.

Hair growth patterns

Hair is the frame for the face. The length, quantity, quality and texture of the hair all contribute to the total image. Fine hair often lacks body; most clients want fullness and volume which will last. Cutting methods to achieve this include volumising techniques where body can be created by using longer layers levelled in line with the client's baselines and face shape. You should also consider proportioning the hair weight. By setting hair or using light perms, you can create bulk and volume which give foundation to shape and style.

The hair's movement refers to the amount of curl or wave within the hair lengths. However, its growth pattern denotes the direction from which it protrudes from the scalp. Natural hair fall can be seen on wet and dry hair and strong directional growth will have a major impact on the lie of the hair when it is styled. So it is essential that it is taken into account during consultation.

Double crown The client with a double crown will benefit from leaving sufficient length in the hair to over-fall the whole area. If it is cut too short, the hair will stick up and will not lie flat.

Nape whorl A nape whorl can occur at either or both sides of the nape. It can make the hair difficult to cut into a straight neckline or tight 'head-hugging' graduations. Often the hair naturally forms a V-shape. Tapered neckline shapes may be more suitable, but sometimes the hair is best left long so that the weight of the hair overfalls the nape whorl directions.

Remember

Always make and maintain eye contact with your client.

Be aware of your client's expressions and react appropriately.

Remember

Give your clients time to consider your suggestions and advice.

Remember

Look at the amount and quality of your client's hair. Remember that clients with fine hair want volume. Look at the proportion, partings and distribution of the hair.

How much natural movement has the hair got? Will it impede the styling plan?

Are there any strong growth patterns to contend with?

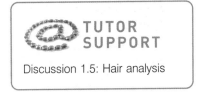

TUTOR SUPPORT

Discussion 1.5: Hair analysis

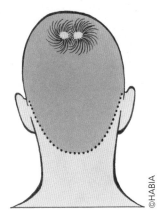

Double crown

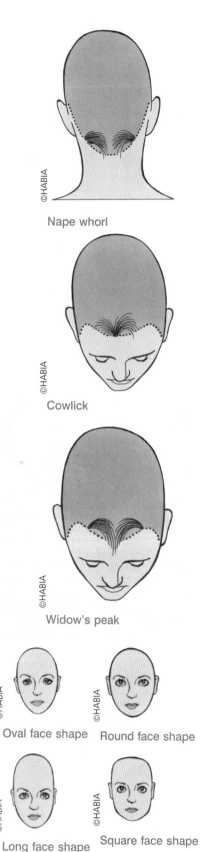

Nape whorl

Cowlick

Widow's peak

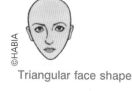

Oval face shape   Round face shape

Long face shape   Square face shape

Triangular face shape

Cowlick   A cowlick appears at the hairline at the front of the head. It makes cutting a straight fringe difficult, particularly on fine hair, because the hair often forms a natural parting. The strong movement can often be improved by moving the parting over so that the weight over-falls the growth pattern. Sometimes a fringe can be achieved by leaving the layers longer so that they weigh down the hair.

Widow's peak   The widow's peak growth pattern appears at the centre of the front hairline. The hair grows upward and forward, forming a strong peak. It is often better to cut the hair into styles that are dressed back from the face, as any 'light fringes' will be likely to separate and stick up.

> **Remember**
>
> Hair growth i.e. the directions in which the hair grows will have an impact on the choice of styling and general style maintenance.

> **Remember**
>
> Head shapes can have a major impact on the final profile of the style you are attempting to create. For example, a flatter crown or back of the head is made more noticeable when a contoured, layered cut is selected as the chosen hairstyle.

Face and head shape

The basic, natural shape of the head, face and features are what form the underlying structure in styling. The proportions of the hair mass and distribution in relation to the face and head are vital in choosing a style. The outer hair shape should fit the face shape to achieve a suitable hair arrangement.

The contours of the head are its focal points. Those on the side of the head are formed by the parietal and temporal bones. Those on the back of the head and nape are formed by the occipital bones, which can be concave or convex: curving inwards or outwards. The frontal bone forms the forehead shape. It is the beginning of the profile, which follows along the nose to the lips and chin. This can vary in shape and may be concave or convex.

The face shape is made up of straight or curved lines, and sometimes a mixture of the two. Straight, fine shapes appear angular and chiselled or firm and solid. They can be triangular, rectangular, square or diamond shaped. Curved line shapes appear soft and may be round, oval, pear-shaped or oblong. Shapes which have some straight and some curved lines are defined as heart shaped or soft square shaped.

To create a pleasant balance, the hairstyle and face shape need to be compatible. An angular hair cut will not suit a soft, rounded face. A soft hair shape will not complement a chiselled face. Hair shape outlines can be made to look quite different from the front by simply changing a parting from side to centre. Side partings tend to make the face appear wider, whilst centre partings close down the width of a wide forehead.

An oval face shape suits any hairstyle. Round faces need height to reduce the width of the face. A centre parting can also help to reduce width. Long facial proportions are improved with short, wider hairstyles. Square-shaped faces need round shapes with texture on to the face to soften them. Longer lengths beyond the jaw line improve the balance and proportion.

Ears, nose and mouth

Often ears are out of balance, which can affect the cut if you use them as a guide. Generally, large ears or even large lobes are accentuated by hair cut short or dressed away from the face. It is often better to leave hair longer over the ears unless it is an essential part of the style's impact.

Your client may wear a hearing aid and this may be a sensitive issue. Some clients wish to have all signs of an aid hidden, but others do not mind and even display it. You should discuss this with your client carefully and with sensitivity; they may feel too embarrassed to bring up the subject themself. The size of the aid will need careful consideration when completing the total image.

The position, shape, size and colour of the nose and mouth are very important in the facial expression. The angles that are created can be softening or harsh and must not be ignored when the image is being planned. Hair shape and make-up can contribute to create the required effect.

Eyes

We already know the importance of maintaining eye contact when communicating with the client, showing that you are listening to each other. But eyes play a major part in the selection of hairstyles too. Heavy fringes can accentuate and frame or they can obstruct vision.

Eye colour is a guide to the natural colouring of the client. This is a useful pointer when choosing hair colour. Eye shape is another element to be considered when choosing which style to create. Ideally, eye, head and face shape should all be complemented by the hairstyle and colour.

The eyebrows frame the eyes. Their shape, size and colour are all significant. A very harsh appearance is created if the eyebrows are removed and various other effects are created by adding shapely lines. Eyelash and brow colouring help to balance facial effects and give the eyes more definition.

Spectacles should be considered when you are deciding on a hairstyle. Frame and lens colour, size and shape have a major impact upon styling and therefore must be taken into account.

Neck and shoulders

The length, fullness and width of the neck will affect the fall of the back and nape hair. Longer necks allow better positioning of long hair. They are complemented by high, neat lines; for example, mandarin collars or polo-neck tops. Short necks need to be uncluttered, with short hair and low collars. Long and thin necks are more noticeable with short styles and will therefore be better suited to longer hair around them. Shorter necks can be counterbalanced with height or upswept hair styles.

Remember

Checklist
- What are the shape, position and size of the client's ears?
- What is the shape and size of the client's nose and mouth?
- Are these features a major concern to your client?
- What shape is your client's facial and head shape?
- Are there any significant features that need to be accounted for?
- Small faces need 'opening up' while larger faces need narrower framing effects.

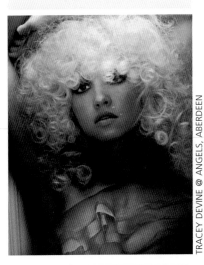

TRACEY DEVINE @ ANGELS, ABERDEEN

Remember

The eyes are the focal point upon the face. Good images in magazines use this aspect to sell everything from clothes to hairdressing. Your client will be drawn to strong images, but are they wearable in everyday life? The majority of 'hair shots' use hair in ways across the eye line to create artistic impact. These snapshots of 'still life' are stimulating but not feasible. You must make a point of this during your consultation.

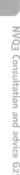

TUTOR SUPPORT

Project 1.2: Influencing factors and features

Remember

The eyes are the focal point upon the face. Use them within the style's construction.

What colour and shape are your client's eyes?

What are the eyebrows like?

Does your client normally wear spectacles?

Remember

How long or short is your client's neck?

How wide or narrow is your client's neck?

Have you taken these features into consideration?

Remember

What is the purpose of the style – fashion, special occasion?

Work, social and leisure pursuits are all factors to be considered.

Different styles suit certain age groups.

Will the final effect suit the lifestyle requirements?

EKU *statement*

G21 (eku18) How the following factors limit or affect the services and products that can be offered to clients: lifestyle

Body shape

The body shape also needs to be considered. You need to carefully balance the amount, density and overall shape of the hair to your client's physical body shape. This is particularly important if your client considers her shape or size a particularly important factor. For example, a small, clinging hairstyle would look wrong on a large body shape.

Lifestyle, personality and age

Remember that people are constrained by what they do for a living or what they like to do in their spare time. Usually, people who work in environments where they have face-to-face contact with clients have to be more particular about the image they portray. This is a very important factor in style selection.

From a leisure point of view, you should find out whether the client does a lot of sport or exercise. If so, the hairstyle will have to be versatile and able to withstand a lot of washing and possibly heat styling. Also, think about how the style could be handled to create a number of different effects when the client is going out. If you are styling for a special occasion, it is worth asking what dress will be worn. A beautiful gown needs to be accompanied by an elegant hairstyle. However, this style will need to be altered for normal wear.

- Many clients want practical and manageable styles for work.
- Nurses, doctors and caterers, among others, may require styles which keep the hair off the face, or they may have to wear face and head coverings at work.
- Dancers, athletes and skaters, among others, need hairstyles which will not get in their eyes and obscure their vision.
- Fashion models may require elaborate styles for special photographic or modelling sessions or displays.

Character and personality can often override physical features when you are choosing a style for your client. A self-confident client will be able to wear looks that a self-conscious client cannot. Make sure you take this into account so that mistakes are not made. Is your client confident and outgoing or shy, timid and retiring, not wishing to stand out in a crowd? Is she professional and businesslike?

And what age group does your client fall in to? There are basic rules that apply to people at certain ages:

Children – simple, practical shapes (although parents often try to suggest fashions).

Teenagers – fashionable, trendy and willing to try new things.

Young married – something suitable for work, attractive easier to maintain styles.

Parents – practical and attractive styles, often shorter styles.

Middle aged – softening shapes to disguise wrinkles.

Senior age – softening shapes.

Young businessmen – fashionable cuts.

Older men – simple, practical styles.

These are only general guides – there will always be exceptions to the rules.

Make-up

Make-up can enhance features, define eyes and mask or disguise features or blemishes. How the client uses make-up may give a clue to her personality, dress sense and style. In business, a well made-up person is seen to be finished, groomed and in control. Lipstick reflects the colour depth of the skin and eyes creates light on the face and defines the lips. Shiny lipstick is most suitable for someone with a glitzy image. Matt lipstick is more suitable for the quieter person, or when a natural look is required. Lip balm or gloss looks natural and keeps lips soft.

Make-up can create a range of images: soft and kind, bold and extrovert. It can make people feel different about their appearance and so boost confidence if it is properly applied.

Manageability (see G21.4 for more information)

Different styles need different amounts of commitment from the client once they leave the salon. You need to take these factors on board when consulting with the client to make sure that they will carry on being happy with the style you both choose until it is time for their next visit.

Using visual aids in consultation

Pictures

Visual aids are essential! Use them and encourage clients to bring in pictures too.

A picture paints a thousand words' – the term is a cliché but very true. Pictures convey aspects of hair styles or effects that are very difficult to put into words. They eliminate ambiguous technical jargon and establish a basis for things that you and the client can confirm.

We know how to speak with clients; we know what to ask and what not to ask. We listen, hear and confirm back to the client. The whole discussion forms a naturally developing contract, an obligation that will be performed, so it is vitally important that we summarise and agree throughout the whole process.

This natural form of check and recheck enables you to move forward. It covers each feature and factor bit by bit. The same feelings are felt by the client. By covering and confirming each aspect, you convey professionalism and competence, which ultimately concludes with you gaining the client's trust.

Pictures are an immensely important visual aid and another form of language that hairdressers understand very well. One reason for this is their understanding of visual/spatial imagery. However, there is a vast difference between what the client sees in a photo and what the hairdresser will see.

A client brings in the photo to the left as an example for her own hairstyle. What aspects of this image does she find appealing? What is the client deriving from the image?

- mood
- colour contrasts
- attitude
- fun 'clubbing' hairstyle
- sex appeal
- perimeter shape.

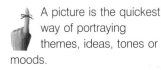

Remember

 Make-Up
How much make up is your client wearing?

What image is she trying to portray: natural, classic and businesslike, dramatic or romantic?

Remember

Personality plays an important factor in style choice. A confident person will be able to wear more effects, colour etc. than someone who lacks confidence.

Remember

How much time will the client have available to style their hair?

How easy is it for them to replicate the same effect?

Are products essential for maintaining the look?

How often do they wash and condition their hair?

Remember

A picture is the quickest way of portraying themes, ideas, tones or moods.

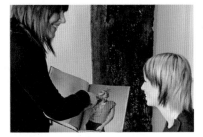

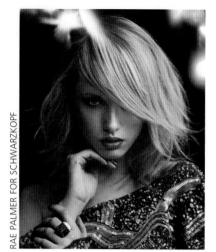

RAE PALMER FOR SCHWARZKOPF

What do you, as the hairdresser, see?

- a textured, above-the-shoulder-length bob
- no fringe
- unrealistic hair across the face
- false inference of hair colour produced by photographic lighting
- limited flexibility for work/social wear.

From this example you can see that great images convey a lot more than hairstyles. We don't expect the client to understand the technical aspects of the style. She doesn't. She is *buying into* an ambience. You see something with a trained eye that is quite different. Yes we all find good imagery stimulating, but as hairdressers we are trained to strip off those *aesthetic* veneers in order to make sense of what we are seeing.

Colour charts

Colour charts are extremely useful for hairdressers. We rely on them every day. However, they are not always a very helpful medium for the client. We tend to treat others as we would want to be treated ourselves. This is a good philosophy, but there are times when our expectation of others is a little over-optimistic. Generally speaking, clients have very little ability for self-visualisation. This could be confirmed another way. Think about shopping. How often do women shop in pairs? Other people's comments, assistance and points of view are very important. The reason is obvious. If we need more reassurance about what we are doing we have to involve someone else; ideally someone else who knows us, our likes and dislikes, and most important of all someone who can objectively comment about our decision-making process.

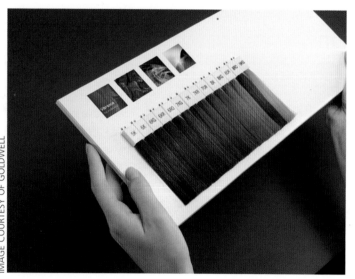

IMAGE COURTESY OF GOLDWELL

Colour chart

The colour chart is a useful tool for hairdressers and a nice colouring book for clients. Unless you can help the client visualise the amount, intensity, density and saturation of the resultant colour, the visual aid will have little or no impact on the decision-making process of whether to buy colour or not.

Remember

A colour chart is useful to show tones and hues, but don't expect your client to be able to visualise an all over effect from a small sample.

Computer-generated images

The internet is a valuable medium for conveying information about hair and hairstyles. Many salons have their own websites. The ease of using computer-generated images and uploading them to salon sites is proving a very cost effective advertising medium. However, there is very little information technology used for graphical purposes within salons. Although many software packages are available for generating makeover effects, very little use is made of this medium at present. The constraints of cost, training and operator time are still barriers to salons that want to harness this technology.

Advising clients relies on a good knowledge of what is available, in order to match products and services to clients' requirements. Acquiring this knowledge is an ongoing process, as products are always being updated.

When you have completed your analysis and identified both your client's wishes and the factors that influence your styling options, you should be able to make your recommendations to the client.

EKU statement

G21 (eku6) The services and products available for use in your salon

G21 (eku9) The duration of services available in your salon

G21 (eku11) The reasons why special advice is necessary for certain services (e.g. could be painful, very lengthy to perform, etc.)

G21 (eku12) Current fashion trends and looks

Remember

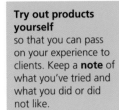

Try out products yourself so that you can pass on your experience to clients. Keep a **note** of what you've tried and what you did or did not like.	**Other people's experiences** are useful to know. You could do some **market research** on clients, friends or colleagues.	**Specialist magazines** often contain adverts and articles about new products on the market. Look at the **features page** to see what's new.

You will need to know

- The ranges of services and products your salon offers.
- The prices and timings of those services and prices of the products available.
- Any services that need particular or special advice prior to implementation.
- Current fashion trends and looks.
- Any situations where referral is needed.

Every salon has its own range of services and products – you must know the ranges of services and products that your salon offers. In most situations, your salon will have a service or product that meets 99% of the client's needs. It would be impractical or impossible to cover *every* type of treatment. Needless to say, you must be familiar with what your salon offers; you need to know what the costs are of these services/products and how long they will take.

Some services also need additional preparation or special conditions – before they can be carried out. For example. Your salon may do hair-pieces for hair-up work; some salons may do added clip-on hair extensions, whereas others offer the complete bonded extensions systems. In any of these cases it would be unlikely that all the necessary materials to do all of these services will be in stock. So you need to be able to tell your client exactly when those items will be available, the differences, benefits and pitfalls, how long it will take how they will look after them and how much it will cost.

There are other special situations too. You may wish to offer a colouring service to a new client, but you know that you will have to conduct your skin test first. So you will need to tell the client what they can expect and also what you need to know and how they should contact you in the event of any adverse, contra-indications (in other words, a positive reaction to a patch test).

(See taking deposits, p. 40.)

Remember

Keep abreast of all your salon's recent additions. If new products are introduced, then it's your job to find out; what they do, how they work and how long they take and how much they cost.

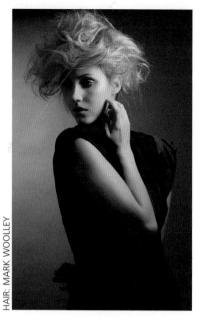

HAIR: MARK WOOLLEY

EKU *statement*

G21 (eku5) Your salon's policy for referring clients to other salons

Diversion (See adverse hair and scalp conditions p. 23)

Remember

If you are not sure what the problem is and it looks medical, refer the client to a pharmacist or their GP.

Remember

If you need to refer clients to a trichologist, you can find a listing through the trichological institute on the internet www.trichologists.org.uk.

Keep abreast of current fashions

Your knowledge should be up to date and there are numerous ways in which you can do this:

- Trade shows and exhibitions.
- Courses and seminars.
- Trade magazines.
- Fashion magazines.
- TV and the internet.

You should keep in touch with what's happening in celebrity world. These well-known icons create fashion; they are prepared and groomed by personal stylists that are employed by production and promotional companies so that they are always in the eye of the public. People are stimulated by the entertainment industries and the media are always following the lives of celebrities from film, TV and music. The success of magazines such as *OK* and *Hello* is due to the attention they pay to these people's lives and what they are up to.

Your customers will expect you to be aware of what is happening in these sectors and you will need to be ready to advise whether these new looks are going to suit them.

Remember

There is always another way of tackling the problems. When you can't provide what the client wants, always offer suitable alternatives.

Referrals

There will be situations where the clients anticipated service can not be provided.

This could be due to:

- adverse hair and skin problems
- your salon not offering that particular service or treatment.

Specialist remedial referral

Some hair and scalp conditions can be treated in the salon, but many more will require specialist, remedial attention. You need to know which ones are handled by the various specialists.

For example, a mother brings a child in for a haircut who obviously has nits: the child cannot be dealt with in the salon. You need to be sympathetic and not over-reactive. Tell the mother that the child is infected and explain what course of action is necessary. Explain the benefits of looking out for infestations on a regular basis and the signs that they would probably see, i.e. small whiteish/grey nodules attached to the hair close to the scalp, generally around the back and nape, evidence of the louse itself or as peppering of brown speckles over the child's pillow at night and itching.

But that is as far as your comment should go. You need to refer them to a pharmacist so that the mother can purchase a remedy and apply it to her child's head.

A client with eczema may be aware of their condition, but you may be concerned that a planned service may aggravate the condition further, a referral to their doctor first, is preferable, if only to eliminate the concern that your planned service won't make the condition worse.

If you find a condition that you are not sure about, tell the client. Say, 'I'm not sure what the problem is but I do think you should get it checked out before we continue our planned services.'

Salon referrals

You need to keep abreast of the salons in your area that offer special services that your salon doesn't. Services such as trichological analysis, hair extensions, hair transplants, wigs and hairpieces may be carried out locally in other salons. But remember, with referrals you must follow your salon's policy for external re-direction.

| G21.4 | Advise clients on hair maintenance and management |

What the clients really want is to be able to achieve the same finished effects that you do in the salon. They don't necessarily appreciate the amount of time that you put into your training to achieve NVQ level 2 or your current training at level 3. You just seem to make it all seem so simple and that's not a bad thing.

You already know the limitations created by adverse hair conditions, hair textures, types and tendencies. But to them, you are the enabler; you create the beautiful effects and now you need to pass on a little advice and a few tips on how the effect can be managed away from the salon between visits.

You need to:

● find out what the client is already doing with their hair
● explain the benefits modifying the care regimen in relation to the new effect
● advise them on the correct product regimen to maintain their hair at home
● tell them how to maintain their hair between salon visits.

EKU *statement*

G21 (eku29) Suitable conditioning treatments and the importance of regular conditioning

EKU *statement*

G21 (eku32) How lifestyle can influence the clients choice of style (e.g. active sports, career and job requirements)

What is the client already doing with their hair?

Rightly or wrongly your client will have some sort of routine in place for washing and fixing their hair into place. This may be a simple affair: a client with little self-respect or self-awareness and washes their hair because they think it needs it, then puts a towel around their head and takes the towel off in an hour or so and runs a brush through it to finish it off!

EKU *statement*

G21 (eku30) The products to use for home care and those to avoid and why

Or, more likely, it is a more involved activity. The client already has a care regimen in place that is designed to meet their current needs. This could involve a treatment shampoo and conditioner and a variety of styling and finishing products which are all carefully used in concert with a range of hairstyling equipment.

Whatever care routine your client has, you need to be aware of what they are doing and how they are doing it. It can have a negative effect on what you are trying to achieve, so you would only be doing yourself in injustice, by not asking.

Explain the benefits of modifying the care regimen in relation to the new effect. Remember this important phrase: 'People are reluctant to change'. Bear this in mind when you make any reference to changing from one care regimen to another. People and therefore your clients will be used to a routine that suits both their

- lifestyle, and
- present hair requirements.

If you create a new effect or, provide a service that has a detrimental effect on their lifestyle requirements. You'll probably find out that it just doesn't work. Whatever, you do for them, it must be *symbiotic* and fit in with lives; i.e. their job, their leisure pursuits and most importantly the time that they can afford to maintain it.

The other aspect relates to what they are already doing with their hair. If the products that they are already using conflict with what you are doing, you must make this known. What is the point of doing half a job? You are *in partnership* with your client. What you do and advise them to do, must be taken on board so that they can have the best possible chance of replicating the effect.

Advise them on the correct product regimen to maintain their hair at home

Products are an essential part of the equation. What they use has a direct effect on the result. For example, if a client is used to a conditioning product for normal-frequent use, and you do a highlighting service for them, do you think that their current conditioner is up to the job? Similarly, if your client has been using defining waxes on their hair for some time because of the texture it achieved on their short hair, do you think it would still be appropriate if they had just had a full head of hair extensions? No, is the short answer.

All modern, fashionable hairstyles involve some form of product care and maintenance. Even casual, carefree styles need the right shampoos and conditioners. But most hairstyles are far more demanding than this. You need to advise your clients on the correct products for their hair, how to use them and what benefits they get from using them.

EKU *statement*

G21 (eku31) How to protect the hair from the effects of humidity (e.g. environmental, sports, related, steamy conditions)

G21 (eku33) How the use of excessive heat can damage the hair

G21 (eku34) How to maintain their agreed style

Tell them how to maintain their hair between salon visits

The advice that you give clients on how to managing the effects themselves is the *real deal*. If they can get a similar effect to that of *just left the salon*, then you will have really made a big difference to their lives.

Remember to cover the obvious things too. It's so easy to forget the basics when you are trying to explain how to make the most out of their hair. Often the simplest of things make all the difference and have a long-lasting effect on the general condition of the hair or how long it will stay in. For example, a client who is always using very hot equipment to style their hair is going find out the hard way that either the hair needs protecting from the heat or, there won't be anything left to protect! Similarly, if their lifestyle involves a lot of sport or going to the gym, then they are going to get hot. Any moisture whether environmental or from the body is going to dampen the hair and this means it won't stay in very long.

Remember

Be positive and suggest ways around problems and if possible find ways to avoid the negative effects altogether. We all want our clients to become regular visitors, if you can tell them what they need to know, and then they will tell everyone else.

G21.5   Agree services with your client

With all other parts of the consultation done, you are almost ready to complete the service. You have:

✔	Identified what the client'wants – your initial part of the consultation had looked at what the client' s expectations were by asking questions and using visual aids.
✔	Identified what the client's needs were – in light of what they wanted, you matched this against their perceived needs and what you saw as the actual needs of the hair following your analysis.
✔	Analysed the hair, skin and scalp – and looked for any adverse conditions, incompatibility issues and conducted, or arranged for any necessary tests.
✔	Made your recommendations – these were based on what you found during the analysis and where this conflicted with client's expectations (because you thought they were unrealistic or they didn't realise that there were other issues to address) you have offered other suitable alternatives in a caring and sympathetic way.
✔	Provided your advice on how the look or effect can be maintained and recreated at home by using the right maintenance routines or purchasing the correct home-care product regimen.

So with all these things done; that must be everything? Not quite. You have made your assumptions based upon the clients needs; your professionalism has ensured that any misunderstandings were made clear. But without seeking confirmation from the client you cannot continue.

The final part of the consultation will require the commitment from the client that confirms that:

✔	They are aware of what the agreed service entails (timings or special conditions).
✔	They have agreed to the services and/or products that you have negotiated.
✔	They understand the costs for the services and/or products and these have been considered acceptable.

EKU statement

G21 (eku9) The duration of services available in your salon

EKU statement

G21 (eku7) Your salon's pricing structure and payment policies e.g. requirements for deposits

And that you:

✔	made sure that all records have been completed and are now up to date
✔	made the necessary appointment(s) or
✔	are now ready to carry out the agreed service.

Final notes

Service timings

Different services have differing durations and timings and in a busy salon; making the most of the available time in an appointment system is a difficult operation. Some special services like hair extensions can take many hours, whereas routine services like cut and blow-dry may take only 45 minutes. Whatever the service you must bear in mind that time is as valuable as money. You need to be realistic when you provide that information to the client.

Their time is precious; if you don't give them an accurate idea of how long things will take or what sorts of things are involved, then you will find that they are going to be rather angry if you run late. If you are unable to give an exact time, don't make it up; give them a range that covers the minimum and the absolute maximum. Let them decide if that is suitable; if not offer alternatives, there is always another day.

Service and product costs

People don't like hidden costs. Hairdressing is a business built on trust, loyalty and most importantly, repeated business. In other words, we want our clients to be satisfied with what we provide. We want them to return again in the future, where we can build on the relationship further and develop a long-term, ongoing business arrangement and this particular factor marks the difference between customers and clients.

With this in mind, you should always provide an honest and accurate cost for what has been agreed. If the client decides that she wants to add other things into the service package, that's fine, providing that no misunderstandings occur.

Taking deposits

You will also need to check to see if a deposit is needed. Often in situations where there is an large investment of salon time or stylist's time, then other preparations need to be arranged in advance and it would be normal practice to take a deposit. This would be done at the time of making the appointment and would be refundable or deducted at the time when the service is finally carried out.

Remember

Taking a deposit
Check what the policy is in your salon. What sorts of services need deposits in advance?

Client records

Keeping proper client records is essential for good salon management and to ensure clients receive a service appropriate for their individual needs. The records also give vital information should there be any subsequent client complaint or worse, if there was any pursuance in a legal case against the salon.

Remember this is personal and private information, it must be handled confidentially and you have a duty to uphold the rights of your clients if you keep their personal information on file. (For more information see the Data Protection Act (1998), Appendix 4.)

Activity
Calculating bills

Using your salon's price tariffs, calculate the cost for client X:

1 A full head of highlights (with bleach or high lift colour) on long hair with a reshape (trim) cut and blow-dry?

2 Now add to this an in-salon conditioning treatment.

What would be the costs of the following services and products in your salon for client Y?

A A restyle cut and blow-dry for a female with long hair

B A retail size shampoo and conditioner for dry damaged hair

C A retail size defining paste

Now add A, B and C together to create the final bill for client Y.

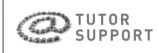
TUTOR SUPPORT

Short answer test 1

TUTOR SUPPORT

Discussion 1.1: Success of the business

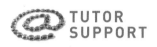
TUTOR SUPPORT

Discussion 1.2: Potential uses for photographic images

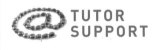
TUTOR SUPPORT

Short answer test 2

Remember
Consultation Checklist

- Listen carefully to what is requested
- Use visual aids to assist the consultation process
- Communicate the possible effects
- Explain why certain effects are not possible
- Give good reasons for suggested actions
- Ensure that the client understands what is being said
- Agree on a final and suitable course of action
- Assure and reassure throughout
- Make it clear if follow-up appointments are necessary
- Carry out the agreed service or treatment
- Encourage the client to rebook the next visit before she leaves
- Maintain the client's goodwill and safety throughout the appointment
- Record the details for future reference

Checkerboard	I know and understand the principles of positive communication	I can communicate positively and professionally with the clients	I always recognise the adverse hair and scalp conditions when I analyse the client's hair
I can identify the range of hair and scalp problems	I know how to negotiate, reaching a mutually beneficial conclusion	I always carry out working practices according to the salon's policy	I've covered most of it!
I always explain technical terms, eliminating ambiguity and false beliefs	I know when and who to refer clients to in situations where external assistance is required	I understand the necessity of personal hygiene and presentation	I always explain the costs, timings and special conditions at the end of the consultation
I know and respect the client's rights, equal opportunities, data protection, anti-discrimination and consumer legislation	I always provide the client with advice on how to maintain their hair themselves at home	I always seek agreement form the client about planned service and products	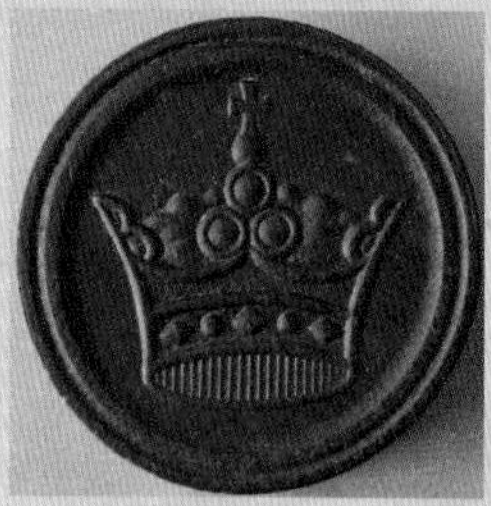

Assessment of knowledge and understanding

Revision questions

Quick quiz: a selection of different types of questions to check your knowledge.

Q1   The three stages of hair growth are anagen, ... and telogen.   Fill in the blank

Q2   The cortex is the outermost layer of the hair.   True or false

Q3   Select all that apply. Which of the following are infectious diseases?   Multi selection

Impetigo	☐	1
Scalp ringworm	☐	2
Alopecia	☐	3
Head lice	☐	4
Psoriasis	☐	5
Eczema	☐	6

Q4   The natural colour of hair depends on the amount of PPD within it.   True or false

Q5   Which of the following is commonly known as split ends?   Multi choice

Trichorrexis nodosa	○	a
Monilethrix	○	b
Tinea capitis	○	c
Fragilitis crinium	○	d

Q6   Dandruff is a condition of the scalp usually caused by fungal infection.   True or false

Q7   Which of the following tests are relevant to semi-permanent colouring   Multi selection
services?

Skin test	☐	1
Strand test	☐	2
Curl test	☐	3
Incompatibility test	☐	4
Porosity test	☐	5
Test cutting	☐	6

Q8   The active part of the root from which hair grows is called the _ _ _ matrix. Fill in the blank

Q9   Which face shape suits most hairstyles and lengths?   Multi choice

Square	○	a
Oblong	○	b
Oval	○	c
Triangular	○	d

Q10 During consultation and hair analysis, any contra-indication found will not   True or false
allow the planned service to be carried out.

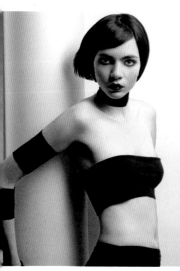

SHARON COX @ SANRIZZ

Chapter**two**
Promote services and products

G18
G18.1
G18.2
G18.3

CREDIT VALUE FOR UNIT G18
6 Credits

More Information
- Consumer Legislation see Appendix 4
- Unit G19 Support customer service improvements

Promoting services/products: quick overview

Unit title

G18 Promote additional services or products to clients

This is an **mandatory** unit and is made up of three main outcomes

Main outcomes

G18.1 Identify additional services or products that are available

G18.2 Inform clients about services or products

G18.3 Gain client commitment to using additional services or products

What do I need to do for G18.1?

- Keep abreast of the salon's services and products
- Check with others when unsure of new services or products
- Spot the products or services that would be useful to certain clients
- Spot the chances to introduce those products or services

What do I need to do for G18.2?

- Choose the right times to introduce services or products with clients
- Choose the right ways to introduce services or products with clients
- Give sufficient, accurate information that would help the client to buy the introduced services and products
- Give the client the time to respond to introduced services and products

What do I need to do for G18.3?

- Know when to close discussions when clients show no interest
- Continue with promotional information when the client is interested

- Establish agreement when the client commits to purchase
- Pass the client on to the relevant service or product provider

What aspects do I need to cover for G18.1, G18.2 and G18.3?

- The ranges of services and products that your salon offers

What do I need to know for G18.1, G18.2 and G18.3?

- The salon's procedures for promoting additional business
- How the services and products will benefit the client
- How the sales of services and products will benefit the salon
- How the features and benefits of services and products are communicated
- How to overcome reservations about services and products
- How to give balanced information to clients

Introduction

The services and treatments that salons provide to their clients are constantly being updated so that they meet an ever-increasing customer expectation. We want clients to enjoy the experience. That experience lasts longer when they can maintain the effects that we do for them in the salon; by taking home the right products to help them achieve the same results.

So by offering new or improved services and products your salon is able to:

- increase client satisfaction
- retain client loyalty for the future.

It is possible to make a really good job of satisfying our clients, but unless they continue to return (and within a reasonable time scale) the financial and ongoing success of the salon is drastically affected. So we need to stimulate the client's loyalty by encouraging them to:

- buy our other services, products and treatments
- return on a regular basis
- share their experiences with other people.

G18.1 Identify additional services or products that are available

Promoting ourselves first

One thing that we as hairdressers and barbers should bear in mind, good communication far outweighs technical excellence. That sounds a little hard to swallow but it's true. You could be an average stylist with reasonable communication skills and you will go far; unfortunately, a brilliant stylist with poor communication skills doesn't have much of a future in a salon setting! Hairdressing is changing very quickly, and not just because of changing fashions and trends.

When it comes to creating success we can only rely on ourselves and the secret is all about communication.

Good customer service is being customer focused. It is centred upon the needs of the client and is reflected within all of the aspects that are involved within routine salon operations: the telephone response times, salon refreshments and magazines, visually pleasing interiors and the polite and friendly staff. It is your duty to be up-beat, outgoing and positive when you communicate with the clients.

Salon services and products

Most salons have tariffs and point of sale material that provide information about the services and products they provide. This is a good way of providing information to clients as they can easily be seen and provide a talking point in the salon. But printed material is not always at hand or available, particularly when services and product ranges are being continually updated.

You need to be aware of changes and additions, so that you can provide advice on available services or products that would benefit your clients. You also need to keep up to date on all the features and benefits of newly introduced services and products. If you find that there are recent additions in the salon that you haven't seen before, you will need to ask your manager or supervisor for more information.

Products are not wallpaper!

Products should never be treated as wallpaper though. They are not decorative items used to cheer up a 'dingy' corner; they have far more important purposes. Retail displays are an expensive investment for the salon and stock resting on shelves is an expensive cost. Products provide a useful, additional input to the salons income and many salons look for a significant proportion of their turnover to be derived from these sales.

There are hidden benefits to the purposes of retailing which may not have thought about. The promotional displays are an integral part in supporting the salon's image. If you think about it another way; the salon *only* purchases products for use and resale that are befitting the quality of services that your salon wants to be identified with. It therefore enables the clients to gain an extension of the salon experience, in the products that they take home.

Features and benefits

In order for you to promote and ultimately, sell your salon's services, treatments and products you need to recognise how they are viewed by clients. To do this you need to consider each service or product in terms of its features and its benefits and how these aspects would meet the needs of your clients:

- 'Features' are the functions; i.e. what the service, treatment or product does.
- 'Benefits' are the results of the functions; i.e. advantages, what the service or products achieves.

For example, suppose you recommend a client to spend £11.50 on a conditioning treatment. Why should she do this? What are the features and benefits of the service?

- The feature is: it re-conditions dry, damaged hair.
- The benefits for her are: it improves the dryness and helps to smooth damaged lengths, thus improving handling, making the hair easy to manage and comb, enhancing the hair further with shine and lustre.

So these benefits justify the investment on her hair.

Knowledge of service and product features enables you to sell your clients the benefits. You thereby create a need, and once the client has accepted the need, you are in a good position to make the sale.

The first step is therefore for you to gain a thorough knowledge of each service and product available in the salon, and to *translate* this knowledge into an understanding of the features and benefits for each one.

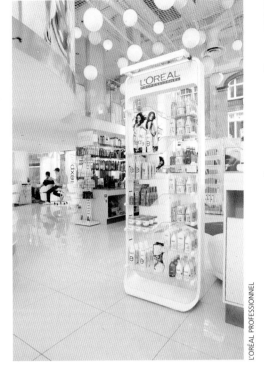

L'ORÉAL PROFESSIONNEL

EKU *statement*

G18 (eku5) How to introduce additional services or products to clients outlining their benefits, overcoming reservations and agreeing to provide the additional services or products

G18.2   Inform clients about services or products

New clients that come in to our salons are part of a very special group. They have probably found us through the network of already satisfied customers. Those satisfied customers feel confident enough in our expertise to promote our skills and services by recommending us to their friends and colleagues.

If recommendation is such a powerful channel of communication, why don't we use it more?

Well we can. The perfect time to talk about the variety of services and treatments available to clients is when they are in the chair in front of us. Recommendation is the simplest way of extending the range of services to our clients and enhancing the professional relationship.

The most effective way of introducing clients to products that will benefit them is to use them on their hair in the salon.

This style of introduction creates a close relationship between:

- something that the client needs (with the added benefit of)
- seeing how it is applied (through to)
- the results that it achieves.

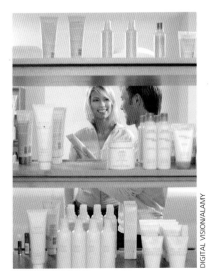

DIGITAL VISION/ALAMY

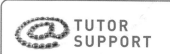

TUTOR SUPPORT

Project 2.1: Features, benefit and cost

EKU *statement*

G18 (eku1) Your salon's procedures and systems for encouraging the use of additional services or products

G18 (eku2) How the use of additional services or products will benefit your clients

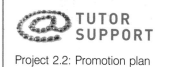

TUTOR SUPPORT

Project 2.2: Promotion plan

This style of promotion is improved further by not only showing the product to the client but by passing it to them so that they can experience the product by:

- holding it and
- smelling the fragrance.

How do we inform clients?

In-salon promotions

An in-salon promotion is the most popular way of conveying *messages* to the clients; it becomes a topic of conversation whilst they are having their hair done. However, any form of salon activity costs money and that outlay has to be budgeted for.

So the first part of the process is to find out what the promotion is about. If it is linked to a new product introduction, then there will be some form of supporting resources to help inform the clients. Whenever a new product or range of products is introduced, the manufacturer will produce a variety of point of sale material that provides people with professionally produced information, posters etc. to help with its launch. The amount of supporting material tends to be distributed in-line with the levels of purchases made by the salon.

Implementation stages of product or service promotion

The following information provides you with a checklist for implementing an in-salon promotion.

✔	Find out the budget.
✔	Make individuals aware of the product's features and benefits.
✔	Let staff know what their roles and targets are.
✔	Implement the promotion.
✔	Evaluate the effectiveness of the promotion.

The budget is set by management and may include the initial outlay figure for purchasing the products as well as the additional cost of setting up the promotional activities. Everyone involved should be informed well in advance of the promotion about the nature and purpose of the event. This provides staff with a clear idea of what the newly introduced products do, their application, how they benefit the clients and the product selling costs.

Usually there is an introductory period to a product launch that may entice customers with special offers or deals.

The most popular promotions are usually in the form of:

- introductory discounts – where products are available for a set period at a lower price
- multi-buys – typically two for ones or get three for the price of two
- special offers – buy all three and get a free beach towel or scarf.

Staff should be made aware of the promotional plan, any incentives linked with the promotion and also their personal targets for the introductory period. Each member of staff could have an individual role to play in the overall team plan. For example, the junior may ask the client if she wants to try the new conditioner on her hair at the basin. From this a client gets the chance to gain her first experiences of the product.

The promotion continues at the styling position where display materials, e.g. show cards or leaflets, inform the client about the benefits from using the product; which is backed up further, by the stylist's recommendation and advice. Other questions would ask if she noticed and liked the *smell* of the conditioner when it was applied; or if she can *see* and *feel* the difference that it has made to her hair.

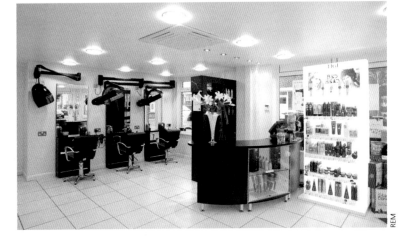

Then finally, before the client leaves, she *connects* again with the promotion and sees a well-put-together display in reception. The receptionist could now ask if she would like to add the product to her bill for her use at home.

You can see from this example that it can be a whole team approach. This is particularly obvious in larger salons where individual staff can lose the continuity as clients are handled by a number of different individuals. In these situations, passed on communications are paramount as useful sales can be lost.

Common senses

When a promotion is implemented, a plan of action is put into effect and all successful promotions have to be a *sensory event*. Effective selling is experiential; it provides the purchaser with a variety of experiences that they can:

- see
- touch
- smell
- hear
- or taste.

Our five senses provide the only ways in which people can be influenced in making a purchasing decision. The more sensory *channels* that are involved in the promotional environment, the more chances are that the customer will buy. At the end of the promotional period the success and impact of the event can be evaluated by team discussion, review of sales reports and feedback from the clients on how the promotion was received.

Activity

The following table lists a number of situations that could occur. Complete the missing information for each one.

Scenario	Which legislation applies?	What action should be taken?
A client returns a pair of electrical straighteners that were bought from the salon at the weekend. She says that they don't work.		
A client is dissatisfied with the colour that her hair has turned out. She feels it is too dark.		
A client is unhappy about a product that she has bought, she says it makes her scalp itch.		
A client feels that her 'special promotion' purchase of a hairdryer is a 'con', because she has seen the same item on the internet at a full price for less money.		

MAHOGANY HAIRDRESSING SALONS AND ACADEMY
WWW.MAHOGANYHAIR.CO.UK

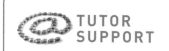

TUTOR SUPPORT

Short answer test

Promotional materials

A typical product promotion will consist of:

- point-of-sale merchandising – central 'island', open cabinet, shelf displays
- shelftalkers – printed promotional slips/cards fixed to/dangling from shelves; 'mobile' ones that bob or bounce deliver best results
- eye-catching displays are instantly informative – locate them where they'll be seen at reception or centrally in treatment areas
- arrangement of popular lines at eye level with price details; use 'price watch' stickers
- linking displays with money off and other special offers – first visit, loyalty, recommend-a-friend discounts and promotional tie-ins with major local stores.

Window displays

Window displays are an essential way of advertising services, their costs and displaying products. They are relatively inexpensive to dress, if they are maintained by salon staff.

New salon customers find us through a variety of different ways and the image of the salon created by the front window is part of that formula; although we shouldn't forget that reputation, location, advertising campaigns and the most important, personal recommendation, all have a major impact too.

Website

In the past the only way for people to locate and find out about businesses was through directory listings. This form of advertising, e.g. *Yellow pages* and *BT Phonebook*, was poor in quality, often badly printed and, if you took out a large display advert; very expensive. This type of business finder is quickly becoming obsolete, as most businesses are turning to more engaging forms of media.

Now the most popular and interesting way to find out about what a business has to offer from a remote location is through its website. Most salons now have an internet presence and as managing the information upon a website gets easier; many salons can upload their own photographs, edit textual content and can provide engaging, interactive and fun ways to sell their services and products. Larger salon chains with greater resources have very attractive websites that not only provide the customer at home with information, but enable them to buy products and make appointments too.

This makes the website a very powerful marketing tool.

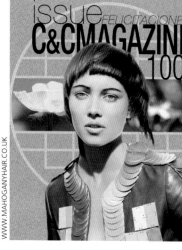

EKU *statement*

G18 (eku6) How to give appropriate balanced information to clients about services or products

---

G18.3 Gain client commitment to using additional services or products

Remember

A client not only shows their interest through body language. They will show their uninterest too!

Recognising interest – buying signals

You need to be able to differentiate between genuine interest and a polite and friendly, but negative response. Just because someone responds in a polite or friendly way is not an indication of 'I want to buy that'.

Genuine interest is expressed in at least two ways:

| ✔ | The client will *ask* how that will benefit them, e.g. 'Would that be suitable for my type of hair?' or 'How does that work?' |
| ✔ | The client will *show* their interest by taking the product and holding it for closer examination, or through their positive body language. |

Therefore when you introduce or recommend the client to a new service or product, you will need to look for the signs of interest above.

Anything other than these signs could indicate a lack of interest and you should be careful how you proceed. There is little point pursuing the issue if you are receiving little or no response; even if you think it's the best product or service that she could have. The last thing that you want to be seen as; is 'pushy' or a 'commission seeker.' It won't help your professional standing and it may tarnish your professional relationship too!

Communication

So from the information already covered in this section you can see that there are many ways in which we communicate with our clients. Establishing an effective communication between you and the client is the most important aspect that determines your success in your role. The relationship between stylist and client is built on quality of service, professional advice, trust, support and a listening ear. Good communication ensures productive and effective action. On the other hand poor communication can lead to misunderstandings, misinterpretation and mistakes.

Verbal communication

Verbal communication is what you say and what others hear, it should always be:

- clear to the listener
- brief, but what you say should create interest and initiate a response
- uncomplicated – your information should be easy to understand, avoid the use of technical terms
- friendly, polite and courteous.

Questioning styles:

- *Open questions* – These are a better type of question to use when you want the client to give you information. Examples are: 'What products do you use when you wash your hair at home?' 'How do you apply the colour when you do it at home?' 'Which way do you style the front of your hair?' 'When was the last time that you had a full set of highlights?'
- *Closed questions* – This type of question should be avoided. Closed questions lead the client to give only simple yes or no responses and yield very little information. Examples are: 'Have you washed your hair with anything different lately?' 'Do you find the colour application at home is easy?' 'Have you always had a centre parting?' 'Did you have your highlights done recently?'

Non-verbal communication

Non-verbal communication (NVC) is commonly referred to as *body language* and this type of communication is an effective way of letting others know what we really mean.

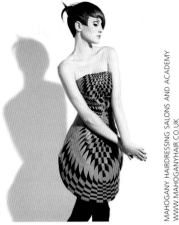

MAHOGANY HAIRDRESSING SALONS AND ACADEMY
WWW.MAHOGANYHAIR.CO.UK

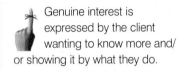

Diversion For more information on this topic see Unit G21, pp 8 & 9

Remember

Genuine interest is expressed by the client wanting to know more and/or showing it by what they do.

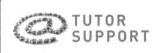

TUTOR SUPPORT

Discussion 2.3: How to recognize when a client might be interested in a product or service

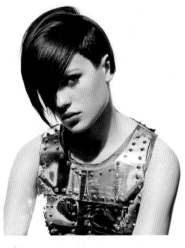

MAHOGANY HAIRDRESSING SALONS AND ACADEMY
WWW.MAHOGANYHAIR.CO.UK

Diversion For more information on this topic see Unit G21 page 11

Physical contact
Most people are embarrassed by physical contact from someone they do not know well.

Body zones - proxemics
Do not crowd or appear over-familiar with your client. Imagine how you would feel if someone came up to you and got a little too close. What do you do? Immediately back off and go on the defensive.

NVC – You're a liar!
Some physical behaviours which may contradict your verbal communication:

- Sweating
- Excessive hand movements
- Biting of fingernails
- Chewing of the inside of the mouth
- Drying up of the mouth
- Lack of eye contact.

Diversion Posture, body position and gestures See Unit G21, p. 9–10

Excellent communicators are good listeners, they understand how to ask the clients the right questions and listen effectively to responses, building on the information given to them and then finally, helping the client to buy.

Activity
The table below lists a variety of different personality traits that could be demonstrated by clients within the salon. Complete the missing information by stating how you would go about handling each of the types.

A client is showing	What signs would they be showing?	How would you handle this trait?
Anger		
Poor confidence		
Uninterest		
Interest in a product		
Disbelief in what you are saying		
Signs of being confused		

Beware, the messages that we provide through body language may be totally different to what we are saying; it may be SHOUTING just the opposite!

We express ourselves with body language through:

- posture
- facial expression
- gestures
- tone and manner of voice.

So it is very important that we send and receive the right messages, particularly when dealing with clients and new customers.

Good selling
- Listening, asking questions, showing interest
- Using the client's name
- Empathising (putting yourself in the client's place), establishing a bond
- Recognising non-verbal cues (dilated pupils = 'I approve'; ear-rubbing = 'I've heard enough')
- Identifying needs; helping clients reach buying decisions
- Knowing your products/services
- Highlighting the results or user benefits; demonstrating these where possible
- Thinking positively, talking persuasively, projecting confidence and enthusiasm.

Bad selling
- Doing all the talking
- Not listening, not 'hearing' unspoken thoughts, arguing
- Interrupting – but never letting the clients interrupt you – thus losing an open opportunity for giving extra information
- Hard selling, 'spieling' (working to a script)
- Threatening – 'You won't get it cheaper anywhere else', knocking the opposition

- Manipulating – 'Oh dear, I'll miss my sales target'
- Knowing nothing about the product
- Treating 'no thanks' as personal rejection
- Blinding clients with science
- Staying mainly silent waiting for an order
- Insisting the client should buy the product.

RUSH LONDON

Consumer legislation

The rights of your customers should not be compromised; they are protected from fraudulent and sharp practice by a variety of consumer legislation. For more information see Appendix 4.

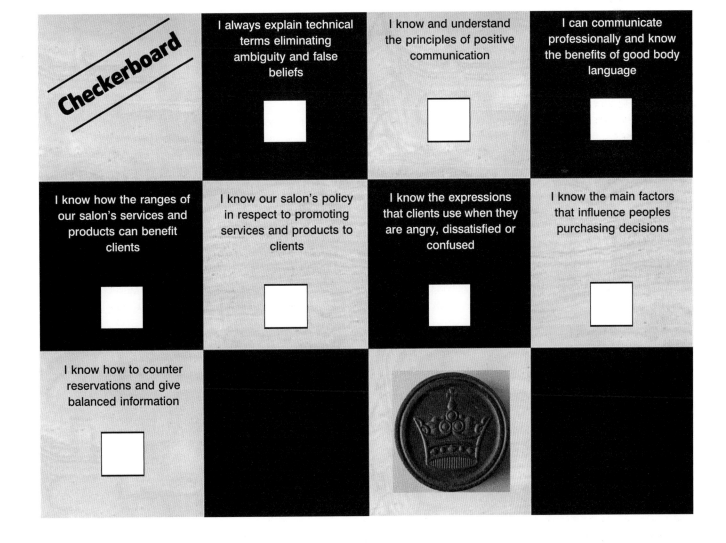

Checkerboard

Checkerboard	I always explain technical terms eliminating ambiguity and false beliefs ☐	I know and understand the principles of positive communication ☐	I can communicate professionally and know the benefits of good body language ☐
I know how the ranges of our salon's services and products can benefit clients ☐	I know our salon's policy in respect to promoting services and products to clients ☐	I know the expressions that clients use when they are angry, dissatisfied or confused ☐	I know the main factors that influence peoples purchasing decisions ☐
I know how to counter reservations and give balanced information ☐			

Assessment of knowledge and understanding

Revision questions

Quick quiz: a selection of different types of questions to check your knowledge

Q1   A product's _ _ _ _ _ _ _ _ are aspects that state what it does.   Fill in the blank

Q2   A key feature of good customer service is being customer focused.   True or false

Q3   Which of the following would be considered as an indication of positive   Multi selection
communication?

Avoiding eye contact?	☐ 1
Smiling?	☐ 2
Standing over the client and talking to them through the styling mirror	☐ 3
Talking with your hand covering your mouth	☐ 4
Sitting at the same level as the client, talking to them face to face	☐ 5
Sitting with folded arms	☐ 6

Q4   People have a comfort zone that is an invisible space around their body.   True or false

Q5   Which of the following is a specific benefit of semi-permanent colour?   Multi choice

It lasts well	○ a
It's quick and simple to use	○ b
It runs and stains easily	○ c
It changes the hair's natural condition	○ d

Q6   A 'shelftalker' is a salesperson.   True or false

Q7   Which of the following are effective forms of promotion?   Multi selection

Point of sale material	☐ 1
Eye catching displays	☐ 2
Dusty shelves	☐ 3
Poorly trained staff	☐ 4
Clever clients	☐ 5
Eye-level product placement	☐ 6

Q8   Excellent _ _ _ _ _ _ _ _ skills are an essential aspect of good   Fill in the blank
communication.

Q9   Which legislation protects the clients from defective purchases?   Multi choice

Data Protection Act (1998)	○ a
The Sale of Goods Act (1979)	○ b
Disability Discrimination Act (DDA 2005)	○ c
The Prices Act (1974)	○ d

Q10 If a client asks how a product would benefit them, then it is a sign of   True or false
genuine interest.

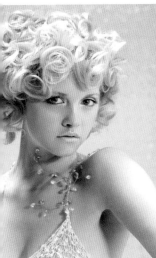

CKY TURNER @ GOLDSWORTHY'S

Chapter**three**
Customer services

G19

G19.1

G19.2

G19.3

**CREDIT VALUE
FOR UNIT G19**
5 Credits

More Information
Legal requirements see
Appendices

- Consumer and retail
  legislation
- Data Protection Act
  (1998)

Improving services: quick overview

Unit title

G19 Support client service improvements

This is an **optional** unit for hairdressing and barbering at level 3 and is made up of three main outcomes

Main outcomes

G19.1 Use feedback to identify potential client service improvements

G19.2 Implement change in client service

G19.3 Assist with the evaluation of changes in client service

What do I need to do for G19.1?

- Gather informal and formalised feedback from clients
- Develop an understanding of the customers' service experiences
- Identify ways in which services can be improved
- Share ideas with work colleagues

What do I need to do for G19.2?

- Present ideas to work personnel who are able to approve your concepts
- Carry out changes to services in line with your concepts
- Inform clients about changes to services
- Collectively support ideas in a positive way

What do I need to do for G19.3?

- Discuss/review changes with team members to evaluate success
- Work collectively to evaluate any negative impacts and explore ways of avoiding them

Keywords

Customer feedback

The information retrieved by a variety of methods, used as a mechanism for evaluating the customer's experiences

Consumer protection

The legislation protecting customers from unlawful sales practices and mishandling of personal information.

Information covered in this chapter

- The purpose and value of making improvements to customer services
- Ways of gaining customer feedback, prior to implementing any changes
- The ways of sharing the findings of feedback and defining a way of implementing change

EKU *statement*

G19 (eku1) How client experience is influenced by the way service is delivered

What aspects do I need to cover for G19.1, G19.2 and G19.3?

- The ranges of services that your salon offers

What do I need to know for G19.1, G19.2 and G19.3?

- How client feedback is obtained
- How the impact of change affects the client's experience
- How to work with others through the planned changes
- Why it is important to give the client a positive impression of the changes to services

Introduction

As hairdressers you provide services to your clients on a daily basis; you are talking about your client's hair, the way that they handle it and providing useful tips and advice along the way. You have your finger on the pulse and (pardon the pun) at the *cutting edge* of what is going on.

This close business relationship provides the salon with a unique opportunity to gain valuable feedback and ideas from listening to real experiences that can have a critical influence in the construction of useful campaigns and promotions that genuinely meet the needs of your clients.

This chapter looks at the activities that salons can undertake to improve their offerings to customers. By undertaking this unit, you will be able to support management in gaining useful feedback from clients, helping to evaluate the findings and take part in the implementation of improved services.

Why change services at all?

Generally speaking, hairdressers do very well in providing good customer service. The way in which services are delivered to clients enables them to keep on top of the constantly changing market that they are servicing. This is where personal service industries have distinct advantages over other service sectors. The close relationship between business and customer enable salons to adapt quickly to changes in requirement and to be responsive to customer needs.

Salons have to change because the demands of the clients are continually changing. However, these changes in customer expectations do not happen to each and every member of the salon clientele at the same time. It is a gradual, creeping, one-way process and for established businesses the constant need for change would be like riding a bike up a long incline. Not a steep hill, where you would quickly run out of puff, but more of a continual pressure that you recognise, but take in your stride.

The main reasons for changing and improving services are:

- marketplace competition
- stimulate more business/better productivity.
- customer expectation

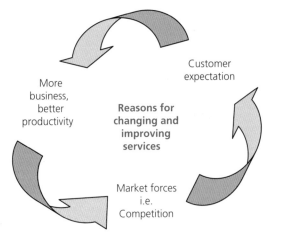

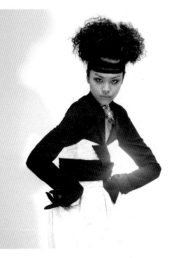

This is a list but not in any order of priority. A better illustration of the reasons is shown in the diagram. Here we see the factors that influence change and they all have an impact, or forces that we can't easily quantify.

We don't know what our competitors are doing, we don't know what our customers will want next month and we don't know how much the business will benefit from improved services.

What we do know is that: competition isn't going to go away, our clients will always continue to expect more from our salons' services and that it will be beneficial for the business in the longer term. How big a benefit in terms of financial gain, better marketplace offerings and perceived image, can all be measured later by evaluation, reports and customer feedback.

Customer expectation

Reasons for changing and improving services

More business, better productivity

Market forces i.e. Competition

What is different about your salon's offerings?

In marketing speak a business *carves out its niche* in the marketplace by developing a unique selling point (USP) for its products or services. This USP is the factor that customers see as the defining aspect that makes them want to buy.

So if you look at what services and products your salon offers compared to others, what is different?

- Do you do a blow-dry or perm that your competitors don't?
- Does your L'Oréal shampoo work differently to the shampoo sold by the salon across the street?
- Do you have technical skills that are unique in your area?

The honest answer to each of these questions is probably NO! But don't give up hairdressing yet, there's more to it than that.

It's not necessarily what you offer that counts it's the *way* in which it is offered

The secret is in the *way* that salons conduct business with their clientele and that is the service. That's the USP, that's why your clients keep coming back and that's the bit that we are going to improve.

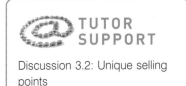

TUTOR SUPPORT

Discussion 3.2: Unique selling points

G19.1	Use feedback to identify potential client service improvements

You can't really find out how to improve services without first finding out how the clients feel about the salon services you already offer. This means that you must find ways to gather feedback information so that some form of evaluation takes place. Then depending on those findings, decisions and courses for action can be determined. You can do this either by formal, i.e. a structured ways, or informally during conversation with the client.

EKU *statement*

G19 (eku1) How client experience is influenced by the way service is delivered

G19 (eku2) How client feedback is obtained

TUTOR SUPPORT

Project 3.1: Client satisfaction

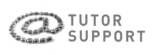

TUTOR SUPPORT

Discussion 3.3: Why clients leave the salon

Before we look at the ways in which we gather data from the clients it would be useful to try to understand the sorts of outcomes that could happen if we do nothing.

Customer feedback

We learn a lot about our services from those people receiving them, or at least we should do. Customer feedback is extremely important. Their likes and dislikes are the first indicators of what works for them and how we should respond. However, customers expect more. Generally speaking, they want to be able to copy what you do; they don't necessarily think that what you do is magic because you make it look so simple.

The feedback that we get from clients must shape what we do in the future. Without change, the continuation of client returns will fall off. We cannot allow the existing service provision to stay as it is. So, unless we accept this fact we will be unable to satisfy the salon clientele in the future.

Why do salons lose clients?

Salons lose customers all the time and this can happen for a number of reasons:

- moving house
- job moves
- a friend's influence
- poor service
- boredom (the client wants a change).

Home moves and job moves are unfortunate for business, but obviously necessary for the clients and their families. This loss of client is a form of churn rate and part of the acceptable percentage that the business has to be prepared for. It is also satisfying when they keep in touch. Most salons will have a few clients who have moved away but can't bear to think of forging new associations with another salon. We love to talk about it too, particularly when others can't understand why they want to travel so far to have their hair styled.

Friends' influence has a powerful yet negative impact on the business. Social groupings have their leaders and followers and this is no good for anyone. When friends pressurise your clients to try their own hairdresser you have a three-to-one odds of retaining the custom, which is fine if you like gambling:

1 The client likes the new experience and you lose.

2 The client doesn't like the new experience but is too ashamed to return and drifts off. You lose again.

3 The client doesn't like the new experience and can't wait to get back to your safety. You win.

Then again your clients are out there busily recommending your great talents. In this situation you can win again. The power of personal recommendation is immense and should be encouraged. Many salons run 'recommend a friend' campaigns. This is a strong business builder so use it.

Poor service – there isn't much too say about this as it is self-explanatory and totally unacceptable. This is the quickest way to lose clients and all those others that they come into contact with. (See client complaints p. 404.)

Boredom is unfortunately the main reason why salons lose clients. It's very hard to predict when boredom will set in, but if you have a strong rapport with your client you should be able to spot the signs. Typically, it will occur when you fall into the trap of regularly doing the same style over and over again. This may not be your fault either. It is human nature to stick to what you know and it is very damaging. There is only a handful of styles that *truly* suit the client. Shocked? This is based on a number of significant factors and mainly physical proportions, client competence/ability and client lifestyle routines. Embarking on other styling routes is an interesting journey, but you will find that the client will gravitate back to the safe home ground of 'tried and tested' at some point in the future. So when a returning client undergoes the same service as the last time or returns back to the style they have had before, you can 'hammer another nail into the coffin of boredom'. You can combat boredom though in the way in which you handle your client's styling preferences. Product manufacturers do exactly the same in marketing. *New and improved!* means we have modified what you have been happy with before and given it a new slant, in either formulation, packaging or both. In marketing terms this is called 'extended product life'. We can invent a new strategy and call it 'extended client life'.

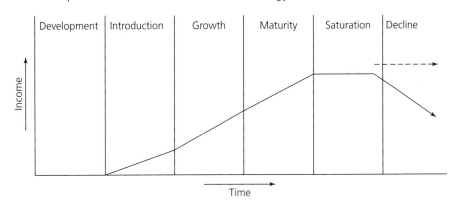

Extending product service/life

From the diagram we can see the typical graph for a newly introduced product. Taking it through the development phase (this can be similar to planning new services or treatments), we move into the introduction phase where sales start to increase following advertising and promotion. Moving forwards, further sales bring steady growth, which leads to the maturity phase. If continued interest is not stimulated, it is soon followed by a fall-off in sales during saturation. It is at this *boredom* point that the marketers reinvent the product with 'new and improved' in order to achieve an extended life of the sales.

Collecting information from the client

You have a unique opportunity to sample the service that you provide to clients by collecting the information and putting it to good use. This can be done openly or discreetly and is purely a matter of choice. However, if you do keep the collected written information on computer etc. you will need to ensure that you keep this confidential and that the salon is not breaching the **Data Protection Act (1998)**.

There are many ways of sampling consumer opinion. In the salon it is often easier to talk to the clients as part of the routine conversation that takes place during visits. If it becomes part of the salon's policy for getting this feedback, a system for collectively discussing and providing this feedback to management needs to be devised. This system should be able to:

- provide fair, unbiased feedback from a wide sample of clients
- welcome contributions from all staff members
- record and 'formalise' the findings of the sampled client feedback
- provide sufficient quantifiable data for future analysis.

Remember

A drop-off in business can be staved off either by introducing new services to your clients or by revival, i.e. reviewing where they are with their present image and ensuring that they are happy with it.

EKU *statement*

G19 (eku2) How client feedback is obtained

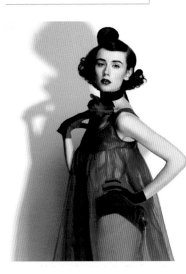

Remember

Make notes of any significant responses, if you notice that a pattern starts to occur then it's time to take action.

Informal information collection

Verbally through discussion

This will happen everyday during the conversations that you have with your clients. You will always be discussing something about their hair, the salon or salon staff, regardless of the other topics that you chat about. This is an ideal time to sample and find out the experiences gained by the clients during their visits, but unless you remember to back this up with some form of recording and documentation, much of what you here will be forgotten.

For example if clients start saying:

1 'I didn't like the new conditioner; it left my hair all flat and lank.'
2 'That new styling mousse makes my scalp itch.'
3 'Have you got something like *OK* to read, instead of *Homes and Gardens*?'
4 'Do you have fresh ground coffee, or just plain instant?'

Then this sort of feedback could be indicating that something is fundamentally wrong and the salon is neither meeting the expectations of clients, nor *reaching* the needs of its target market.

Through non-verbal means

People will often show their innermost feelings by the way in which they express themselves through mannerisms gestures and their body language. If a client is not happy about a certain part of the service they may not tell you directly, but you will get the general impression by what their body language is *telling* you.

EKU *statement*

G19 (eku3) How to work with others to identify and support change in the way service is delivered

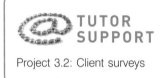

TUTOR SUPPORT

Project 3.2: Client surveys

Formal collection of information

The simplest way of collecting useful data from the client would be through a client suggestion box or alternatively via client questionnaire. These are very useful systems but they do need a lot of preparation and planning. If not carefully focused they can create too much information.

Before looking at the method of collection it would be useful to review the techniques of asking questions.

Questioning styles

Open/closed questions The choice of questions used within your survey technique will depend on how you will evaluate the data. However, the simplest way of indicating opinions is by objective type questioning and the simplest way of doing this is by asking for a straight forward 'yes' or 'no' answers. In this scenario, the client is asked to give a clear response with a definitive positive or negative answer; the drawback with this type of questioning is that it doesn't prompt for any additional information. So, the framing of the questions has to be carefully considered so that it elicits the right form and amount of feedback.

On the other hand, open style questions allow the client to elaborate in their answers. This may be more difficult to quantify as the range of responses can be quite diverse and evaluation can be more complex or ambiguous.

Leading questions Leading questions are focused in their style, they force people to answer within a narrow band of options and provide easily quantifiable data for management. However, although they may retrieve the information that the salon wants, it doesn't necessarily provide a useful mechanism for getting the customers real feelings.

Multiple choice questions using Likert scale See example of a multiple choice type questionnaire below.

Shampooing and conditioning

Q. The newly introduced, complementary head massage has been a useful addition to the backwash service.

- Strongly agree   • Disagree
- Agree   • Strongly disagree
- No opinion

Multiple choice using the Likert scale

Activity

Competitor comparison

You need to put your services and products to the test, which will mean making like-for-like comparisons between your salon and the competition. The table shows the types of information that you should address.

Service attributes	Worse (–3, –2, –1)	Same	Better (+1, +2, +3)	How vital is this attribute (essential, preferred, other)?
Service availability				
Range of services/treatments				
Ranges of products				
Communication standards				
Presentation/appearance				
Quality of work output				
After-care and advice				
Consultation				
Time allowed				
Refreshments + costs				
Payment options				
Salon image and location				

Much of this information is available through your clients from their feedback and general discussion, but beware the difference between useful data and idle gossip.

Client surveys

These are a particularly useful way of formally collecting client feedback. If you choose to keep the feedback anonymous you may find that the client will provide a really true perspective on the services she has experienced. If the survey is well constructed, it will be easy to quantify the feedback and sort the customer data.

Suggestion boxes

These can collect a lot of feedback data. However, with so many diverse comments it may be a little unwieldy to attempt to address every client's innermost thoughts. However, it is worth remembering that this type of feedback does point to *real* client feelings and give clear indications and directions towards clients' expectations.

Questionnaires

These are very useful tools for collecting customer feedback. They do pinpoint customer feelings and provide sufficient data for analysis. This is because well-drafted consumer surveys are designed to 'steer' responses into clear, specific, quantifiable areas. They need a lot of thought in their construction and will often use the multiple choice type of question as a way of channelling the answers. The favoured style of question for eliciting the strength of people's feelings about a specific issue is shown in the figure above showing an example using the Likert scale.

Telephone survey

Another way of gathering feedback is through telephone surveys, although they can be quite time consuming to organise and implement during normal salon hours. Bearing in mind the amount of unsolicited calls that people receive at home, you may find that the clients consider this to be an intrusion of privacy and may respond to you accordingly. As most people are fed up with being called by all and sundry, this may be your last option for obtaining feedback.

Salon website

This is a useful way of getting people to provide comments at a time that suits them. If people are allowed more time to give their feedback then the resulting data may be a little more focused (and therefore more useful) than simply asking clients to answer questions whilst they are sat waiting in reception.

If a salon does have a website the feedback technique doesn't have to be too sophisticated or technically demanding either. Larger salons and chains may have database-driven websites which can enable question and answer interactions; a simpler e-mail response through a site's 'Contact Us' button will be fine for standard HTML-type websites.

What are your competitors doing?

Knowing your business well is fundamentally crucial to its ongoing success. When a business is started its whole operation and the way in which it is planned to engage with its market are mapped out within a business plan. The climate in which the business operates is constantly changing though. Therefore the originally drafted business plan also needs to change. There are many reasons that necessitate the change, but the main one is competition.

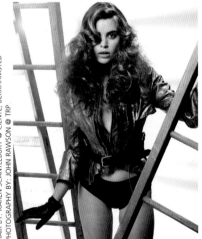

HAIR BY: KAREN SCANTLEBURY @ CIENTE, BERKHAMSTED
PHOTOGRAPHY BY: JOHN RAWSON @ TRP

Your salon's market position is constantly being undermined by the increased pressures that your competitors bring to bear. *Your competition wants your customers, just as much as you want theirs*. The success of your business is dependent upon increasing:

- service quality and value
- market share
- prices for services and treatments
- levels of staff abilities/skills.

Therefore, in order to achieve these goals, better understanding and knowledge about your competition are essential. Competitor analysis is big business. There are a growing number of specialist companies offering a wide range of 'undercover' services designed to infiltrate and make comparisons between service quality levels. The types of information that competitors want varies, but the most pointed attacks will elicit your pricing policy and service standards.

You will have seen this at work already. How often does a bogus client contact the salon to find out the current costs for particular services or stylist availability? Even if you are sure that another salon is trying you out for size, it would be difficult to decline the information. Pricing policy depends on many things though, so in isolation the information is meaningless. Only when other aspects of service are brought into play can a far more useful customer comparison be made. The pricing of salon services is linked to:

- labour costs
- business fixed costs, i.e. rent, rates, light, heating, insurances
- costs of materials
- expected profit margins
- target client market.

So if these factors relate to the total viability of the business, what would happen if the information fell into the wrong hands? The only additional costs that they will incur are those involved in trying to attract your clients through marketing, promotion and advertising. Management guru Michael Porter indicates that there are five forces which act upon any business:

- power of competitors
- power of buyers in the market
- power of suppliers to the business
- threats posed by potential entrants
- threats posed by substitute products.

1 Other businesses know what they should be paying staff.

2 Business costs in relation to salon location are public domain information. Local authorities keep a rateable value listing for all commercial properties.

3 If your competitor knows what products you use, then he knows what he would have to pay for them.

4 From the tariffs you charge, your competitors know which socio-economic category you are trying to attract.

The one thing that they have to calculate is the profitability of the service and whether it is something they can match or even beat on price.

You need to put your services and products to the test, which will mean making like-for-like comparisons between your salon and the competition. The table in the activity 'Competitor comparison' shows the types of information that you should address.

The other popular method for collecting service quality information is the mystery shopper, or in this case 'mystery client'. In this method of collecting useful feedback; an unknown person is employed to go and sample the services of your salon or a competitor. They are given a brief beforehand and will be looking for specific aspects of the

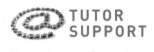

TUTOR SUPPORT

Discussion 3.1: Influencing factors

Remember

Making competitor comparisons

If your competitors know part of this formula, then your salon is vulnerable. The shocking thing is they do!

TUTOR SUPPORT

Discussion 3.4: Competitor services

Remember

Much of this information is available through your clients from their feedback and general discussion, but beware of the difference between feedback that provides useful data and that of cynical, idle gossip.

salon service during their visit. They will pay at the end of the service as normal and would provide their feedback at some later time. They will not make themselves known to you at any part of the process and this is an ideal way of making comparisons between your offerings and those of the competition.

G19.2 — Implement change in client service

Salon survey – customer satisfaction

1. How well do you think that you were received when you arrived at the reception of our salon today?

Very well	Good	OK	Not well	Poorly
23	17	11	0	0

2. Does this reflect the usual way in which you are received at our salon?

Yes	No
40	11

Salon Survey form

EKU statement

G19 (eku3) How to work with others to identify and support change in the way service is delivered

Sharing the information

After collecting the feedback, the data need to be sorted or collated in line with the answers received. This could be done by the creation of a master document that contains all the questions and after each question; the range of responses numerically received for each of the responses provided.

After collating the information, it may be more beneficial to share this with all the salon team, particularly as this becomes an open forum and provides a basis for discussion. However, where responses could be targeted at individuals then a little sensitivity should be employed or alternatively where negative feedback relating to individuals occurs, it should be taken up with the person on an individual basis as part of their performance appraisal.

Activity

Care should be taken in quantifying data. In the example shown in the salon survey on customer satisfaction shown above, the two questions seem to be targeted at the quality of service received on entering the salon.

1 Is question 1 in the example a useful question?

2 Why?

3 Is question 2 in the example a useful question?

4 Why?

5 What does question 2 indicate if several people are responsible for reception duties?

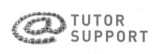

TUTOR SUPPORT

Project 3.3: How client feedback is analysed and can make changes

Identifying possible changes to services

Following the collection of data and the subsequent collation, there are two obvious reasons for making changes to services:

- customers are dissatisfied with some part of the existing provision
- the salon wishes to improve the existing provision.

If clients are dissatisfied with some aspects of the existing service, then it would be pointless if this is not addressed and corrected for the future. However, it is worth bearing in mind that sometimes the further improvements may not be feasible. When customer expectations exceed the salon's resources then a management decision needs to be taken. For example: imagine that a salon has always provided complementary drinks to its clients in the past. Then following a survey it has been noted that clients want a freshly ground cappuccino coffee instead. The management is now confronted with three possible options.

- they continue to offer the poorer quality, less expensive complementary service as they have always done in the past
- they decide to invest in an expensive, commercial ground coffee machine and choose to charge the clients for the service in the future
- they invest in the new machine, continue to offer an enhanced complementary service and foot the bill themselves.

You can see the dilemma; they now know that the client doesn't like their existing complementary service, but does that mean that the clients would like to pay for a premium service in the future? *Not necessarily!*

Other improvements to services are far clearer cut. If a client complains that a gown smells of perfume, it is both negligent and poor service by the staff for not removing it from the salon and putting it in the laundry.

So, where services are not meeting the expectations of clients, something needs to be done; as this is a true reflection of what is already happening and these things need to be addressed immediately, just so that things can stay the same!

More importantly is the improvements to existing services and this means changing the salon's provision to enhance what is already offered.

Presenting and sharing your ideas

Where you have found a useful contribution and enhancement for the salon's services, you need to prepare your case. It doesn't matter how small the changes are, as they all have value and have obviously been found to be less than expected (sub-standard) during the data collection process. However, you do need to justify your reasons for change, think about the impacts that your suggestions will have on others and the salon. Quite simply, if you present your idea to someone who can approve it and it can make a significant difference to what already takes place then, providing it can be afforded, there shouldn't be too much opposition.

Decide if you need the support of others first. If you need to gain the assistance of your fellow staff (as your ideas might directly affect what they already do) then you may find that you would be better off presenting it to them first. This is particularly useful as they may have views or opinions that could help you shape and hone down your final presentation to authority.

In many situations a change to services needs a supporting programme of training too. For example, if after a survey it was found that the salon should provide some sort of outreach service for weddings then those involved in delivering the service to the bride and entourage at home would need to be proficient at all sorts of special occasion hair work.

TUTOR SUPPORT

Project 3.4: Improving services

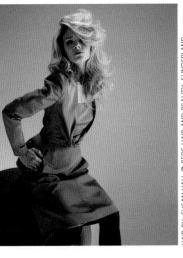

HAIR BY: SUSAN HALL @ REDS HAIR AND BEAUTY, SUNDERLAND
PHOTOGRAPHY BY: JOHN RAWSON@TRP

EKU *statement*

G19 (eku3) How to work with others to identify and support change in the way service is delivered

G19 (eku4) Why it is important to give a positive impression to your client about the changes made by your salon even if you disagree with them

Remember

'Mighty oaks from small acorns do grow.'

In other words, many new avenues for stimulating new business can occur from small beginnings.

When you have decided what changes need to take place, you need to make sure that all the staff is made aware of how improvements will be implemented. There are several ways of doing this (see below).

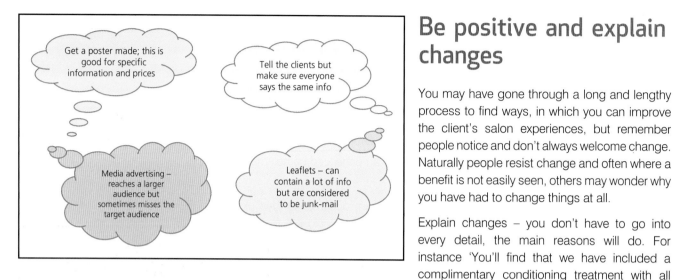

Get a poster made; this is good for specific information and prices

Tell the clients but make sure everyone says the same info

Media advertising – reaches a larger audience but sometimes misses the target audience

Leaflets – can contain a lot of info but are considered to be junk-mail

Be positive and explain changes

You may have gone through a long and lengthy process to find ways, in which you can improve the client's salon experiences, but remember people notice and don't always welcome change. Naturally people resist change and often where a benefit is not easily seen, others may wonder why you have had to change things at all.

Explain changes – you don't have to go into every detail, the main reasons will do. For instance 'You'll find that we have included a complimentary conditioning treatment with all our clients who have colour services Mrs Green. We have found that our clients were not taking up this particularly beneficial part of the service, so we now include it as part of a total service package.'

Be positive – if you are enthusiastic, your clients will be far keener to take the changes on-board. If you aren't positive, then you will find a general reluctance from everyone.

Remember

When changes have been made to existing services you need to do two things:

1 explain the changes and give the reasons why it was necessary to do this

2 be positive when you discuss the changes with clients, be 'up-beat' and enthusiastic – have a positive body language.

Activity

With your fellow staff/students; discuss the various methods/systems of communication that your salon could use to find out what clients think and feel about the current services provided.

Record the details of your findings in your portfolio.

G19.3 Assist with the evaluation of changes in client service

EKU statement

G19 (eku3) How to work with others to identify and support change in the way service is delivered

After the implementation there must be some form of evaluation of the impact that the newly introduced changes have made. Feedback can be gathered informally from the client during routine salon services, but what you do with this feedback is vitally important.

A group discussion should take place and someone – possibly you – should record the main outcomes of the team meeting so that there is some documented information being fed back to the management. Each member of the team will have varied feedback so be ready to take on-board comments from all the team.

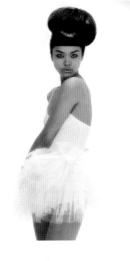

HAIR BY: HAYLEY WELLING @ CIENTE, BERKHAMSTED
PHOTOGRAPHY BY: JOHN RAWSON@TRP

Negative comments

Not all feedback is positive. There will be occasions when all the best-made plans aren't received too well! There isn't any easy way to give negative feedback; no one likes criticism but there is some constructive ways to go about it.

It is easy to sound arrogant, flippant and off-hand so you need to be tactful in your delivery. If possible don't weed out individuals, they wont find it an endearing strategy and all you'll end up doing is alienating yourself away from the rest of the team. Accentuate the positive; find ways of tempering and balancing the feedback with an equal amount of positives as well as negatives. Constructive criticism can be a useful learning experience; just think how supportive it can be when looking at someone's areas for improvement in appraisal.

When the negative feedback is coming your way, think about the ways in which you can adapt and change to accommodate the improvements. Be mature, it's impossible to get new strategies right on every occasion and there will be plenty of opportunities for the future. Remember learn by mistakes and then move onwards and upwards.

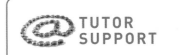

TUTOR SUPPORT

Discussion 3.5: Criticising ideas and agreeing on a compromise

Remember

Service improvement is the core aspect for taking a business in the right direction. Be motivated by it and make plenty of contributions towards it.

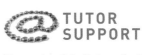

TUTOR SUPPORT

Discussion 3.6: Data collection handling and storing

Salon and legal requirements

Before any of these information collecting activities can be put into practice, make sure that there are no contraventions to your salon's policy or that which jeopardises the salon where there may be breaches of the law.

Remember

Clients have rights too; don't make the mistake of contravening the law when it comes to handling personal information. The appendices at the end of the book address all relevant legislation and give an idea of what each area covers and who it refers to.

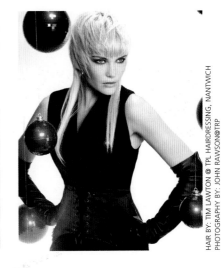

HAIR BY: TIM LAWTON @ TPL HAIRDRESSING, NANTWICH
PHOTOGRAPHY BY: JOHN RAWSON@TRP

EKU *statement*

G19 (eku4) Why it is important to give a positive impression to your client about the changes made by your salon even if you disagree with them?

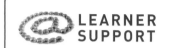

LEARNER SUPPORT

Support client service improvements puzzle

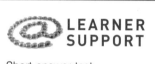

LEARNER SUPPORT

Short answer test

Activity

Customer service

With the help of your receptionist you can conduct a simple survey to find out when salon customers want to come in. Create a simple graph displaying the days of the month along the bottom axis and a range of times (say 8.00 am to 8.00 pm) along the vertical axis. When customers call the salon, mark each point on the graph to show when they want to come in as opposed to what is available. Each plotting point could be colour coded to refer to different staff members. Run the exercise over a complete calendar month to see what happens.

- Are there any specific days that people would like?

- Are there any specific times that people would like?

- Do the findings of the survey highlight any shortcomings or inefficiencies with the present work systems and time scales?

Checkerboard

	I know and understand the principles of positive communication	I can communicate positively and professionally with the clients	I always carry out working practices according to the salon's policy
I am knowledgeable in the services, treatments and products that the salon offers	I know the techniques of gaining client feedback	I know how to evaluate the feedback data	I know how to present data to others and share in their ideas
I know how to gain client feedback for service improvements	I know how to receive negative feedback in a constructive way		

Assessment of knowledge and understanding

Revision questions

Quick quiz: a selection of different types of questions to check your knowledge.

Q1	A _____ question style prompts a simple yes or no response.	Fill in the blank
Q2	A leading question forces people to answer within a narrow band of options.	True or false
Q3	What would provide strong reasons for changing or improving services?	Multi selection

Competition by other salons?	☐	1
Manufacturer's sales pressure?	☐	2
Customer feedback	☐	3
Too much stock on the shelves	☐	4
Good sales and turnover	☐	5
Friends and family feedback	☐	6

Q4	Client boredom leads to lost custom.	True or false
Q5	Which style of questioning provides the most effective way of finding out how strongly a client feels about salon services?	Multi choice

Open questions	○	a
Closed questions	○	b
Multiple choice (Likert scale)	○	c
Leading questions	○	d

Q6	Customer feedback has little importance in shaping a business's future.	True or false
Q7	Which of the following responses indicates that the newly introduced complementary head massage has been a useful addition to the salon's services?	Multi selection

Strongly agree	☐	1
Agree	☐	2
No opinion	☐	3
Disagree	☐	4
Strongly disagree	☐	5

Q8	A formal collection of client information could be made through questionnaires or a _____ box.	Fill in the blank
Q9	In multiple choice (Likert scale) question type, the middle option shows what sort of response?	Multi choice

A strong agreement	○	a
A mild agreement	○	b
Neither agreement or disagreement	○	c
A mild disagreement	○	d

Q10	A negative feedback from a client questionnaire is a useful indicator.	True or false

Part**two**
Hairdressing technical services

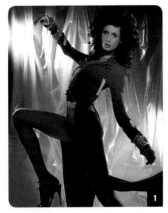

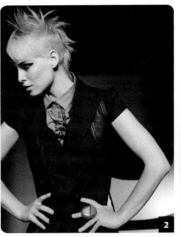

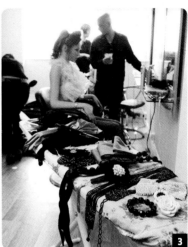

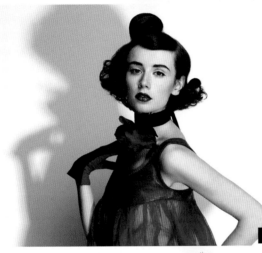

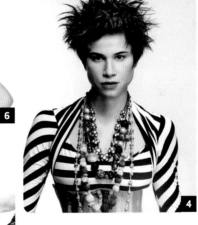

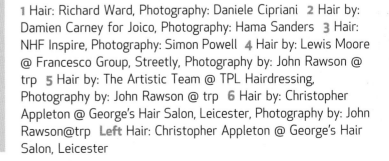

1 Hair: Richard Ward, Photography: Daniele Cipriani 2 Hair by: Damien Carney for Joico, Photography: Hama Sanders 3 Hair: NHF Inspire, Photography: Simon Powell 4 Hair by: Lewis Moore @ Francesco Group, Streetly, Photography by: John Rawson @ trp 5 Hair by: The Artistic Team @ TPL Hairdressing, Photography by: John Rawson @ trp 6 Hair by: Christopher Appleton @ George's Hair Salon, Leicester, Photography by: John Rawson@trp **Left** Hair: Christopher Appleton @ George's Hair Salon, Leicester

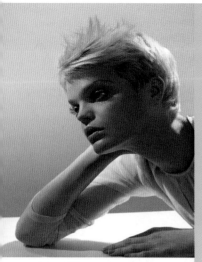

Chapter**four**
Creative cutting

GH16

GH16.1
GH16.2
GH16.3

CREDIT VALUE
FOR UNIT GH16
8 Credits

More Information See Units:

- G21 Provide hairdressing consultation services
- G22 Monitor procedures to safely control work operations

Diversion See appendices for Electricity at Work Regulations

EKU statement

GH16 (eku4) Your responsibilities under the Electricity at Work Regulations

---

Creative cutting: quick overview

Unit title

GH16 Creatively cut hair using a combination of techniques

This is a **mandatory** unit for Hairdressing at level 3, it is made up of three main outcomes

Main outcomes

GH16.1 Maintain effective and safe methods of working when cutting

GH16.2 Creatively restyle women's hair

GH16.3 Provide aftercare advice

What do I need to do for GH16.1?

- Make sure that the client is adequately covered and protected
- Make sure that your working position is comfortable and safe
- Keep the work area clean and tidy and make sure that waste materials are disposed of properly
- Work without causing risks to you or your client's health and safety
- Work efficiently and effectively

What do I need to do for GH16.2?

- Choose suitable visual aids to help with style selection for your client
- Prepare your client's hair before cutting
- Seek confirmation of the desired look before starting
- Cut your client's hair using a variety of creative cutting techniques
- Check that the final effect is; accurate, that it compliments the client's features, their personal image and that the client is satisfied with the results

What do I need to do for GH16.3?

- Give accurate constructive advice on how the client can maintain the look

What aspects do I need to cover for GH16.1, GH16.2 and GH16.3?

- A variety of cutting tools and equipment
- A range of factors that influence or limit the choice of styling
- Different types of cutting techniques that are used to create creative effects

What aspects do I need to know for GH16.1, GH16.2 and GH16.3?

- Your salon's requirements for preparation, timings and standards of service
- How to work safely, effectively and hygienically when cutting hair
- Factors about hair that affect styling choice, suitability and durability
- The ways of methodically cutting wet or dry hair to achieve the desired effects
- How to correct commonly occurring problems that can occur during cutting
- The aftercare advice and recommendations that you should give to clients

Introduction

The content in this chapter looks particularly at the aspects of creative cutting and the techniques that will enable you to construct a variety of fashionable styles. It aims to provide you with new alternatives that should encourage you to think more *laterally* about style design and style visualisation; it will hopefully give your existing skills a boost and find new ways of applying them.

Creative cutting design is about deciding what needs to be done; making the right choices and selecting the visual images that will not only suit the client, but also enable them to see ideas of what is achievable for them.

Building on from the basics

As you became more skilled in styling hair, your confidence and willingness to explore new ways of doing things has developed into true professionalism. This

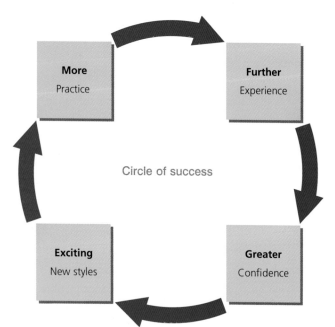

More
Practice

Further
Experience

Circle of success

Exciting
New styles

Greater
Confidence

whole process has a simpler, single word that is unfortunately often overused and something that many new stylists think they already possess. It is *experience*.

Level 3 work is a continual process of building on from the basics and practising a range of techniques, gaining more experience, building up your confidence and producing a wider variety of new effects.

That's the principle in a nutshell. The rest of this chapter breaks this down into the following essential aspects:

- preparation and maintenance
- client consultation
- identifying the influencing factors that affect style choice
- cutting techniques and accuracy
- good customer care.

GH16.1 Maintain effective and safe methods of working when cutting

Preparing the client

Your salon has its own policy and codes of practice for preparing clients and you must observe these. Some things are general common sense and courtesy, whereas others are client or salon specific. But at the very least your salon will have a procedure for: gowning and protecting the client from spillages or hair clippings, methods for preparing tools and equipment and the expectations for personal standards in relation to technical ability and hygiene.

You may be an experienced operator but don't forget the basics.

Above all you do need to remember the client's personal comfort and safety throughout the salon visit i.e:

- Cover the client with a clean, laundered gown and place a cutting collar around the shoulders – Make sure that the gown is on properly and fastened around the neck. It should cover and protect their clothes and come up high enough to cover collars and necklines. Don't make the fastening too tight, but it should be close enough at least to protect the client's clothes and stop hair clippings from going down their neck, which is both uncomfortable whilst they are in the salon and irritating if they are returning to work or doing things for the rest of the day.

- Make sure that the hair is clean – You can't cut hair well if it is loaded with hairspray or it has product build-up. If the client uses a lot of finishing products on their hair you will need to make sure that this has been thoroughly washed out before you start. The quality of the finish that you can achieve is directly proportional to the freedom required to complete the job without the hair locking together with grease or gum. You should be able to comb hair freely during sectioning so that you can achieve the correct holding angles and cutting angles without tangles or binding,

- Adjust the working position and height – Client working height has a lot to do with your safety too. If a client is slouched in the chair, they are a danger not only to themselves but to you too. Client comfort should extend to the point where it makes the salon visit a welcome and pleasurable experience. Clients shouldn't clutter the floor around the styling chair with bags, magazines and shopping. Anything that can safely be stored away should be: it is not only a distraction; it's a safety hazard too.

- Position in relation to the mirror – The positioning of the client in front of the mirror is very important. Any angle of the head other than perpendicular to the mirror and the angle of the head to the seated position will affect the line and balance of the haircut.

Many salon workstations have built-in foot rests and there are good reasons for this. The foot rest:

1 is there to improve the comfort for the seated client at any cutting height

2 helps balance the client and encourages them to sit squarely in front of the mirror

3 tries to discourage the client from sitting cross-legged

4 promotes better posture by making the client sit back properly with their back flat against the back of the chair.

All of the above factors are critical for you and the client in ensuring their comfort throughout, and that you are not hindered in doing your task. For example, if your client sits with crossed legs, it will alter the horizontal plane of their shoulders and this will make your job of trying to get even and level baselines more difficult.

- Rough-dry the hair so that you work with damp hair throughout the cut – Dry off the client's hair so that they are not sat with saturated hair, it is uncomfortable for them as wet hair soon feels cold even if it doesn't drip onto the gown and their clothes. During cutting it enables the natural tendencies, movements and directions of the hair to be seen. This is extremely important for cutting hair with the wave movement and hair growth patterns all being considered as the style develops.

Your personal hygiene

Personal hygiene can't be stressed enough; it is vitally important for anyone working in personal services. Your personal hygiene or lack of it, will be immediately notice-able to everyone you come into contact with. You may have overslept, but if you haven't showered it will be very uncomfortable for you, your colleagues and the clients as BO is unpleasant in any situation. Other strong smells are offensive too; the smells of nicotine and smoking are very offputting to the client, particularly if they are a non-smoker.

EKU *statement*

GH16 (eku38) The importance of keeping the hair damp throughout the wet cutting process

GH16 (eku36) The importance of considering weight distribution and working with the natural growth patterns of the hair

Remember

Salon chairs are designed with comfort and safety in mind; your client should be seated with their back flat against the back of the chair, their legs uncrossed and the chair at a height at which it is comfortable for you to work. You need to be able to get to all parts of the head, so the chair's height should be adjusted to suit the particular height of the client. Don't be afraid of asking the client to sit up: it is in their best interest too!

Remember

Always dry the client's hair well to remove the excess water before combing, blow-drying or finger-drying.

EKU *statement*

GH16 (eku16) The importance of personal hygiene

Hair science: Did you know?

We all carry large numbers of micro-organisms inside us, on our skin and in our hair. These organisms, such as bacteria, fungi and viruses, are too small to be seen with the naked eye. Bacteria and fungi can be seen through a microscope, but viruses are too small even for that.

Many micro-organisms are quite harmless, but some can cause disease. Those that are harmful to people are called pathogens. Flu and cold sores, for example, are caused by viruses, thrush and athlete's foot by a fungus and bronchitis often by bacteria. Conditions like these, which can be transmitted from one person to another, are said to be infectious.

The body is naturally resistant to infection; it can fight most pathogens using its inbuilt immunity system, so it is possible to be infected with pathogenic organisms without contracting the disease. When you have a disease, the symptoms are the visible signs that something is wrong. They are the results of the infection and of the reactions of the body to that infection. Symptoms help you to recognise the disease.

Infectious diseases should always be treated by a doctor. Non-infectious conditions and defects can be treated with products available from the chemist.

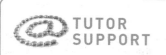
TUTOR SUPPORT

Project 4.1: Risk assessment for cutting services

EKU *statement*

GH16 (eku9) The safety considerations which must be taken into account when cutting hair

---

Remember

Bad breath is offensive to clients too. Bad breath (halitosis) is the result of leaving particles to decay within the spaces between the teeth. You need to brush your teeth after every meal. Bad breath can also result from digestive troubles, stomach upsets, smoking and strong foods such as onions, garlic and some cheeses.

EKU *statement*

GH16 (eku3) Your salon's and legal requirements for disposal of sharps and waste materials

Preparing the tools and equipment

Get your own scissors, razors, clippers, combs and sectioning clips ready beforehand – and that doesn't mean as the client arrives in the chair from the basin! You must be prepared; your tools and equipment must be hygienically clean and safe to use. You would have needed to have removed your combs from the Barbicide™ or steriliser prior to use. These would be rinsed and dried and put near to your work station. All cutting tools would need to be checked and maintained on a daily basis.

Plastic and rubber cutting tools

- Never use dirty or damaged tools. Germs can breed in the crevices and corners and can cross-infect other clients.
- Clean or wipe all tools before disinfecting or sterilising.
- Cutting collars should be washed and dried before use.

Other cutting tools

- Some disinfectants can corrode metal and blunt edges. Check the manufacturer's instructions before using them.
- If corrosion or rusting occurs the equipment is rendered unsafe. Always make sure that this doesn't happen.
- Take special care when cleaning and lubricating scissors.
- All electrical repairs should be carried out by professional people. Do not attempt to undertake them yourself.

Remember

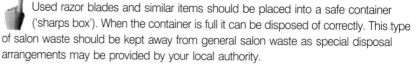
Disposal of sharp items
Used razor blades and similar items should be placed into a safe container ('sharps box'). When the container is full it can be disposed of correctly. This type of salon waste should be kept away from general salon waste as special disposal arrangements may be provided by your local authority.

What is your salon policy for disposing of sharp items?

Contact your local council offices' environmental health department for more information.

Preventing infection

A warm, humid salon can offer a perfect home for disease-carrying bacteria. If they can find food in the form of dust and dirt, they may reproduce rapidly. Good ventilation, however, provides a circulating air current that will help to prevent their growth. This is why it is important to keep the salon clean, dry and well aired at all times, and work areas free from clutter or waste items. This includes clothing, work areas, tools and all equipment. Some salons use sterilising devices as a means of providing hygienically safe work implements. Sterilisation means the complete eradication of living organisms. Different devices use different sterilisation methods, which may be based on the use of heat, radiation or chemicals.

Ultraviolet radiation

Ultraviolet (UV) radiation provides an alternative sterilising option. The items for sterilisation are placed in wall- or worktop-mounted cabinets fitted with UV-emitting light bulbs and exposed to the radiation for at least 15 minutes. If your scissors or combs are sterilised in a UV cabinet, remember to turn them over to make sure both sides have been done.

Chemical sterilisation

Chemical sterilisers should be handled only with suitable personal protective equipment, as many of the solutions used are hazardous to health and should not come into contact with the skin. The most effective form of salon sterilisation is achieved by the total immersion of the contaminated implements into a jar of fluid. For more information on disinfecting and sterilising, see Unit GH22, p 388.

Autoclave

The autoclave provides a very efficient way of sterilising using heat. It is particularly good for metal tools although the high temperatures are not suitable for plastics such as brushes and combs. Items placed in the autoclave take around 20 mins to sterilise. (Check with manufacturers' instructions for variations.)

Your work position

The client's cutting position and height from the floor have a direct effect on your posture too. You must be able to work in a position where you do not have to bend 'doubled up' to do your work. Cutting involves a lot of arm and hand movements and you need to be able to get your hands and fingers into positions where you can cut the hair unencumbered, without bad posture.

1 You should adjust the seated client's chair height to a position where you can work upright without having to over-reach on the top sections of their head.
2 You should clear trolleys or equipment out of the way so that you get good all-round access (300°) around the client.

Working efficiently, safely and effectively

Working efficiently and maximising your time is essential so making the most of the resources available should occur naturally. One way of making the most of the salon's resources is being careful in the way that you handle the equipment and the products that

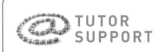

TUTOR SUPPORT

Project 4.2: Cleaning and sterilising of tools for cutting

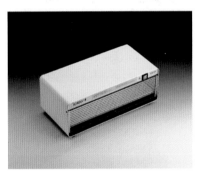

UV sterilisation

EKU *statement*

GH16 (eku10) Why it is important to avoid cross-infection and infestation

GH16 (eku12) Methods cleaning, disinfecting and or sterilisation used in salons

EKU *statement*

GH16 (eku11) Why it is important to keep your work area clean and tidy

GH16 (eku13) Methods of working safely and hygienically and which minimise the risk of cross-infection and infestation

GH16 (eku15) Why it is important to position your cutting tools for ease of use

EKU *statement*

GH16 (eku2) Your salon's expected times for cutting hair to shape

EKU *statement*

GH16 (eku5) Your salon's image and expected standards of service

Remember

Look out for ways and things that can make your client's visit more comfortable and pleasurable. This is the first step in providing a better customer service.

EKU *statement*

GH16 (eku8) How the position of your client and yourself can affect the desired outcome and reduce fatigue and the risk of injury

you use. Always treat the salon's materials in the same way that you would look after your own equipment; always try to minimise waste, being careful of how much product you use.

You need to work in an orderly environment; you need to have the materials that you need at hand and the equipment that you want to use in position and ready for action. What would be the point of starting to cut the client's hair without any scissors, or combs? You can't keep disappearing to go and get something else that you have forgotten; you need to be thinking about all of the things that you need *before* you need them. This is a good exercise in self-organisation and shows others that you are a true professional.

Keep an eye on the clock; you must remember that you need to be working to time and that means providing the service in a commercially acceptable time. Don't forget your client is expecting to go home at some point too. If their time constraints seem unreasonable or unrealistic, make sure that you tell them beforehand. For example; if they are expecting to be back within their lunch-hour and you need to restyle cut, dry and finish long hair in that time, let them know how long you will overrun by.

Activity

Every salon has their own way of doing things. Write down in your portfolio under the following headings what your salon's practices in respect to:

- disposing of sharps
- conducting client consultation
- preparing clients for wet and dry cutting
- preparing and maintaining tools and equipment

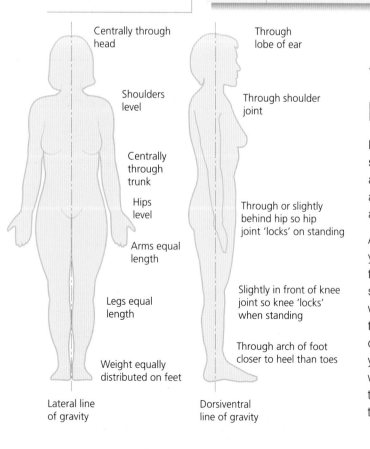

Centrally through head

Shoulders level

Centrally through trunk

Hips level

Arms equal length

Legs equal length

Weight equally distributed on feet

Lateral line of gravity

Through lobe of ear

Through shoulder joint

Through or slightly behind hip so hip joint 'locks' on standing

Slightly in front of knee joint so knee 'locks' when standing

Through arch of foot closer to heel than toes

Dorsiventral line of gravity

Your working position and posture

Hairdressing, as you already know, involves a lot of standing and because of this you need to be comfortable in your work. You should always adopt a comfortable but safe work position and sometimes comfortable and safe are not necessarily the same thing.

A naturally comfortable position for work should allow you to stand close enough to the styling chair without touching it, this should allow you to position your shoulders and torso directly above your hips and feet with your weight evenly distributed. You shouldn't have to twist at any point as you can easily work around the chair or get your client to turn their head slightly towards you. You should wear flatter shoes, so that your body weight is comfortably supported on the widest parts of the feet. This will allow you to work for longer periods of time without risk to injury or fatigue.

Always make a point of lifting your arms to check the working height for your client. If you have to raise your arms anywhere near horizontal during your work, you will find that your arms will start to ache very quickly. Make your adjustments to the styling chair, either up or down to suit your needs. Don't forget to tell the client that your are adjusting the chair as it might be a little shocking if they found themselves unexpectedly being 'jacked' up to the ceiling!

Consultation

Effective communication with the client, as in any service, is an essential prerequisite to cutting hair. Consultation is not just a process that takes place before a service; it is a continual process of reconfirming *what* is taking place *whilst* it is taking place. So, during your discussions, you must determine what the client wants and weigh this against the limiting factors that will influence what you need to do.

You need to understand your client fully and be able to negotiate and seek agreement with her throughout the service.

Using visual aids

Visual aids such as style magazines, internet downloads and trade publications are an excellent source for fashionable effects. Pictures are a universal language and this is one simple way of collecting ideas and themes and working out what sorts of things work and those that doesn't.

The haircutting style that you choose with your client should take into account each of the following points about the client's

- face and head shape
- physical features and body shape, size and proportion
- hair quality, abundance, growth and distribution
- age, lifestyle and suitability
- purpose
- ability or time to recreate the effect herself.

General styling limitations

The proportions, balance and distribution of the hairstyle will be a frame for the head and face. Therefore you need to examine the head and face carefully, if you look at the outline of your client's face, you will see that it's either round, oval, square, heart shaped, oblong or triangular. Only an oval face suits all hairstyles, so all the others listed present some form of styling limitations; in other words they become a styling choice influencing factor.

Physical feature	How best to work with it
Square and oblong facial shapes	Are accentuated by hair that is smoothed, scraped back or sleek at the sides and top. The lines and angles are made less conspicuous by fullness and softer movement.
Round faces	Are made more conspicuous if the side and front perimeter lengths are short or finish near to the widest part of the face. This is made worse if width is added at these positions too. Generally this facial shape is complemented by hair length beyond the chin.

EKU statement

GH16 (eku17) The importance of consulting with the client throughout the cutting process

EKU statement

GH16 (eku18) How to clearly present information, advice and recommendations and to assist your client to come to an informed decision

Remember

Be sure to listen to your client's requests. Many mistakes can be avoided if you achieve a clear understanding of what the client is asking for.

Diversion For more information see Unit G21 Provide hairdressing consultation services – Using visual aids in consultation pp. 33–34.

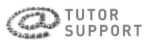TUTOR SUPPORT

Project 4.4: Consultation for a restyling cutting service

EKU statement

GH16 (eku27) How the factors in the range can affect the way the hair is cut

Physical feature	How best to work with it
Square angular features, jaw, forehead etc.	Is improved with softer perimeter shapes, avoid solid, linear effects around the face. Shattered edges and texturising will help to mask these features.
Flatter heads at the back	Are improved by graduation, creating contour and shape that is missing from having a flatter occipital bone.

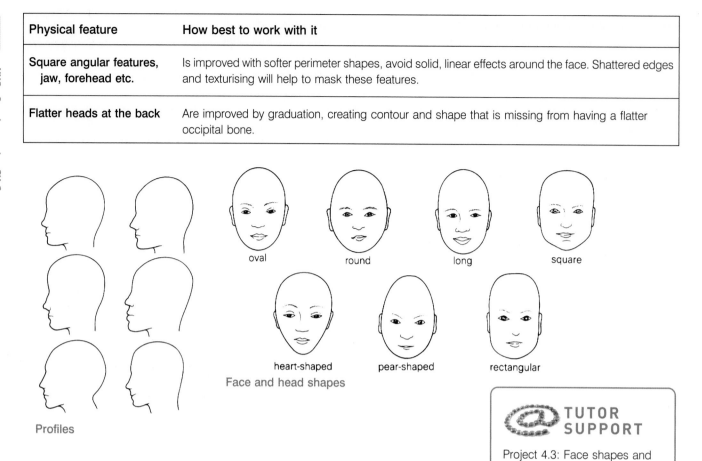

Profiles

oval   round   long   square

heart-shaped   pear-shaped   rectangular

Face and head shapes

TUTOR SUPPORT

Project 4.3: Face shapes and profiles

Head, face and body physical features

Physical feature	How best to work with it
Prominent nose	Hair taken back away from the face accentuates this feature, while hair around the face and forehead tends to diminish the feature.
Square jaw line	Is softened by longer perimeter lengths either coming around and on to the face or styled with fullness. Conversely, shorter side lengths will have an opposite effect.
Protruding ears	Are better left covered rather than exposed. Sufficient hair should be left to cover and extend beyond their length if at all possible.
Wrinkles around the eyes	Are made more obvious by hair being scraped back at the temples or straighter more angular effects.
Narrow foreheads	Are disguised by softer fringes and side partings, whereas they are made more obvious by hair taken back away form the face.
Larger body shapes	The overall effect is balanced and improved with longer, fuller hairstyles; they are made much worse by short, sleek, layered shapes.
Small faces	Can be swamped if the hair is left long with a centre parting and no fringe.
Large faces	Are accentuated by short cropped or sculpted hair.

Physical feature	How best to work with it
Shapes of glasses	There are so many available and are a definite fashion accessory. Generally people will have had assistance in the selection and suitability of their frames. Therefore they should not work against the hairstyle that you want to create as they should already suit the shape and size of the face.
The way the head is held	Many people tilt their head to one side or forwards. Sometimes this is because they are tall and want subconsciously to reduce their height; sometimes they hide behind their hair because they lack confidence or they think it makes them more alluring.
	You need to look out for this natural posture but not make any comment other than asking whether they have any preference to finished lengths, fringes and partings.

Reason or purpose for hairstyle

The reason or purpose for the hairstyle is a big factor in deciding what is suitable or otherwise.

- A style suitable for a special occasion will differ from one that is selected for work. The requirements for competition or show work are quite different from those for general daily wear. But versatility needs to be considered for everyone: people want styles that they can dress up or down.

- Some jobs have special conditions about hair lengths and styles; for example, people working in the armed services or police have to wear their hair above the collar while at work. Men have easily accommodated this by using clippers for very short styles. Women have either had to have short layered styles or hair that is long enough to wear up and out of the way.

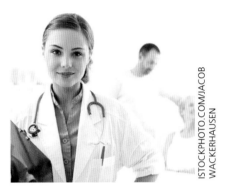

ISTOCKPHOTO.COM/JACOB WACKERHAUSEN

Remember

The success of any hairstyle is based on the information that you get during the consultation. Be thorough: an extra five minutes spent discussing the final effect could make all the difference!

Quality, quantity and distribution of hair

- Good hair condition is an essential prerequisite for great hairstyling. It doesn't matter how much work has gone into the thought and design of a hairstyle, if the hair is in poor condition to start with, it still will be after. Some aspects cannot be altered by cutting alone; for instance, if the hair is dry, dull and porous when the client enters the salon, it still will be when she leaves.

- Regular salon clients in the UK – the ones you tend to see more often than the others – tend to have something in common. Difficult hair. It can be difficult for a number of reasons; it can be fine or unmanageable, lank and lacking volume or just not responsive to styling without force. Thin, sparsely distributed hair is always a problem: if there isn't enough hair to get coverage over the scalp, then there is not a lot you can do about it. One thing that you should remember though is not to put too much texturising into it; this will only make the problem more noticeable. Fine hair presents many problems too. Very fine hair is affected by dampness and quickly loses its shape. This type of hair always benefits from moisture repelling styling products so get your client used to using them.

- Dry, frizzy hair can also be a problem, as the more thermo styling it receives, the more moisture is lost and the less it responds to staying in shape – in other words, the harder it is to style. The problem just keeps going on like a merry-go-around. Dry, unruly thick hair needs to be tamed and most clients with this problem would like their hair to look smoother and shinier. Again this is a conditioning issue and you need to attack the problem before tackling the style.

EKU *statement*

GH16 (eku19) The factors that must be taken into consideration prior to and during cutting (e.g. hair density, hair growth patterns, etc.)

Sometimes this type of hair benefits from finishing products so put them on as you finish and define the hairstyle.

- Very tight curly hair can be difficult too, particularly if your client wants it to appear straight. It is possible to smooth and straighten hair, particularly when you use ceramic straighteners or thermal styling. But keeping it straight is another matter, and you may want to consider other options instead.
- Cutting wavy hair presents some problems but not if it is looked at carefully before it's wet. Avoid cutting across the crests of the waves; you can't change the natural movement in the hair so try to work with it.
- Straight hair, particularly if it is fine textured, can be difficult to cut. Cutting marks or lines can easily form if the cutting sections and angles are not right. Make sure that you only take small sections of hair and remember to crosscheck after, at 90° to the angle in which you first cut, to avoid this happening to you.

Hair positioning, type, growth and tendency

The perimeter outline formed by the hair in relation to the shape of the face is the first thing most people see. It is this effect that people make decisions upon and comments about; for example, 'That's a beautiful haircut.' 'I think that really suits you.' The complete hairstyle is based upon the frame that the hair creates for the face. How you 'fill in' the detail – the movement, direction, colour and placement – is down to your interpretation, understanding, technical ability and experience.

Hair growth direction and distribution should be a major consideration for what is achievable within a hairstyle. You need to make allowances for strong movement, high or low hairlines, natural partings, hair whorls, cowlicks, widow's peaks and double crowns. Look for these before shampooing. The client cannot compensate for these, so when the hair is in need of washing, they will be plain to see. After the hair is washed the degree and strength of the feature can be seen and then you can reconsider how you will tackle it.

(For more information on growth patterns, see Unit G21 Provide hairdressing consultation services pp. 19–20.)

Style suitability

Style suitability refers to the effect of the hair shape on the face, and on the features of the head and body. A hairstyle is, quite simply, suitable when it 'looks right'. But this is a difficult or certainly a subjective thing to quantify.

Aesthetically and artistically speaking, the client's 'hair will look right' when the hairstyle does one of two things. It either *harmonises*, i.e. fits the shape of the face and head – and is therefore a backdrop to an overall image; or *contrasts*, i.e. it accentuates features of the face and head – by creating a prominent frame for the overall image.

Age

As much as you would like to demonstrate your creative ability on everyone who walks through the salon door, bear in mind that some styles are inappropriate for certain clients. Beyond the physical aspects of style design, age does create some barriers to suitability.

Remember

When you choose a suitable hairstyle, always allow for the natural fall of the hair.

TUTOR SUPPORT

Discussion 4.1: Influencing factors effecting choice of style to recommend to the client

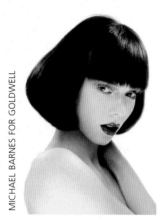

MICHAEL BARNES FOR GOLDWELL

- Younger children (7–11-year-olds) are better suited to simpler hairstyles that don't require too much maintenance. More often than not, and certainly from a hair health and hygiene point of view, they are better off with shorter hairstyles. The next age banding (12–16-year-olds) want to have fashionable looks and many want colours too! Unfortunately, these are still minors and the paying parent and educational establishments must have the last say.

- Young men and women can get away with anything. Fashion will always dictate, and, more often than not, even if there are reasons for not doing a particular style, they will insist on it. This group can enjoy more extreme and dramatic effects and what's more they can get away with it. There are more styles applicable to this age group (16–25-year-olds) than to any other. This is because of the diversity of music, TV and social cultures; these people are influenced by the music they buy, the celebrities they follow on TV and the people they mix with.

- Professional men and women tend to go for watered-down versions of young fashion. Thinking this in another way: in the clothing fashion world the designs that are seen on catwalks in Paris, London and New York are always the catalysts and precursors for what the high street shops will sell. Dozens of the haute couture fashion houses demonstrate their season's offerings at the pre-season shows, but not all designs are picked up by the buyers of commercial high street fashion chains, who usually go for the lesser extreme. People want to appear to be trendy and in touch, but not look ridiculous.

- Older woman require greater consideration. Often the signs of ageing in the skin show quite clearly and therefore they must influence the way in which you select only appropriate and suitable effects.

EKU *statement*

GH16 (eku19) The factors that must be taken into consideration prior to and during cutting (e.g. hair density, hair growth patterns, etc.)

GH16 (eku20) The factors which should be considered when cutting wet and dry hair

Balance

Balance is the effect produced by the amount, fullness and weight distribution of hair throughout the style. The opposite, imbalance, is lack of those proportions. Symmetry or symmetrical even balance occurs when the hair is distributed equally as in a mirrored image through a vertical or horizontal plane. Asymmetry or asymmetric effects occur when the overall shape does not have the same distribution on either side. However, both symmetrical and asymmetrical shapes can be balanced – see the illustration 'Aesthetic balance' (p 358) and see Unit G21 Provide hairdressing consultation services for more information on factors that influence styling choices.

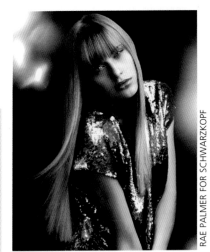

RAE PALMER FOR SCHWARZKOPF

Activity
Complete the table below to say why each of these consultation factors are important and what might happen if these aspects are ignored.

Factors	Why is this important?	What might happen if this is ignored?
Client's requirements		
Hair growth patterns		
Hair texture		
Hair density		
Lifestyle		
Physical features		

Diversion Unit GH21
Develop your creativity

HAIR BY: THE ARTISTIC TEAM @ JACKS OF LONDON
PHOTOGRAPHY BY: JOHN RAWSON@TRP

EKU *statement*

GH16 (eku29) Which tools can be used on either wet or dry hair or both

GH16 (eku14) The correct use and maintenance of cutting tools

Cutting tools

Scissors

Scissors are and will always be the most important piece of hairdressing equipment that you will ever own. Your future income, popularity and success will rely upon this relatively inexpensive item. If you look after them you will be surprised how long a single pair will last. Scissors can be used on either wet or dry hair and vary greatly in their design, size and price. There isn't any single way of choosing the correct pair for you; however, there are a number of aspects that you should consider. Scissors should never be too heavy or too long to control; heavy scissors become cumbersome in regular use and if they are too long you will not be able to manipulate them properly for precision, angular work. Long blades are really good for cutting solid baselines on longer hair, but a real nuisance for precise work around hairlines and behind ears!

To judge a pair of scissors' balance and length, put your fingers in the handles as if you were about to use them. When the scissors are held correctly the pivotal point should just extend beyond the first finger. This allows the blades to open easily and means that the thumb is in an ideal position to work them.

The more expensive scissors will often have one single blade that has small serrations throughout the length. This is really beneficial as this becomes the lower blade in cutting grips the hair and stops it from being pushed away by the closing blades. Sharpening of this type of scissor blade is not recommended though as this factory finish will be removed immediately.

Cutting comb

Get into the habit of only using quality cutting combs. You will find that by spending only a little more you will get so much more out of them. The design of a cutting comb for hairdressing is different to that of barbering.

The hairdressing cutting comb is parallel throughout its length whereas the barbering comb is tapered. There are two sorts of cutting comb. The first and by far the most popular have two sets of teeth, one end to the middle is fine and close together the other end is wider and further apart. This allows you to do fine sections on fine hair and wider sections on coarser hair. The second type of cutting comb has uniform teeth throughout the length of the comb.

The length of cutting combs varies greatly. Again, what's best for you depend on the size of your hands and what you can manage and manipulate quite easily. The normal length of a cutting comb is around 15 cm but longer ones are now very popular and give a better guide for cutting baselines, these can be 2 or 3 cm longer. The quality of combs and the materials they are made from varies greatly. The best-quality combs are made from plastics and have the following properties:

- They are very strong but flexible; the teeth do not chip or break in regular use.
- They remain straight in regular use and do not end up looking like a banana after a couple of weeks!
- They are constructed by injection moulding and do not have sharp or poorly formed edges (as opposed to combs that are made from pressings and have flawed seams and tend to scratch the client's ears and scalp).

Remember

Use quality combs
The comfort of quality combs and in particular cutting combs is the most important factor.

Your professionalism will be inferred from the comb that you use. There is nothing worse than using cutting combs on clients when each time you take a section you scrape and scratch the client's scalp! You will also find that, in regular use, if you persist in using cheap combs your hands will become sore as the teeth will scratch you when you pass the comb into your hand on every section that you take!

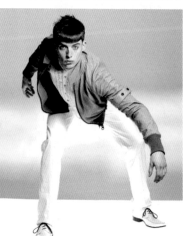

- They are resistant to chemicals making them ideal for cleaning, sterilisation and colouring (as they will not stain).
- They have anti-static finishes that help to control finer hair when dry cutting.

Thinning scissors

Thinning scissors can be used on dry or wet hair and can have either one or two serrated blades. These cutting surfaces will remove bulk or density from the hair depending on the way in which they are used. This has two useful applications for cutting:

1 the tips of finely serrated scissors provide a quick way for texturising the perimeter edges of hairstyles;

2 the whole blades can be used for removing weight (tapering or thinning) from sections of hair but closer to the head.

Thinning scissors with both blades serrated will remove hair more quickly than those with serrations on just one side, and this is more noticeable on scissors that have broader notches in them as opposed to fine teeth.

Razors

The open or 'cut-throat'-style razor used to be made out of a single steel blade which was hinged and closed into a protective handle.

The modern counterpart for this has disposable blades which can be removed and discarded after use. (Blades are discarded after each client to avoid cross-infection. They are disposed of safely into the salon's sharps box.) Razor cutting is carried out on wet hair and *always* with sharp blades. Because of the way in which razors are used, razoring should never be done on dry hair as it will pull and tear the hair even if the blades are new.

Electric and rechargeable clippers

Clippers consist of a moulded, easy-to-handle body with a pair of serrated cutting blades. For more information on this topic, see Unit GB8, p 117.

Clipper attachments

Clippers are purchased with a range of plastic attachments. These enable the clippers to be used safely in cutting wet or dry hair to a uniform layered length. These attachments vary the cutting depth from:

- Grade 1 – extremely short leaving a shadow of hair across the scalp.
- Grade 2 – very short allowing the skin to still be seen on all but very thick hair.
- Grade 3 – moderately short, the first grade length that enables the skin not to be seen on most but very finer hair types.
- Grade 4 – short, but a very popular length, leaving enough hair to resemble very short layering.
- Grades 5–8 – longer grades that produce layered effects that could be achieved by club cutting techniques.

Remember

Never keep scissors in your pockets: it is unhygienic but, more importantly, it is a dangerous thing to do.

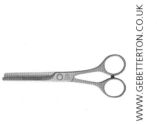

WWW.GEBETTERTON.CO.UK

Remember

Check the clipper blade alignment regularly to make sure that the blades are parallel and have not been knocked or loosened. If they are loose or out of alignment get someone to check and make the adjustments.

Diversion For more information on this topic, see Unit GB8, p 117.

Remember

When new scissors are bought they come in a protective case, get into the habit of keeping them in it. This will make them easy to identify when there are plenty of other pairs about and will also provide useful protection when they are carried around.

EKU *statement*

GH16 (eku22) The potential risk of ingrowing hair resulting from the continual close cutting of curly hair

GH16 (eku21) The average rate of hair growth

Maintain your tools

Clippers – a little clipper oil should be applied last thing so that the lubrication can provide a protective coating overnight. Then, before use, they can be cleaned, any excess oil removed, and made ready for the next day's use.

Scissors – carefully wipe over the blades at the end of the working day to remove any fragments of hair and then apply a little clipper oil to the pivot point to prevent any corrosion around the fastening screw. This will prolong their life and stop them from binding or getting stiffer to use.

Avoid ingrowing hairs

Ingrowing hairs are an uncomfortable aspect of closely cut wavy or curly hair. When hair is razored or clippered close to the skin; say at the neckline, the action of the cutting implement tends to slightly pull the hair within the follicle. After the hair is cut, the hairshaft tends to retract back into the follicle giving a very close, a smooth finish to the touch. Unfortunately, if the area isn't kept thoroughly clean the open area of the follicle can become partially blocked with dead skin cells or dirt. This will change the growing direction of the hair within the follicle, often allowing it to find a new position within the skin. Bearing in mind that the average rate of hair growth is about 1.25 cm per month; if allowed to continue, an ingrowing hair will result. The physical effects of this will not be noticed until:

- It starts to create a raised area often accompanied with a mild infected spot.
- It begins to itch as it causes irritation beneath the skin.

If the ingrowing hair is not brought to the surface or removed from the skin, a longer-term, more serious condition/infection will result.

Activity

Note: this activity should be carried out with the electric clippers removed from the power supply or rechargeable clippers 'rundown'.

Knowing how to remove, replace, realign and maintain a clipper's blades is an essential part of hairdressing. Get your supervisor to show you how the lower blade-retaining screws are undone and removed. This will give you access to both cutting blades and the area below the armature (the vibrating arm that works them) for cleaning purposes.

When you have dismantled the blades, check them for signs of corrosion. If a rusted area exists it will look like blackened areas around the blade edges. If blades have been allowed to get to this stage they should be replaced by new ones as their ability to cut cleanly without friction has been greatly reduced.

With the blades stripped down, you can now use clipper oil to lubricate the two blades, wiping any excess away. Now you can replace the blades (the right way up) and partially re-tighten the retaining screws. Finally, readjust the alignment of the blades and tighten the screws. Check the alignment once more: the lower cutting blade should extend around 3 mm further than the upper cutting blade with the clippers adjusted fully forwards to the shortest cutting length.

Hand them back to your supervisor so that your maintenance can be checked.

Neck brushes, water sprays and sectioning clips

Neck brushes will remove loose hair clippings from around the neck and face. Get used to passing the neck brush to your client when you are cutting dry hair as the small fragments are irritating when they fall onto the face. Neck brushes usually have synthetic bristles and these are easily washed and dried before they are used.

Water sprays are used for damping down dry or dried hair, to assist you in controlling the haircut. Stale water is unhygienic, so make sure that the water is emptied out and refilled on a daily basis.

Sectioning clips are usually made from plastic or thin alloys. They are used to divide the hair and keep bulk out of the way whilst you work on other areas. They are sterilised by immersing them into Barbicide™ solution for the manufacturer's recommended length of time.

Cutting checklist

✔	Make sure that the client is protected adequately first.
✔	Always gain agreement before attempting anything new or different.
✔	Make sure you consider the reasons and the purpose for the style.
✔	Assess the style limitations, hair problems or physical features.
✔	Avoid technical jargon or style names. If jargon is used, by you or the client, always clarify in simple terms what it means to avoid confusion.
✔	Don't just do the style if you think that it's wrong. If there are reasons why you think it will be unsuitable, you will be doing the client a big favour in the longer term if you tackle the issue straight away.
✔	Always give the client some advice on how to handle the style themselves.
✔	Give the client an idea of how long it will take to do

GH16.2   Creatively restyle women's hair

Accurate sectioning

In order for you to be able to manage sizeable amounts of hair at any one time, you must organise and plan the haircut. The planning bit becomes automatic; it's the few moments that you spend thinking:

- How do I go about this?
- Where do I start?
- What is the finish going to be like?

So, if the planning is automatic it's the organisation bit that you have to address. Quite simply, being organised is about working in a methodical way. It is the way in which you routinely start at one point, divide and secure all the rest of the hair out of the way, finish that bit and then take down the next part to work on, and so on. Each part or section that you work on should be small enough for you to cope with, without losing your way and continuing on blindly! It seems a strange term to use, but 'blindly' is exactly the right word. If the sections are too deep or too wide you will not be able to see the cutting guide that you need to work to. Accurate sectioning guarantees that every cut is addressed to the same length every time.

EKU *statement*

GH16 (eku31) How to create and follow guidelines

Cut hair with natural fall

Being aware of and cutting with natural fall is extremely important. Looking for the directions of growth within the hair is an essential part of consultation as it is within the execution of the haircut. If you work with the natural fall i.e. partings, nape hair growth,

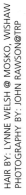

HAIR BY: LYNNE WELSH @ MOSKO, WISHAW
PHOTOGRAPHY BY: JOHN RAWSON@TRP

Remember

As previously covered in the section on preparation, always try to wash the hair, even if it is only a dry haircut. This way when you dry the hair off, you will be able to see the natural fall far easier and be able to work with it.

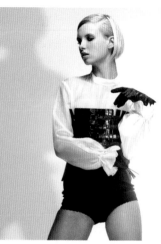

EKU *statement*

GH16 (eku30) The reasons for establishing and following guidelines

GH16 (eku31) How to create and follow guidelines

GH16 (eku37) The importance of applying the correct degree of tension to the hair when cutting

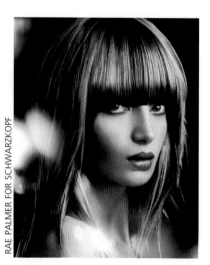

double crowns etc. you will be compensating for these anomalies and be able to produce an easier to manage result. Ignore these factors and you will be giving both you and the client a hard job in styling it.

Remember

Cutting baselines/perimeter outlines

A baseline is a cut section of hair, which is used as a cutting guide for the following sections of hair. There may be one or more baselines cut: for example, a graduated nape baseline may be cut; another may be cut into the middle of the hair at the back of the head. Other baselines may be cut at the sides and the front of the head. The baselines will determine the perimeter of the hairstyle, or part of the style, and may take different shapes according to the effects required.

Symmetrical: The baseline for evenly balanced hair shapes in which the hair is equally divided on both sides of the head. Examples are hairstyles with central partings or with the hair swept backwards or forwards.

Asymmetrical: The baseline to be used where the hair is unevenly balanced, for example where there is a side parting and a larger volume of hair on one side of the head, or where the hair is swept off the face at one side with fullness of volume on the other.

Concave: The baseline may be cut curving inwards or downwards. The nape baseline, for example, may curve downwards.

Convex: The baseline may be cut curving upwards and outwards – the nape baseline, for instance, may be cut curving upwards.

Straight: The baseline may be cut straight across, for example where you wish to produce a hard, square effect.

Controlling the shape

There are three aspects of cutting that you must get right on every haircut:

- *The holding angle* – the angle at which the hair is held out from the head.
- *The cutting angle* – the angle at which the scissors, razor etc. cuts the hair.
- *The holding tension* – the even pressure applied to sections of hair when it is held.

That doesn't seem much to guarantee success, but it does take a lot of practice and concentration. Even if you start well in the haircut you cannot afford to lose it in the closing stages.

Cutting lines Also known as perimeter lines, these are the outline shape created when layered hair is held directly out with tension (perpendicular) from the head. The curves and the angle in relation to the head, determines the shape of the cut style. The main ones are:

- the contour of the shape from top to bottom
- the contour of the shape around the head, side to side.

Cutting guides These are prepared sections of hair that control the uniform quality of the haircut. When the cutting guide is taken and first cut, it is to this length and shape that all the other following sections relate. In preparing this cutting guide you need to take all the client's physical features and attributes into consideration, i.e. eyes, eyebrows, nose, bone structure, head shape, neck length, hairlines etc.

Cutting the lines and angles Comb the hair and hold the sections with an even tension. The tension ensures that accuracy is maintained throughout the cut and the position in which you hold and cut the hair determines the position the cut sections take when combed back on the head. The angles and lines of cutting depend on the different lengths required by the style. The first cutting line – the outer perimeter line – may be related to the nape (when starting at the back). The second cutting line – the inner perimeter line – depends on the different lengths required throughout the style.

Activity

The table below contains a list of terms used within cutting.

Recreate the table within your portfolio and then for each one:

(a) give an explanation of each term

(b) find examples or draw a sketch of the effects

Cutting term	What does this term mean?	Examples of the effect
Graduation	*layer the hair out*	
Fading	*to blend into haircut*	
Reverse graduation	*starting large from front to bc*	
Disconnection	*disconect front section from back section.*	

EKU *statement*

GH16 (eku34) The importance of cross-checking the cut

GH16 (eku35) How to cross-check and balance the cut

Cross-checking the cut

Possibly at different points during the cut, but certainly after the cut you will need to recheck what you have already done. This is done by taking and holding sections at a plane which is at right angles (90°) to the original cut sections. (In other words if you originally cut the hair in vertical meshes; your cross-check will be done with horizontal meshes.)

Cross-checking provides a final technique for checking the continuity and accuracy of the hair cut. Where you find an imbalance in weight or extra length that still needs to be removed, it provides you with the opportunity to create the perfect finish.

EKU *statement*

GH16 (eku39) The types of problems that can commonly arise when cutting women's hair and ways in which they can be remedied, if possible

Dealing with cutting problems

A lack of attention during the cut or a missed detail or aspect during the consultation can lead to cutting mistakes. The variety of mistakes is too varied to cover, but normally result in an imbalance in weight proportions or a difference in perimeter lengths.

If, on finishing a symmetrical cut, you feel that one side seems to be slightly longer than the other; you need to stop before taking anything off the apparently longer side. If it is obviously longer and the client has commented too, you need to put your comb and scissors down and recheck through the fingers.

Standing behind the client you take a small piece of hair from the same position on the head at either side with your forefingers and thumbs. Then slowly slide your fingers down either side until you get to the ends. Looking at the length through the mirror, see if the ends terminate at the same lengths either side; if they do, the cut is fine. Often a cut can seem wrong and the more you look at it the worse it seems. By putting the scissors and

TUTOR SUPPORT

Discussion 4.2: Cutting problems and solutions

comb down you break the fixation and blind panic and have a chance to review it again calmly, with your hands empty. (Most hairdressers make the fatal mistake of immediately taking some off the apparently longer side; only to find that the other side then seems wrong and then as they continue, each side gets shorter and shorter!)

If, however, there is a difference in both lengths, then you now have the chance to redress the balance.

Clients are particularly attached to their fringes; (pardon the pun) if a fringe is taken too short the client generally feels very conspicuous. So how can you replace hair that is already too short? Well you can't replace the hair but you can reduce the effect by reducing a solid fringe line by slightly *point cutting* to 'break up' the density and reveal a little skin of the forehead through the hair.

What really bothers people is the stark contrast of between the solid line of the fringe and the skin; this focuses even more attention on the area. Therefore the solution is to reduce this contrast by softening the demarcation line. (This technique of reducing obvious mistakes can be used throughout the perimeter of hairstyles as it works in most cases.)

Finally, another popular cutting fault is caused by an imbalance of weight in layering on one side to the other. Again, if you get to a cross-check situation and find that the layer pattern on one side seems different to the other side, stop.

You need to find out if it is due to:

- one side being longer than the other or,
- a greater reduction in weight by texturising on one side rather than the other.

If it is length then you can easily re-cut the longer side to match. But if it is due to weight reduction, you will see a 'collapse' in the overall style shape on the side that has had the greater amount of texturising. You can then remedy the fault by further texturising the hair from the thicker side.

Cutting and styling techniques

Club cutting

EKU *statement*

GH16 (eku28) How and why to use all the cutting techniques in the range on women's hair

This is the method of cutting hair bluntly straight across. It systematically cuts all the hair, at an angle parallel to the first and middle finger, to the same length. It is the most popular technique and often forms the basis or first part of a haircut, before other techniques are employed.

Club cutting is used in both layered and one-length cuts and is therefore a particularly suitable choice for maintaining or creating bulk and volume. It is an ideal way to cut finer hair types or for use with people who have sparser (less dense) hair.

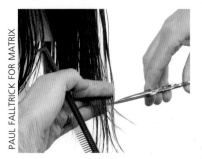

Holding with an even tension.

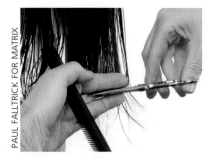

Cutting with the scissor blades parallel to the fingers.

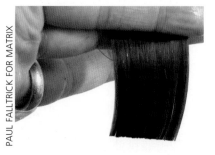

A completed 'club cut' section.

Freehand cutting

Freehand cutting is mainly used on straighter hair for creating the profile or perimeter shape. The technique is used on straighter hair because curlier hair needs more control, through holding and tensioning, if you are to make an accurate cut. As the name suggests, freehand cutting relies upon one hand holding and combing the hair into position, and the other controlling the scissors to make the cut. More often than not, when cutting longer, one-length hair, the comb is used to create the guide for making the cut. This technique is more widely used in cutting fringes that, when you are particularly cautious about what the exact finished length of the fringe is. It is easier to comb the length into position and create a profile shape that flows with the client and follows or covers the eyebrows. This would be harder to do if the hair were held between the fingers and cut, because the width of your fingers might interfere with the exact length and position you are trying to cut.

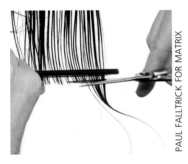

Freehand cutting using the comb to hold the hair.

Rechecking the accuracy of the line.

A completed freehand 'club cut'.

PAUL FALLTRICK FOR MATRIX

Scissor over comb

This technique has been traditionally a barbering technique. In recent years there has been a move in hairdressing generally towards easier-to-manage hairstyles, so therefore this technique is widely used in hairdressing for cutting short styles on both men and women.

Scissor over comb cutting is ideal for producing contoured, layered shapes and close-cut, 'fade-out' perimeters. Faded or graduated perimeters have no set cut length (i.e. baseline); they rely upon the hairline profile and are graduated out from that into the rest of the hairstyle. The technique is used with either wet or dry hair as it uses the comb as a guide instead of the fingers.

Clipper over comb

Clipper over comb involves exactly the same technique as scissor over comb; instead of using scissors the clippers whisk away the hair. Again, this technique enables you to cut hair far closer than you would be able to if you were holding it between your fingers.

Thinning

Thinning is a technique which can be done with scissors or a razor and can be used for reducing or tapering bulk from thicker hair without reducing the overall length, or as a way of texturising the profile of hairstyles to remove lines and angular shapes to create softer, faded, more ambiguous effects.

Remember

Cutting combs used for scissor over comb need to be very flexible. You may want to buy a barbering, tapered comb as this makes cutting easier and quicker. This does not apply to clipper over comb techniques. Because of the weight and bulkiness of electric clippers it is easier to use a standard parallel cutting comb.

EKU statement

GH16 (eku32) How to personalise and adapt cutting techniques

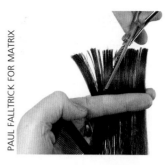

Point cutting with thinning scissors.

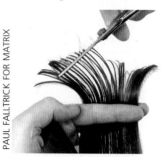

Removing the bulk from the ends.

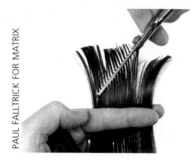

Maintaining the same cutting angle throughout the technique.

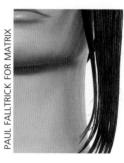

Finally removing any definition to the previously club cut lengths.

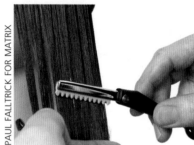

Razor tapering.

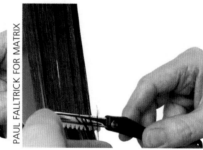

Removing weight from the ends.

The tapered effect.

Texturising technique # 1

Texturising by **point cutting** or **pointing** is a technique where the angle of the cut changes to become almost parallel with the held hair. It is a way of reducing lines and bulk from the ends (1–2 cm) of the hair in order to create softer, more textured edges. It uses the point ends of the scissors and is more successful on straighter hair than wavy; it does not add any value to curly hairstyles at all. If curlier hair is point cut it can often make it more difficult for the client to manage: the hair would lose perimeter density and the curl would increase, making the hair fluffier.

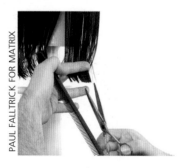

Note the scissor position, parallel to the held lengths.

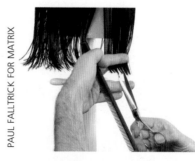

Point cutting to 'shatter' the club cut lengths.

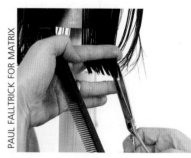

Continue the technique until the weight is removed.

Texturising technique # 2

Texturising by **brick cutting** is similar to point cutting in that it only uses the point ends of the scissor blades, but is intended to remove 'fine chunks' of hair from the mid-length and nearer the root of hand-held sections. Its main advantage is when cutting shorter hair to create stiffer sections that support the outer hair perimeter shape. Put another way, it can produce volume whilst creating spikier edges.

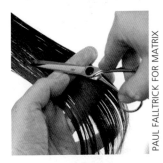

Removing mid-length hair with the point of the scissors.

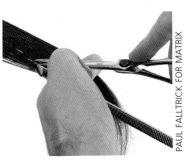

Change positions within the length to avoid any cutting lines.

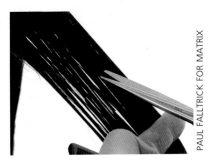

Weight reduces quickly.

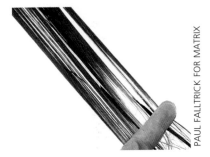

The tapered effect.

Texturising technique # 3

Texturising by **slicing** is a technique for either very sharp scissors or razors. Slicing will produce a tapering effect in a hair section without reducing the overall length. It is always done with the hair held at an angle slightly downwards. The scissors or razor is introduced to the hair nearer the root and then, in one continuous and angled, downward motion, it takes a longer slice out and towards the ends of the held hair.

The finished effects will produce 'shattered' looks with irregular, tousled appearances that can be dressed with product to create texture and definition.

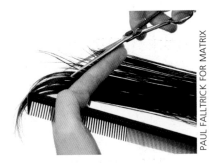

Positioning the scissors safely away from the fingers.

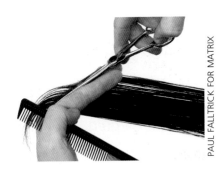

Scoop away the hair without totally closing the blades.

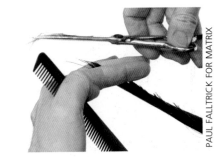

The final part of the movement.

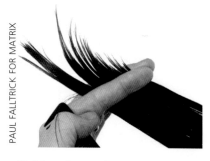

PAUL FALLTRICK FOR MATRIX

Holding the section.

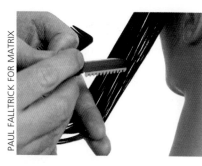

PAUL FALLTRICK FOR MATRIX

Offer the razor to the hair almost parallel to the angle of the hair.

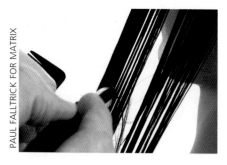

PAUL FALLTRICK FOR MATRIX

Draw down the razor, through the held section.

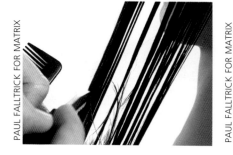

PAUL FALLTRICK FOR MATRIX

Continue the action further down the section.

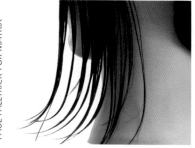

PAUL FALLTRICK FOR MATRIX

The tapered effect achieved by the razor.

Disconnection

Disconnection is used to create a demarcation area between two different levels. It is a deliberate style or styling feature that draws attention to the different levels and can be done on all one length hair or layered effects. Typical examples for this would be a classic bob with a fringe; in this style, where the fringe stops, the sides continue down to the perimeter length creating a 'step' in the hairstyle. But this is not the only type of disconnection; a contemporary bob can have deliberate steps within the sides, this could be to draw attention to cheekbones or a jaw-line. Other examples of disconnection are regularly used on short layered styles that have longer hair over-falling the shorter perimeters.

> **Remember**
>
>
>
> **One-length cuts, layering and graduation**
> The techniques above create a comprehensive palette or toolbox of skills that are used to create all of the final cutting effects. You choose from the outset the *tools* that you need to craft the final effect.
> A *one-length cut* is achieved by combing vertically down and cutting straight across.
> A *graduation* or *graduated cut* is achieved by creating a layered shape that is longer on the upper sections and shorter underneath.
> A *reverse graduation* is achieved by creating a layered shape that is shorter on the upper sections and longer underneath.

Combining the techniques

None of the above techniques are used in isolation by the creative cutter. A precision or artistic cutter will use a combination of these cutting disciplines to create a finished effect. As you become more experienced in your work you will probably find that you would need to use at least 30–50 per cent of these in each hair cut in order to achieve satisfactory fashionable results.

Sources for more information on cutting

You need to keep abreast of what is happening in fashion and creative circles: style magazines, websites on the internet and music and TV are all sources for what is happening now, but that is only part of the story.

Fashion predictions and forecasts are created by clothes designers well in advance of the current season. Each couturier will be showing their fashion collections up to 12 months in advance. This provides a good source of information for you, as the designers are always attempting to create a total look involving the hair and hair styling too.

Fashions have to start somewhere too. Every new theme can be tracked back to images, textures and differing cultures from the past. It's not that originality has died; it's more of reworking and amalgamation of older themes in a new, exciting and interesting ways.

Historical collections in museums are a good source for new ideas as well as the internet. Look for the themes created by tribal and ethnic cultures too; many of these such as dreadlocks, corn rows and etched scalp patterns may be commonplace now but have their roots; definitely cemented in the past.

Activity

The table below contains a list of terms used within cutting. For each one give an explanation of the term and what effect they achieve within a haircut.

Cutting term	What does it describe?	What effect(s) does it achieve?
Pointing		
Chipping		
Slider/slice cutting		
Feathering		

Checklists

Before the cut

✔	Communicate with your client and discuss the requirements.
✔	Use visual aids to help interpret the client's wishes or to show ideas and themes.
✔	Examine the hair – its type, length, quality, quantity and condition. Look for factors that influence the choice of style and cutting methods.
✔	Explain if there are any limitations that will affect the result.
✔	After your analysis, agree or negotiate with the client the suitable courses of action to take.
✔	Try to show the hair length to be removed.
✔	Discuss the time that will be taken and the price that you will charge.
✔	Proceed only when all checks have been made and the client has agreed to your proposals.
✔	Ensure that you choose the correct tools and techniques for achieving the variety of effects.

Remember

The most important factor in cutting hair Very few people can do two things at the same time! You will have to learn very quickly that you need to hold a conversation with the client without losing your way and concentration on the haircut. This is the biggest single cause of poor quality hairdressing! (If you cannot do this yet, tell your client that you need the time to focus on the task ahead. Believe it or not, they won't mind.)

Remember

Always ask how much the client wants cut off.

- A trim is a trim, in other words a *reshape* or *reshaping cut*, whereas a different or new cut is a *restyle* or *restyling cut* (if the client is not used to these words explain the difference).

- An inch to one person may be a centimetre to another. Don't be ambiguous, find out exactly how much needs to be cut off!

Remember

Far more customers are dissatisfied as a result of the stylist not listening and taking too much off than because of poor or inaccurate haircuts.

During the cut

✔	After shampooing and towel drying, dry off the hair so that any previously masked tendencies can clearly be seen.
✔	Try to keep the hair damp but not saturated so that any newly added technical features can easily be seen.
✔	Take care with your precision or accuracy by checking each angle at which the hair is taken and held from the head.
✔	Create your baselines and guideline cuts first, so that there is a continuity within the section patterning.
✔	When preparing baselines and guide sections, make sure that you attend to the features of your client's face and head. Use these as guides for accurate directions in the cut lines.
✔	Remember always that the first cuts you make often determine the finished shape of the style.

After the cut

✔	Cross-check each of the sections of the side, nape, top and front for accuracy and finish.
✔	Check the density, texture and features of the haircut.
✔	Position, place and mould the hair where necessary to see the shape clearly.
✔	When all the loose hair clippings have been removed and the client is prepared and comfortable, continue to blow-dry, set and finish the style.

Step-by-steps

Cut disconnection with shattered edges

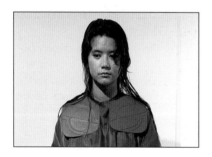

Step 1 Before

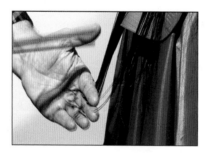

Step 2 Cut perimeter to required length

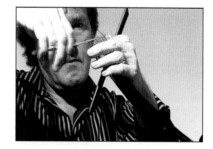

Step 3 Reverse graduate layers to approximate length

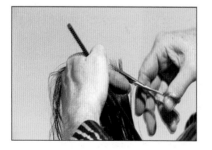

Step 4 Cut layer shaping for top to length whilst creating a disconnection to retain long hair density

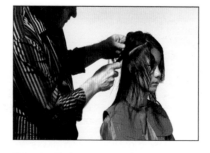

Step 5 Take a horseshoe section to mark out layered area from perimeter length

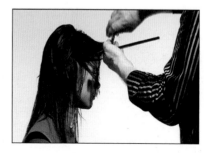

Step 6 Over-extend layering forwards to finish off the facial frame

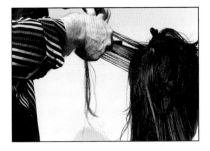

Step 7 After scissor cutting, razor out the density to shatter the layers and disconnection

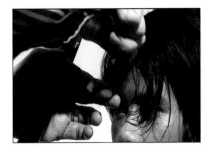

Step 8 Texturise the fringe with light razoring

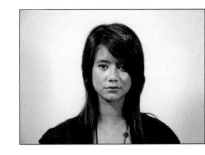

Step 9 Final effect

Concave cut graduation

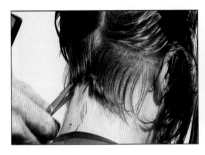

Step 1 Section off lower nape to create concave perimeter

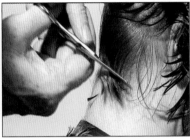

Step 2 Balance the shape the other side

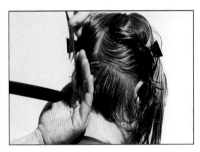

Step 3 Start by holding a vertical guide at the centre of the back

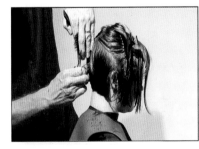

Step 4 Cut to the required length

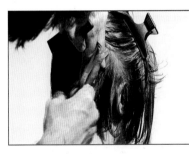

Step 5 Continue the layer pattern by over-extending each vertical mesh back towards the centre

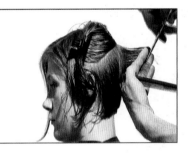

Step 6 With both sides complete, continue up the back to continue the previously cut line

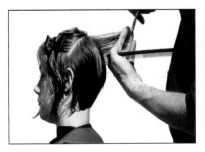

Step 7 Continued from step 6

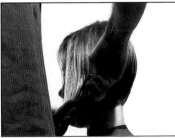

Step 8 With the back done take a horizontal section through to the face and cut to length

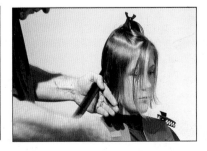

Step 9 Marry up the other side before starting to layer

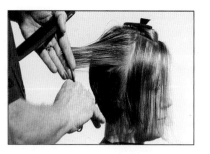

Step 10 With perimeter length cut, over-extend each mesh backwards to find the previously cut guidelines

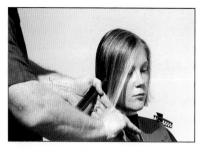

Step 11 Tidy up any slight unevenness

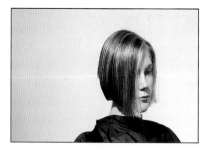

Step 12 Finished cut

Long hair concave grad with square layers

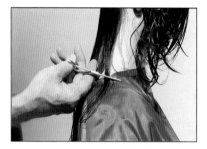

Step 1 Remove cutting collar and cut perimeter to sit on shoulders

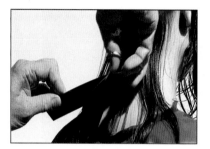

Step 2 Use the cutting comb as a guide to create the angle

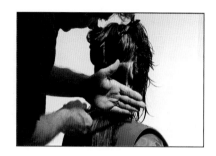

Step 3 Take down next section and cut to the same perimeter length

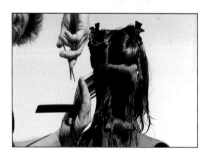

Step 4 Start layer pattern by holding a vertical guide at the centre of the back

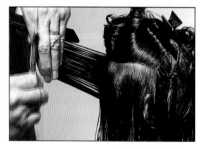

Step 5 Club cut lengths first to maintain your accuracy

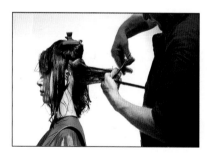

Step 6 Over-extend backwards to create the concave shape

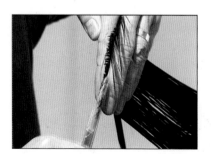

Step 7 Keep your sectioning neat

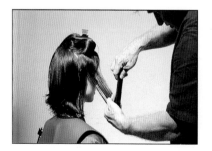

Step 8 Section off at the side to create your perimeter frame

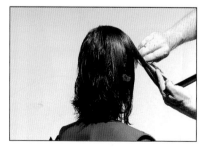

Step 9 Continue up the sides; over-extending the meshes to retain weight at the sides

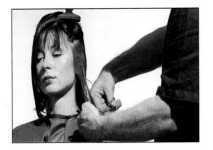

Step 10 Cut the other side to match up the profile length

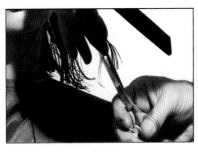

Step 11 Point cut the ends throughout the layering to texturise the shape and increase movement

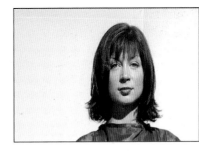

Step 12 Final effect

Graduated bob

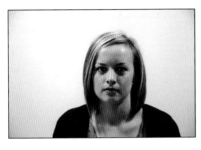

Step 1 Before

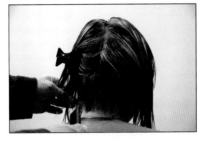

Step 2 Section the hair off at the nape

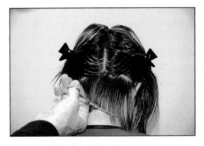

Step 3 Create the outer perimeter shape

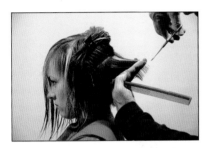

Step 4 Start layer pattern by holding a vertical guide at the centre of the back

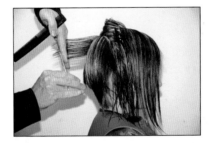

Step 5 Continue the guideline up through the back

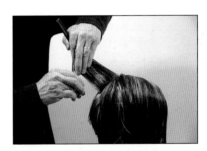

Step 6 Break the layer shape by creating a new guideline at the crown

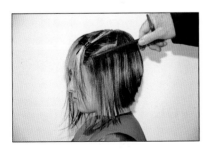

Step 7 Take a section through to the front and secure the remainder out of the way

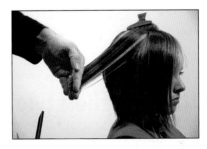

Step 8 Continue up the sides, over-extending the meshes to retain weight at the sides

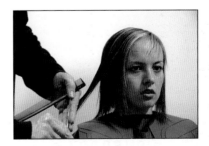

Step 9 Tidy the edges and check your balance

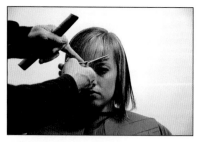

Step 10 Freehand cut the fringe into shape

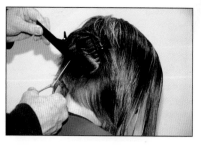

Step 11 Retrace your cut by razoring into the shape

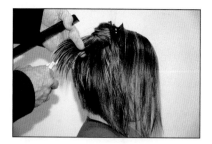

Step 12 Break the density at the points by chipping into the lengths

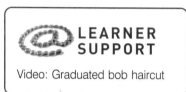
LEARNER SUPPORT

Video: Graduated bob haircut

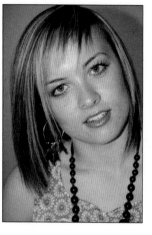

Step 13 Final effect

GH16.3 Provide aftercare advice

EKU *statement*

GH16 (eku40) The recommended time interval between cuts

Good service is supported through good advice and recommendation. The work that you do in the salon needs to be cared for at home by the client too. What would be the point of creating something if the client doesn't know how to achieve and maintain the same effects at home?

Home-and aftercare checklist

✔	Talk through the style as you work; that way the client sees how you handle different aspects of the look.
✔	Show and recommend the products/equipment that you use so that the client gets the right things to enable them to get the same effects.
✔	Tell the client how long the style can be expected to last and when they need to return for reshaping.
✔	Demonstrate the techniques that you use so they can achieve that salon hair look too.

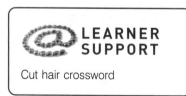
LEARNER SUPPORT

Cut hair crossword

Talk through the style as you work

Make a point of talking through your styling techniques as you go as:

(a) it eliminates long periods of silence whilst you are working and, more importantly,

(b) it is really useful to the client as they get useful advice on how to recreate a similar effect at home.

Styles need to suit their purposes too and you need to bear this in mind in your summing up with the client. If the client's routines or lifestyle is going to have an impact upon their hairstyle then you should make a point of telling them this. If they work in a hot, steamy kitchen then their hair is going to look rather flat and sad when they take their head covering off. Similarly, someone who does a lot of sport is constantly in and out of the shower, so their hairstyle needs to reflect this. Sometimes if the hair is long it can easily be tied back out of the way, but if it's short you need to make some other suggestions.

EKU *statement*

GH16 (eku24) The types of products available finishing women's hair

GH16 (eku42) Products for home use that will benefit the client.

Show and recommend the products/ equipment that you use

As you talk about the ways in which you have styled the hair, make a point of talking through the products that you have used as well. You know by experience the products that you would use on their hair to achieve different results and you also know the ones that you would avoid! Well make a point of telling the client too, because they haven't had the benefit of your training and they don't know.

So when you use a particular product, why not hand it to them so they can have a closer look. This way they get to see, smell and feel the product too and, subconsciously, this has a very powerful effect on them. By doing this you are involving the client in what you are doing by giving them a greater experience of the service.

This way they will be able to see a direct link between the effects that you are achieving on their hair, with the added benefits of buying those particular products that will help them to recreate a similar effect.

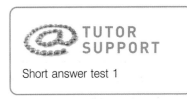

TUTOR SUPPORT

Short answer test 1

EKU *statement*

GH16 (eku41) How to use tools and equipment to maintain the look

Explain how routine styling tools can have detrimental effects

Only hair in good condition is easy to maintain. You know how difficult it is to make dry, damaged hair look good. It tends to be lifeless, dull and sits there just like a wig! Your clients can recognise the difference between good and poor condition and given the choice, they will always choose hair that has lustre, shine, flexibility and strength.

With these known facts, you would be doing an injustice to your clients if you didn't warn them of the pitfalls of repeatedly using hot styling equipment, so make a point in asking them if they use them at home too. If they say that they use straighteners or tongs on a daily basis then tell them about the benefits of using heat protection sprays.

Remember

The condition of their hair is directly proportional to the amount of heat applied to it. So if they are locked into using these styling tools their hair is going to need all the help it can get.

Demonstrate the techniques that you use

Clients want to be able to recreate the effects that you achieve in the salon and this is your chance to show them how to do it. Clients haven't had the benefit of your training; they don't know the little tricks and techniques that make it seem so simple. Show them how to do things; correct combing, blow-drying or positioning of brushes. We have all seen the effects when these are not done properly, so make a point of giving them a few tips on how the can achieve a similar result themselves and how long they can expect it to last.

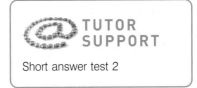

TUTOR SUPPORT

Short answer test 2

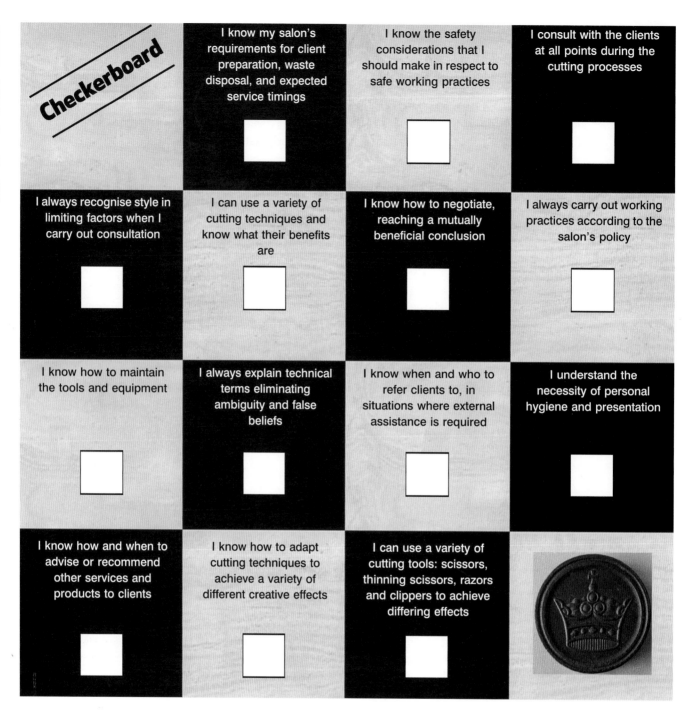

Checkerboard

I know my salon's requirements for client preparation, waste disposal, and expected service timings ☐

I know the safety considerations that I should make in respect to safe working practices ☐

I consult with the clients at all points during the cutting processes ☐

I always recognise style in limiting factors when I carry out consultation ☐

I can use a variety of cutting techniques and know what their benefits are ☐

I know how to negotiate, reaching a mutually beneficial conclusion ☐

I always carry out working practices according to the salon's policy ☐

I know how to maintain the tools and equipment ☐

I always explain technical terms eliminating ambiguity and false beliefs ☐

I know when and who to refer clients to, in situations where external assistance is required ☐

I understand the necessity of personal hygiene and presentation ☐

I know how and when to advise or recommend other services and products to clients ☐

I know how to adapt cutting techniques to achieve a variety of different creative effects ☐

I can use a variety of cutting tools: scissors, thinning scissors, razors and clippers to achieve differing effects ☐

Revision questions

Quick quiz: a selection of different types of questions to check your knowledge.

Q1 Accuracy is achieved by _ _ _ _ _ _ _ _ and cutting the hair at the correct angle. Fill in the blank

Q2 A razor should be used on dry hair. True or false

Q3 Select the texturising techniques from the following list. Multi selection

Club cutting	☐ 1
Graduation	☐ 2
Slice cutting	☐ 3
Fading	☐ 4
Point cutting	☐ 5
Chipping	☐ 6

Q4 Symmetrical styles produce outline shapes that are equally balanced. True or false

Q5 Which of the following is not a cutting term? Multi selection

Crosschecking	☐ 1
Thinning	☐ 2
Free hand	☐ 3
Free style	☐ 4

Q6 Disconnection is a term defining a continuous outline shape or layer patterning. True or false

Q7 Which of the following hair growth patterns does not affect the way that hair lays after it is cut? Multi selection

Nape whorl	☐ 1
Double crown	☐ 2
Widow's peak	☐ 3
Low hairline	☐ 4
Cow lick	☐ 5
High hairline	☐ 6

Q8 A _ _ _ _ _ _ _ _ line or perimeter outline forms a guide line for a bob-shaped haircut. Fill in the blank

Q9 Which of the following cuts would easily describe a disconnection? Multi choice

Graduation in a long hairstyle	○ 1
Reverse graduation in a long hairstyle	○ 2
A fringe in a shoulder-length bob style	○ 3
Texturising in a short cropped style	○ 4

Q10 'Personalising' is the term that refers to any technique that is used to complete a style, tailoring it to the client's specific needs. True or false

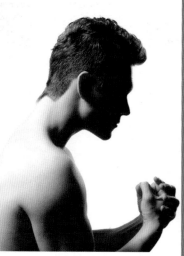

LEE MORAN @ SANRIZZ

Chapter**five**
Creative barbering

GB8

GB8.1

GB8.2

GB8.3

**CREDIT VALUE
FOR UNIT GB8**
5 Credits

More Information See
Units

G22 Monitor procedures
to safely control work
operations

G21 Provide hairdressing
consultation services

Diversion See
Appendices for Electricity
at Work Regulations

EKU *statement*

GB8 (eku4) Your
responsibilities under the
Electricity at Work
Regulations

Creative barbering: quick overview

Unit title

GB8 Creatively cut hair using a combination of barbering techniques

This is a **mandatory** unit for barbering at level 3, it is made up of three main outcomes

Main outcomes

GB8.1 Maintain effective and safe methods of working when cutting hair

GB8.2 Creatively restyle men's hair

GB8.3 Provide aftercare advice

What do I need to do for GB8.1?

- Make sure that the client is adequately covered and protected
- Make sure that your working position is comfortable and safe
- Keep the work area clean and tidy and that waste materials are disposed of properly
- Work without causing risks to you or your client's health and safety
- Work efficiently and effectively

What do I need to do for GB8.2?

- Choose suitable visual aids to help with style selection for your client
- Prepare your client's hair before cutting
- Seek confirmation of the desired look before starting
- Cut your client's hair using a variety of creative cutting techniques
- Check that the final effect is; accurate, that it compliments the client's features, their personal image and that the client is satisfied with the results

What do I need to do for GB8.3?

- Give accurate constructive advice on how the client can maintain the look

What aspects do I need to cover for GB8.1, GB8.2 and GB8.3?

- A variety of cutting tools and equipment
- A range of factors that influence or limit the choice of styling
- Different types of cutting techniques that are used to create creative effects

What aspects do I need to know for GB8.1, GB8.2 and GB8.3?

- Your salon's requirements for preparation, timings and standards of service
- Any salon or local limitations relating to the use of fixed blade razors
- How to work safely, effectively and hygienically when cutting hair
- Factors about hair that affect styling choice, suitability and durability
- The ways of methodically cutting wet or dry hair to achieve the desired effects
- How to correct commonly occurring problems that can occur during cutting
- The aftercare advice and recommendations that you should give to clients

Introduction

Over the past 20 to 30 years contemporary men's hairstyling in Britain has been based around suitability and purpose. This has meant that the decisions that men make about their hair reflect upon what they do in their working lives, how they spend their leisure time and how much hair they have got.

In many other cultures hair styling is part of an intricately crafted process that has its roots in tribal history and personal status.

Hair and hairdressing have always been an essential part of the females' appearance and they have now become a major issue for men too.

Keywords

Fading
A cutting term that refers to the smooth blending of two different hair lengths within a hair cut; or alternatively as a tapering technique where very short hair is faded out to the perimeter skin, for example at the nape area where clippered hair lengths are blended down to a length of grade 1.

Disconnection
An area within a hair cut where there is a distinct difference between two levels within the layering patterns or perimeter base lines (the simplest example of disconnection is a fringe cut into long one length hair).

Texturising
also known as **Personalising**
A name given to a range of techniques such as; chipping, pointing, slicing etc. that can create lift, movement, texture or produce definition within a hairstyle.

Freehand
A method of cutting without holding between the fingers, or below or above a comb.

Scissor over comb
A technique of cutting hair with scissors, using the back of the comb as a guide, especially when the hair is at a length that cannot be held between the fingers.

Clipper over comb

A technique of cutting hair with electric clippers, using the back of the comb as a guide, especially on very short hair and hairline profiles.

Information covered in this chapter

● The tools and equipment used during cutting and barbering

● The preparations that you should make prior to cutting

● The factors that influence hair cutting decisions

● Creative cutting and barbering techniques

● The aftercare advice that you should give

Beyond basic barbering

Creative barbering at level 3 uses all the cutting techniques available within the salon, so there's lots to learn. Your experience with clients will enable you to offer far more than the basic 'quick cut' services and you should therefore optimise these opportunities by using the creative cutting techniques as a 'springboard' to a range of other exciting and profitable styling services.

Remember

Cutting men's hair (as with colouring) uses many of the principles of cutting women's hair. Review other chapters in this book for more information.

Remember

A finished hairstyle always looks better if it is cut wet. Try to educate your own clients into booking for a wet cut at least.

● It will be easier for you to create new effects.

● They will be able to see a better, more professional result.

● You will generate a better professional service with your clients.

● You will break the habits of men expecting a quick, cheap, hair cut.

● It is more hygienic for everyone concerned.

GB8.1 Maintain effective and safe methods of working when cutting hair

Diversion Many of the skills required in creative barbering are also techniques covered in creative cutting. So in an effort to save a few trees, you will find diversion signposts to other areas in this book that already cover these disciplines.

Other material that is specific to barbering skills is covered in this chapter, under the following topics:

● preparation and maintenance

● client consultation

● identifying the influencing factors that affect style choice

● cutting techniques and accuracy

● good customer care.

The preparatory outcome for this unit is very similar to other technical services although there are variations that relate to:

● specific differences for doing male and female clients

● the individual salon policy where you work

● the differences in the tools and equipment used.

As client protection is the first aspect that you must consider, a quick reference for cutting dry or wet is listed below along with the essential knowledge components.

Protect the client

Gowning for the client can either take place before or after the consultation, it really depends upon the salon's policy. In either event, client protection must always take place before a dry cut is started or, if the service is a wet cut, then before the client is shampooed.

For dry cutting	Use a clean fresh cutting gown and put it on your client while he is sitting at the styling location. Make sure that the back is fastened and that any open, free edges are closed together, keeping any loose clippings away from the client's clothes. Place a cutting collar around his neck to ensure that any bumps or lumps in his clothing don't present any false, physical baselines for the haircut and that the collar edges fit snugly against the neck, so that there are no irritating hair fragments that will leave the client itching until he gets home.
For wet cutting	Gown the client as for dry cutting, but when your client is at the basin, place a clean fresh towel around his shoulders before positioning him back carefully and comfortably. Make sure that the basin supports the client's neck properly and that the flanged edges of the basin nestle comfortably on to the client's shoulders which are protected from any spills or seepage by a clean fresh towel.

Like all other practical services in hairdressing, it is essential that you work safely when cutting hair. In doing this you must take the time to prepare and protect the client adequately.

This means that you have:

- pre-selected all the equipment that you are going to use: gowns, towels, combs, scissors, razor and clippers etc.
- checked that they are prepared for use e.g. new blades for the razor, freshly laundered towels and gowns, washed cutting collars, cleaned and sterilised combs, brushes, clipper blades and scissors
- have them all at hand at the work station and ready for use
- ensured that the client is comfortable and in a position where you can work safely.

More information can be found elsewhere here is a quick reference guide to other parts in this book covering the essential information.

EKU *statement*

GB8 (eku1) Your salon's requirements for client preparation

Topic	Related information	Knowledge reference	See page
Client preparation and protection	Unit GH16 Creatively cut hair using a combination of techniques	EKU GB8 7) The range of protective equipment that should be available for clients	74–75
		EKU GB8 8) Why it is important to protect clients from hair cuttings	
Working position and height		EKU GB8 9) How the position of your client and yourself can affect the desired outcome and reduce fatigue and the risk of injury	75,77 and 79
Preparing tools and equipment		EKU GB8 10) The safety considerations which must be taken into account when cutting hair	76 and 77–78
		EKU GB8 16) Why it is important to position your cutting tools for ease of use	
Working efficiently, safely and effectively		EKU GB8 2) Your salon's expected times for cutting hair to shape	78
		EKU GB8 12) Why it is important to keep your work area clean and tidy	
		EKU GB8 14) Methods of working safely and hygienically and which minimise the risk of cross-infection and cross-infestation	
Personal hygiene		EKU GB8 17) The importance of personal hygiene	75–76

EKU *statement*

GB8 (eku6) Your salon's image and expected standards of service

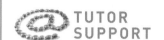

TUTOR SUPPORT

Project 5.1: Risk assessment for cutting services

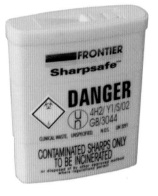

Remember

Disposal of sharp items
Used razor blades and similar items should be placed into a safe container ('sharps box'). When the container is full it can be discarded. This type of salon waste should be kept away from general salon waste as special disposal arrangements may be provided by your local authority.

EKU *statement*

GB8 (eku24) Why hair products should be removed from the hair prior to cutting

---

Activity
Every salon has their own way of doing things. Write down in your portfolio under the following headings what your salon's code of practice in respect to:

(a) meeting and greeting clients

(b) gowning

(c) maintaining tools and equipment

(d) disposal of sharps

(e) hygiene and preventing the spread of infection or infestation

(f) expected standards of service.

Disposal of waste and sharps

Salons also use a lot of chemicals and many of these such as shampoos, conditioners and styling products, are not necessarily potential hazards. In fact much of the other chemical waste created by salons ends up being rinsed down the sinks too and unless this form of disposal is legislated against within local bye-laws, then these chemicals shouldn't present a disposal hazard either.

But sharp items such as disposable razor blades do need to be handled with extreme care. Used sharps must be disposed of carefully to prevent any injury or cross-infection. They should be put in the sharps box and sealed properly before refuse collection.

(See notes below for special conditions for disposal of sharps with certain authorities.)

Activity
Find out and write down in your portfolio:

(a) your shop's policy

(b) the local authority's policy

for the safe disposal of sharp items.

Fixed blade razors

Different local authorities have environmental health bye laws that apply to their region alone. Some authorities do not permit the use of fixed blade razors in barber shops/salons as they are considered to be a likely risk to public health. Find out whether there are any local bye laws that apply to you.

Prevent infection

Infection and disease are brought into the salon/barber shop either:

- by a 'carrier' visiting the salon who then cross-infects other people within the salon or,
- as the result of poor hygiene and cleanliness within the salon.

Most of the preparatory aspects covered in this chapter aim to keep the standards of hygiene within your working environment very high. But there is little point in maintaining the healthy environment unless you check your clients for contra-indications during consultation.

Remove product build-up before attempting to cut

You can't cut hair well if it is loaded with hairspray or it has product build-up. If the client uses a lot of finishing products on their hair you will need to make sure that this has been thoroughly washed out before you start. The quality of the finish that you can achieve is directly pro-portional to the freedom required to complete the job without the hair locking together with grease or gum. You should be able to comb the hair freely during sectioning so that you can achieve the correct holding angles and cutting angles without tangles or binding.

Preparation checklist

✔	Make sure that the styling section and chair is clean, safe and ready to receive clients.
✔	Make sure that the seat is lowered, providing easier access for the clients whether they be young, old or with physical constraints.
✔	Make sure that the client is well protected with a clean fresh gown and a close-fitting cutting collar.
✔	Find out what the client wants. Men can often be more difficult during consultation as they are often reluctant to use a technical term that they are not sure about or express themselves clearly to people they don't know (see the section on communication below).
✔	Style books/files provide lots of male looks to help the diagnostic process.
✔	Make sure you consider the reasons and the purpose for the style. Hairstyles required for professional purposes have more restrictions on freedom and expressions than fashionable, trendy looks or more general wear.
✔	Assess the styling limitations – hair and skin problems or physical features.
✔	Avoid technical jargon or style names; if you do use them, always clarify in simple terms what you mean to avoid confusion; this will help to educate your clients for the future.
✔	Don't just do the style if you think that it's wrong. If there are reasons why you think it will be unsuitable, you will be doing the client a big favour in the longer term if you tackle the issue straight away.
✔	Always give them some advice on how to maintain their hairstyle; men often need products to help them achieve similar effects themselves. Make sure you show them how they can use and apply any new product at home to maintain their own hair/skin condition or styling effect.
✔	Give them an idea of how long it will last and remember to re-book their next appointment before they leave. Alternatively, if they prefer just to pop in on the off chance tell them when they should expect a revisit.

Diversion See also Unit GH16 'Prevent infection' section, pg. 76

EKU *statement*

GB8 (eku3) Your salon's and legal requirements for disposal of sharps and waste materials

EKU *statement*

GB8 (eku5) Any limitations placed on your use of fixed blade razors by local bye-laws and legislation

EKU *statement*

GB8 (eku11) Why it is important to check for infestation and avoid cross-infection

GB8 (eku13) Methods of cleaning, disinfecting and or sterilisation used in salons

EKU *statement*

GB8 (eku45) The importance of consulting with clients throughout the cutting process

GB8 (eku46) How to hold a discussion with a client and assist your client to come to an informed decision on a new look

GB8 (eku47) How to present information and recommendations on looks clearly to clients

HAIR BY: THE ARTISTIC TEAM @ JACKS OF LONDON
PHOTOGRAPHY BY: JOHN RAWSON@TRP

Diversion For more information see Unit G21 Provide hairdressing consultation services – Using visual aids in consultation pp. 33–34.

TUTOR SUPPORT

Project 5.5: Consultation for a restyling cutting service

Consultation

Clear communication

Above all, clear communication is the key to successful barbering. Poor communication is the complete opposite: its biggest barrier. This doesn't just go for men's hairdressing either; many people try to use the names of styles or techniques (technical terms) when they try to describe what they want. Sometimes it works but generally, more often than not, the terms that they (and sometimes the stylists too!) use are incorrect!

This at the very least will lead to an unexpected result and general dissatisfaction. At the worst it could lead to a disaster! In any event this should be avoided at all costs. When you consult the client try not to use jargon or technical terms; it's not clever and definitely won't impress either.

Use visual aids

Men are often very poor at expressing what they want; they need your help in finding the right solutions that suit them and their needs. Try to find different ways of putting things or use pictures to show what you mean. Often a pictorial illustration will express far more than just a cutting style or technique. It creates an overall finished impression too.

Gain confirmation throughout the service

Make a habit of summarising the main points as you go through the consultation by saying:

'So you would like to keep the overall length at the back although you don't mind it shorter around the ears?'

'Do you want me to reduce the thickness in the sides so that it isn't so wide?'

'You want to keep the parting where it is because you find it doesn't lie very well elsewhere?'

It is also worth remembering that other people have a huge impact on the styles that we choose and that goes for your male clients as well. Many men have no *real* opinions about their self-image and this makes it difficult for barbers to contend with. This is because it's hard enough to consult and analyse the needs and requirements of the client who is sitting in the styling chair; it is almost impossible to satisfy someone who is sitting in a chair at home. You need to know what you are trying to achieve and *for whom* you are trying to achieve it. Communication on a one-to-one basis is problematic, but *telepathy* is a skill only afforded to a very select few.

Intelligent communication

Clear communication goes beyond speech too, because as well as using words we show our interest, attitude and feelings by our bodily expressions. Body language is just as clear to others as speech, so you need to remain professional at all times, regardless of how difficult this can be.

We express our innermost feelings via our body posturing, our eyes and mannerisms. Collectively, these can be *saying* something quite different to our mouths. As an experienced barber, you will be well aware of the issues addressed here; you will have seen this daily in a busy salon. Normally, the people that you supervise in your work will still be trying to come to terms with it and that goes for many of the clients too.

As a barber you are already capable of learning by observation and not everyone can do this.

In fact, when you started your training, it was a bit like 'one step forwards and two backwards'. That didn't last for ever, though, you soon got to the point where you didn't keep making mistakes and you didn't need constant help. Once you had grasped the fundamental skills, you found that you could adapt these in new ways to achieve different effects. When you arrived at this point, you were able to analyse what methods and techniques are used in creating any number of given styles.

Activity

Complete the table below to say why each of these consultation factors are important and what might happen if these aspects are ignored.

Factors	Why is this important?	What might happen if this is ignored?
Client's requirements		
Hair growth patterns		
Hair texture		
Hair density		
Lifestyle		
Physical features		

Influencing factors affecting style choice

Male pattern baldness

Your consultation will cover a wide variety of factors that influence what happens next and male pattern baldness (MPB) or the early signs of it should be high upon your list of things to look for.

MPB is a balding or thinning condition that; regardless of claims, is still eluding the scientists. The cause for it is due to high levels of the male hormone testosterone within the body. Many treatments have been developed with little or no long term remedial effects. Hair transplants have been a possible option in the past, but this type of treatment is expensive and needs a lot of upkeep.

Depending at what stage the MPB is, you need to find out how your client feels about it. If the hair loss is relatively slow; there is no need to rush immediately for the clippers and a grade 2. There could be some considerable time before the condition requires a focused attention and therefore; you need to provide advice and reassurance with a range of styling alternatives.

If however, the MPB is at an advanced state then it is obviously going to impact on what styles are achievable. For example; if there is a significant general thinning or hair loss on top, (MPB type 1) then your

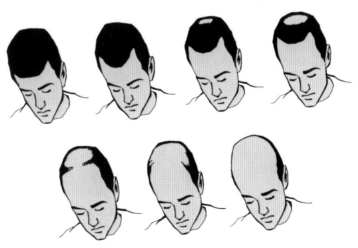

Remember

As many men have shorter hair, their nape hair growth patterns will have far more impact on what hairstyle you choose.

Remember

Personal hygiene is especially important to hairdressers. You work in close proximity to the client so make sure that you eliminate body odour, bad breath or dirty hands and nails by taking the appropriate action.

EKU *statement*

GB8 (eku19) The factors that must be taken into consideration prior to and during cutting (e.g. hair and scalp disorders, presence of male pattern baldness, etc.)

GB8 (eku22) The known causes of male pattern baldness

EKU *statement*

GB8 (eku23) The typical patterns of male pattern baldness

©HABIA

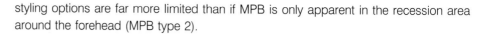

TUTOR SUPPORT

Project 5.4: Face shapes and profiles

styling options are far more limited than if MPB is only apparent in the recession area around the forehead (MPB type 2).

If your client has lost their hair and wears a toupee, you must account for this in your styling. Obviously, there has to be some blending between the natural, remaining hair and the added hair. Be careful not to leave the hair either too long or too short around the blend area. If there is any imbalance in lengths between the two, it is definitely going to show.

If, however, the client wears a full hairpiece then they might just prefer to keep whatever remaining hair very short beneath it. This makes fitting and positioning of the hairpiece easier and will be more comfortable to wear over long periods of time.

Facial shapes

Facial shape	How best to work with it
Square and oblong facial shapes ©HABIA	Square and oblong are typically masculine and provide a perfect base for traditional classic well groomed looks on shorter hair. These facial shapes have less impact on longer men's hairstyles.
Round faces ©HABIA	If shorter, more classic styles are required, the round face is improved by the introduction of angular or linear perimeters. Conversely, if the hair is to be worn longer the roundness of the face will be reduced, as more will be covered.
Square angular features, jaw, forehead etc. ©HABIA	Again these are traditionally accepted as a feature of masculinity. They do not really pose any limitations for classic type work. They also work well with longer hair too. Squarer more angular features are softened with beards and moustaches.
Flatter heads at the back ©HABIA	Are improved by contoured graduation; this creates shaping and tapering that is missing from having a flatter occipital bone. Sometimes the head is both flat and wide and this can make the problem harder to deal with. Wider flatter heads are made less noticeable by longer hair, if this is not possible then explain what the effect will look like if taken very short.

Physical feature	How best to work with it
Prominent nose	Hair taken back away from the face accentuates this feature, whilst hair around the face and forehead tends to diminish the feature.
Protruding ears	Are better left covered rather than exposed. Sufficient hair should be left to cover and extend beyond their length if at all possible.
Narrow foreheads	Are disguised by softer fringes and side partings, whereas they are made more obvious by hair taken back away form the face.
Bushy, thick eyebrows	If the eyebrows are a different colour to the natural hair, the feature will be even more prominent. The hairstyle will be improved with some form of light trimming and grooming.
Large faces	Are augmented by classical, short-cropped or sculpted hair.
Shapes of glasses	Generally people will have had assistance in the selection and suitability of their frames. Therefore they should not work against the hairstyle that you want to create as they should already suit the shape and size of the face.
Long side burns	Are made more prominent with shorter hairstyles, make sure that this is acceptable to your client first as he might be rather attached to his facial hair feature.
Beards	Make sure that the client's beard is still going to be balanced to the amount of hair on top of his head in the finished effect. If an imbalance is going to occur, mention it first and give him the option of taking the beard shorter to compensate.

Remember

Avoid ingrowing hairs

Ingrowing hairs are an uncomfortable aspect of closely cut wavy or curly hair. When hair is razored or clippered close to the skin, say at the neckline, the action of the cutting implement tends to slightly pull the hair within the follicle. After the hair is cut, the hairshaft tends to retract back into the follicle giving a very close, smooth finish to the touch. Unfortunately, if the area isn't kept thoroughly cleaned the open area of the follicle can become partially blocked with dead skin cells or dirt. This will change the growing direction of the hair within the follicle, often allowing it to find a new position within the skin. Bearing in mind that the average rate of hair growth is about 1.25 cm per month; if allowed to continue, an ingrowing hair will result. The physical effects of this will not be noticed until:

- it starts to create a raised area often accompanied with a mild infected spot, or
- it begins to itch as it causes irritation beneath the skin.

If the ingrowing hair is not brought to the surface or removed from the skin a longer term, more serious condition/infection will result.

EKU *statement*

GB8 (eku21) The potential risk of ingrowing hair resulting from the continual close cutting of curly hair

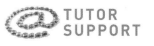

TUTOR SUPPORT

Discussion 5.1: Influencing factors effecting choice of style to recommend to the client

Examination of hair and scalp

While you are looking at the client's hair and scalp, be particularly aware of the texture of the hair. If it is coarse and tightly curled, you will need stronger combs to stretch the hair

EKU *statement*

GB8 (eku20) The average rate of hair growth

EKU *statement*

GB8 (eku26) How the factors in the range can affect the way the hair is cut

out from the head before cutting, and firmer movements will need to be applied. The density of the hair is important too: if it is thick, then styles with varied hair lengths are possible. Conversely, sparse hair, particularly if it is fine, requires a great deal of attention and expertise. If finely textured hair has to cover sparse area of the head, it will have to be longer than hair of coarser texture. The amount, type and growth patterns of hair are all-important too. Younger men may have distinctly higher forehead hairlines than women of similar age. Thinning crowns and decreasing density of hair marks many male patterns, though these are not usually seen in women until much later in life. Hair growth, at a rate of about 1.25 cm each month, is more noticeable with shorter layered styles. To keep them tidy, regular trimming is essential.

Hair growth patterns

Hair growth pattern	How best to work with it
Thinning hair/baldness DR A L WRIGHT	Younger men can be quite sensitive about thinning hair. Be tactful and try to find solutions that are realistic and sympathetic to the problem. When dealing with male pattern baldness most men will tend to opt for shorter 'close cropped' or clippered hairstyles rather than long.
Double crown	A double crown is particularly problematic when it is cut short. It sticks outwards and will not lie down until it grows longer. This is improved if the hair is left longer to over-fall the opposing growth movement and sometimes benefits for a little thinning if the hair is thick.
Nape whorls	Nape whorls can occur on either or both sides; the movement caused by this growth pattern forces the hair to flatten and move towards the centre. This growth pattern is not necessarily a problem for short clippered lengths or longer over-falling hair, it affects shorter layered shapes that need to keep a perimeter baseline.

Hair growth pattern	How best to work with it
Cowlick 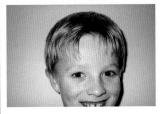	A cowlick appears at the hairline at the front of the head. It makes cutting a straight fringe difficult, particularly on fine hair, because the hair often forms a natural parting. This strong movement can often be improved by moving the parting over so that the weight over-falls the growth pattern. Sometimes a fringe can be achieved by leaving the layers longer so that they weigh down the hair.
Widow's peak 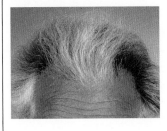	The widow's peak is a hair growth pattern that appears at the centre of the front hairline. The outline shape protrudes downwards in a 'v' shape and the hair grows upwards and forwards, forming a strong peak. It is often better to cut the hair into styles that are dressed back from the face, as any light fringes will separate around this area.

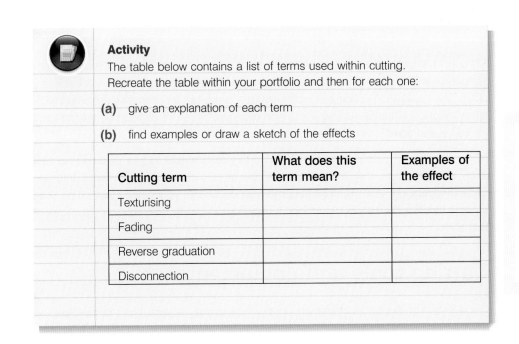

Activity

The table below contains a list of terms used within cutting.
Recreate the table within your portfolio and then for each one:

(a) give an explanation of each term

(b) find examples or draw a sketch of the effects

Cutting term	What does this term mean?	Examples of the effect
Texturising		
Fading		
Reverse graduation		
Disconnection		

Remember

Always look for contra-indications for styling and shaping; these could relate to infections, infestations, poor hair/skin condition, difficult hair growth patterns, face shape and physical features.

Finding out what the client wants

Finding out what the client wants is fundamental to achieving a satisfactory result. Factors such as practicality, suitability and the client's ability to cope with his hair are aspects that you should never overlook.

EKU statement

GB8 (eku38) The importance of considering weight distribution and working with the natural growth patterns of the hair

Remember

How often do you find people using the wrong expression or term to explain what they want? Always make a point of correcting misused terms; it will show that you:

- listen to the client and you are hearing what he says
- have a professional knowledge of your craft and its skills and techniques
- have pride and professional interest in your work.

Diversion For more information on looking after your tools, see Chapter 4 (Unit GH16 Creatively cut hair using a combination of techniques) pp. 84–85.

EKU statement

GB8 (eku29) Which tools can be used on either wet or dry hair or both

GB8 (eku15) The correct use and maintenance of cutting tools

The final effects will be influenced by other considerations too:

- the amount of hair
- the distribution of the hair over the scalp
- the texture of the hair
- the condition of the hair and scalp
- the tendency of the hair, i.e. the amount of wave or curl.

Unless you do take all these factors into consideration, you could have an unhappy, disgruntled client on your hands.

Look out for	Why is it a concern?
Hair density	Scalps with densely populated hair can always be reduced, thinned or controlled in some way, whereas thinner hair or male pattern baldness create a range of limitations that you will need to both express and contend with.
Hair tendency	Curly hair has more styling limitations than straighter hair. Wavy hair is always easier to direct or position than straight hair. Point these factors out before you start.
Hair texture	Fine hair is always difficult to handle, whereas coarser hair when straight will often appear spiky or blunt. Conversely, coarse, wavy hair can often appear dry regardless of natural condition. Each hair texture type creates a different problem.

Although men can wear longer hair as well as short a whole range of modern contemporary styling effects has developed since the basic and traditional short back and sides. The application of hair products will often 'dress up' an otherwise professional or classic-looking hairstyle, turning it into something with a more distinctive 'fashion look' for social and special occasions.

Now and again a men's named style becomes fashionable. Some of these names, such as 'crew cut', the 'mullet', the wedge or a mohawk, have passed into the general vocabulary. Always make sure that you know what your client means if he uses a name to describe a style, remember, it may be completely different from your idea of that style.

Cutting tools and equipment

Good care and regular maintenance of your tools are an essential part of hairdressing and barbering. This covers

- scissors
- thinning scissors
- combs, neck brushes and sectioning clips.

As clippers and razors are mainly associated with men's barbering techniques the relevant information is below.

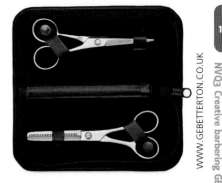

WWW.GEBETTERTON.CO.UK

Clippers

The electric clippers cut hair by oscillation: the side-to-side movement of a upper metal blade passing over a lower rigid or fixed one. On each pass of the upper blade, the hair caught between the teeth of the lower blade is cut and falls away.

Regular cleaning and lubrication will prolong the blades' useful life and keep the cutting edges sharp. Without this care the constant friction of one blade passing over another will affect their ability to work properly, i.e. electric clippers generate quite a lot of heat and, if they have not been maintained, their ability to cut cleanly and efficiently deteriorates over time. New blades are relatively expensive, as they can often cost half the price of a new pair of clippers. If the clipper blades are unable to cut keenly you will not be able to trim, shape and style neck or facial hair shapes accurately.

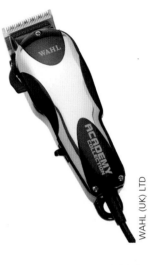

WAHL (UK) LTD

You should always take care not to drop them, as this can easily cause damage to the cutting teeth or even break! Any missing areas of teeth along the blades will be extremely dangerous and could easily cut the client if they were used. So when they are not in use, hang them up out of the way or replace them back in the charger unit.

Clipper blades should always be checked for alignment before each time they are used. The fixed lower blade is adjustable and this allows for small adjustments to be made backwards, forwards or even side to side.

Loosening the small retaining screws underneath allows the blades to be adjusted. This also provides access to the upper blade, for removal, cleaning out the fragments of hair and essential oiling/lubrication.

When the blades are replaced the retaining screws must be retightened properly, if this is not done, the vibration will dislodge the alignment and this could easily take a chunk out of your client's hair, or worse, even cut him!

Well-maintained clippers will cut either wet or dry hair with equal ease, although many stylists prefer to remove the hair first, and then wash the hair after to remove any small fragments and make any final checks.

Remember

Always take care when using any sharp items of equipment. Your safety and the safety of the client are in your hands; take care not to be distracted while you are working.

Razors

The open or 'cut-throat' style razor used in shaving is made out of a single steel blade which is hinged and closed into a protective handle. The modern counterpart for this has disposable blades which can be removed and discarded after use. (Blades are discarded after each client to avoid cross-infection. They are disposed of safely into the salon's sharps box.)

The razor used for hair styling is called a shaper; it too has disposable blades which are fitted into a hinged sheath that provides a handy, safe styling tool. Razor cutting is *always* carried out on wet hair and with sharp blades. This is because of the way in which razors are used; and the angle at which they cut through the hair, razoring should never be done on dry hair as this it will pull and tear the hair; causing it to split, even if the blades are new.

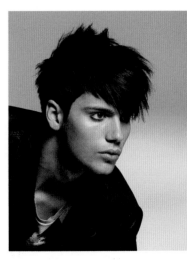

HAIR BY: THE ARTISTIC TEAM @ JACKS OF LONDON
PHOTOGRAPHY BY: JOHN RAWSON@TRP

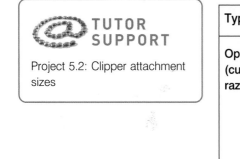

TUTOR SUPPORT

Project 5.2: Clipper attachment sizes

Type of razor		Description
Open (cut throat) razor	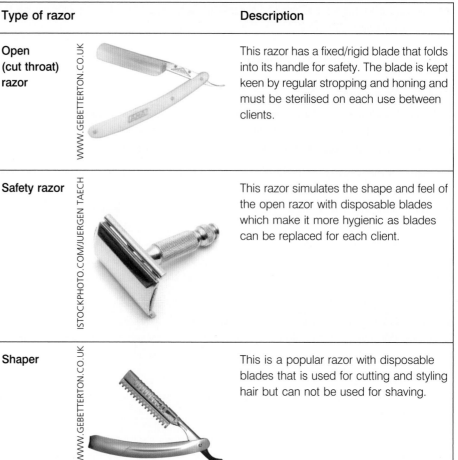 WWW.GEBETTERTON.CO.UK	This razor has a fixed/rigid blade that folds into its handle for safety. The blade is kept keen by regular stropping and honing and must be sterilised on each use between clients.
Safety razor	ISTOCKPHOTO.COM/JUERGEN TAECH	This razor simulates the shape and feel of the open razor with disposable blades which make it more hygienic as blades can be replaced for each client.
Shaper	WWW.GEBETTERTON.CO.UK	This is a popular razor with disposable blades that is used for cutting and styling hair but can not be used for shaving.

TUTOR SUPPORT

Project 5.3: Cleaning and sterilising of tools for cutting

Activity

Clipper maintenance

Note This activity should be carried out with the electric clippers removed from the power supply or rechargeable clippers 'rundown'.

Knowing how to remove, replace, realign and maintain a clipper's blades is an essential part of hairdressing. Get your supervisor to show you how the lower blade-retaining screws are undone and removed. This will give you access to both cutting blades and the area below the armature (the vibrating arm that works them) for cleaning purposes.

When you have dismantled the blades, check for signs of corrosion. If a rusted area exists it will look like blackened areas around the blade edges. If blades have been allowed to get to this stage they should be replaced by new ones as their ability to cut cleanly without friction has been greatly reduced.

With the blades stripped down, you can now use clipper oil to lubricate the two blades, wiping any excess away. Now you can replace the blades (the right way up) and partially re-tighten then retaining screws. Finally, readjust the alignment of the blades and tighten the screws. Check the alignment once more: the lower cutting blade should extend around 3 mm further than the upper cutting blade with the clippers adjusted fully forwards to the shortest cutting length.

Hand them back to your supervisor so that your maintenance can be checked.

Cutting tools and techniques

Cutting tools	Techniques that can be achieved	Explanation of technique
Scissors (straight or flat parallel blades)	Club cutting (blunt cutting)	The most basic and most popular way cutting sections of hair straight across, parallel to the index and middle finger. The blunt, straight sections of cut hair that it produces are ideal for precise lines. The different angles that the hair is held will produce square, graduating and reverse graduating layer patterns.
	Freehand cutting	Cutting without holding with the fingers is known as freehand cutting. It is a technique that allows for cutting with natural fall and without tension. Its main uses are at the perimeter edges around ears, fringes and trimming awkward growth patterns.
	Pointing (point cutting)	Pointing is a texturising technique that reduces bulk from the ends (2–3 cm) of the hair in order to create softer, more shattered, textured edges. It uses the point ends of the scissors and is more successful on straighter hair than wavy, and does not add any value to curly hairstyles at all.
	Deep chipping	Another texturising technique that reduces fine sections of hair from much deeper, closer to the root (1–3 cm from the scalp). It will add texture but is better for creating and adding lift in medium to thicker hair types.
	Brick cutting	A texturising technique that is a combination of pointing and chipping to gain benefits of both forms of cutting techniques. The cutting action would resemble the position of bricks in a wall
	Disconnection	Disconnection is used to create a demarcation area between two different levels. It is a deliberate style or styling feature that draws attention to the different levels and can be done on all one length hair or layered effects. An example of disconnection is regularly used on short layered styles that have longer hair over-falling the shorter perimeters.
'Japanese style' scissors (Hollow ground edges)	All of the above plus slicing or slider cutting (a technique only suitable for extra sharp scissors or a razor)	Slicing is a texturising technique where the hair held at an angle away from the head and slightly downward. Then a single blade of the scissors or a razor cut through the hair in one continuous and downward motion, this reduces the weight from within the hair forming a tapered effect.
Thinning scissors	Thinning/ texturising	Thinning scissors will remove uniform bulk from any point between the root area and ends. However, they have more creative uses when they are used to 'feather' the perimeter edges of hairstyles (which is often more difficult with straight bladed scissors).

WWW.GEBETTERTON.CO.UK

WWW.GEBETTERTON.CO.UK

Cutting tools	Techniques that can be achieved	Explanation of technique
Razors WWW.GEBETTERTON.CO.UK	Tapering	Tapering produces a similar effect to that produced by thinning scissors. Razors are often a better choice, as when used correctly they will produce a non-uniform effect.
	Slicing/slider cutting	See above under 'Japanese style' scissors.
Electric clippers WAHL (UK) LTD	Clippering with grade attachments	Clipper grades (the attachments that provide uniform cutting lengths) are made in a range of sizes for different purposes, and are numbered accordingly they will provide closely cut uniform layering or if differing grades are used; they can provide graduation on hair that is too short to hold between the fingers.
	Fading	A way of blending short hair at the nape or edges of a hairstyle down or 'out' to the skin. It is achieved by using the clippers with the blade 'backed off' creating a very short, tapered effect with a smooth blended effect without any lines.
	Clipper over comb and (scissor over comb)	Both techniques are a popular way of layering very short hair into styles that can't be held between the fingers. The hair is held and supported by a comb and the free edges protruding through are removed.

Combining the cutting techniques

Diversion For information on accurate sectioning, controlling the shape and cross-checking the cut see pp. 123.

As covered throughout this book (see GH16, Chapter 4), there are a variety of cutting techniques: club cutting, freehand cutting, pointing, deep chipping, brick cutting, slicing or slider cutting, thinning/texturising and tapering. None of these techniques are used in isolation; a precision or artistic cutter will use a combination of these cutting disciplines to personalise a finished effect. As you become more experienced in your work you will probably find that you would need to use at least 30–50 per cent of these in each hair cut in order to achieve satisfactory fashionable results.

GB8.2   Creatively restyle men's hair

EKU *statement*

GB8 (eku40) The importance of keeping the hair damp when wet cutting

EKU *statement*

GB8 (eku33) The circumstan-ces in which you might cut into the natural hairline

Cutting rules

Keep the hair damp throughout the cut

Rough-dry the hair so that you work with damp hair throughout the cut so that the client is not sat with saturated hair, it is uncomfortable for them as wet hair soon feels cold even if it doesn't drip onto the gown and their clothes.

More importantly, working with damp hair during cutting enables the natural tendencies, movements and directions of the hair to be seen. This is extremely important for cutting hair with the wave movement and hair growth patterns all being considered as the style develops.

Outline shapes

Many short, layered cuts are graduated at the sides and into the nape sometimes by clipper over comb or, when left slightly longer, by scissor over comb techniques. On shorter hairstyles the neck- and hairlines become the main focal perimeters of the hairstyle. These require careful attention as it is very easy to infringe into the hairline and remove hair that is needed for the outline shape.

Where possible always use the natural hairlines as the limit for the hairstyle. This produces a smoother effect on the eye and produces styles that look balanced and right. If you ignore the natural hairlines and cut above them, you will find that the hair below will grow back very quickly and produce a stubbly effect within a few days. Or, if done on dark hair, it will produce a 'shadowed' effect within 24 hours.

However, natural necklines often lack consistency; the growth is often uneven, intermittent or sparse. Therefore the outline shapes for these men wearing shorter hair need to be defined. The more natural the nape line, the softer and less severe will be the look.

Round neckline	Tapered/faded neckline	Square neckline

The shaping of front hair into a fringe can produce variety of facial frames and the focal point it creates changes the overall effect dramatically. In many men the front hairline recedes and this is often a sign of MPB. This influences the choice and positioning of perimeter fringe shapes. Always give this some thought before cutting the hair.

In men, the side hairlines, sideburns or sideboards bridge the hairstyle and beard shape. These need to fit, and care must be taken in shaping them. Lining the hair above the ears and along the sides of the nape is usually carried out with the scissor points or carefully angled inverted clippers.

Common cutting problems

Necklines

All of the classic perimeter neckline shapes above can easily be ruined if a lack of care and attention occurs. The detail of the outline of very short hair can easily be spoiled by careless layering or clippering. Every millimetre counts. You need to make sure that your outlining with the clippers is even and smooth throughout. If you do make a mistake and find that you have encroached on the outline shape you would be better off re-cutting the outline slightly shorter to eliminate the fault.

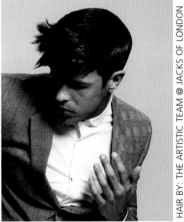

EKU *statement*

GB8 (eku32) The importance of cutting to the natural hairline in barbering

HAIR BY: THE ARTISTIC TEAM @ JACKS OF LONDON
PHOTOGRAPHY BY: JOHN RAWSON@TRP

EKU statement

GB8 (eku27) The range of traditional and current men's hair shapes

Remember

Always check the clipper blade alignment before using them for each client.

EKU statement

GB8 (eku41) The types of problems that can commonly arise when cutting men's hair and ways in which they can be remedied

Remember

Removing cutting marks
The thinning over comb technique can be used as a corrective method on most clipper cut or scissor cut lengths to 'join' areas of differing grades/lengths or to remove cutting marks on fine, medium and coarse hair textures.

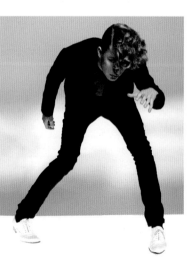

Blending from clipper lengths to scissor length

Another common problem on short hair is found at the blend area between different clippered grades, or between the clippered and hand-held cut lengths. If a careful blending hasn't been made it will show cutting marks at the point where the two areas combine.

There are two ways of tackling this problem:

1 If the hair is still too long on the hand-cut/held side, you can re-fade the two zones together by scissor over comb methods. Be careful not to undercut the longer lengths as this will mean that you will have to re-cut all the clippered area.

2 If the lengths of hair between the two areas are slightly uneven it will definitely show unless you correct it. In any area where clippers fade out to club cut lengths you can re-surface the hair by using thinning scissors over comb just on the very tips of the hair. A light blending of thinned hair produces an optical illusion that cheats the eye by softening the two hard cut edges and the final effect appears correct.

Ears

Nature does not guarantee symmetry, and this is particularly true with faces. One side of the face is not exactly the same as the other and this applies to ears too. One may be larger than the other; they may be irregular in shape or at different heights; you need to make sure that you have considered this before you start. Unevenness on long hair doesn't matter, but when it's on short hair the imperfections will be made clear.

Remember

Men's short hairstyles often benefit from washing again after cutting. This removes all the shorter clippings and makes them more comfortable.

Tapering and thinning encourage the hair to curl at the ends, while club cutting increases density and reduces that tendency.

Feathering and texturising can produce extra lift and bounce.

If your client has a build up of wax, gel or moulding crème on their hair you must insist that the hair is washed to get it out or off the hair before you attempt the hair cut.

You need to find out how your client feels about his facial features. Sometimes these natural imperfections are not a concern, they are merely a characteristic of the client's personality. Don't forget to check on whether your client wears glasses or a hearing aid; take all of these factors into your assessment.

Finally you and your client will be able to agree exactly what look is required, and you will then have a basis on which to decide how the work is to be carried out.

Hair type

If your client's hair is very curly, do remember that it will coil back after stretching and cutting. Similarly, wavy hair, when cut too close to the wave crest, can be awkward to style as it tends to spring out from the head. Very fine straight hair will easily show cutting marks or can disclose unwanted lines from clippering if you take too large sections. Make sure that the sections you take are accurately divided and sectioned.

Final points to remember

1 If the hair is dirty, then for hygienic reasons it must be washed before you cut it. Wet hair is a necessity for blow-drying and finishing, but not necessarily a convenient arrangement for a quick trim before work or during lunch.

2 Clean, dry hair should not be cut with a razor because of the discomfort to your client due to the tearing and dragging action of the razor on the hair.

3 Accurate sectioning and **graduation** produces fine layering. This is partly determined by how much hair there is to cut. Longer lengths can be sectioned with the comb and taken between the fingers, while short lengths are best tackled either by clipper over comb or scissor over comb techniques. A section (that cannot be held between the fingers) is lifted with the comb and a guideline is created by cutting straight across. Subsequent lifting with the comb to the guideline length produces the next section to be cut.

4 Clippers must be used to tidy the necklines on short styles, graduating from the natural line out from the head. How far up the head and how short the cut needs to be is determined by the style and shape agreed with your client. If longer lengths are required higher in the back hair, then the clippers need to graduate away from the head sharply.

5 Cross-checking is an essential part of cutting. It's your way of including a quality control. As you progress through the cut, you obviously need to change your stance, holding position and holding angle. These factors can lead you to go wrong. Typically problems might be that the back section doesn't integrate with the sides properly or the top doesn't blend with the sides, or the fringe doesn't fit with the top. Whatever the potential problem the easiest way to compensate for this is to crosscheck to make sure that the cut works well in different planes.

EKU statement

GB8 (eku25) The types of products available for finishing men's hair

GB8 (eku30) The reasons for establishing and following guidelines

GB8 (eku31) How to create and follow guidelines for the looks in the range

GB8 (eku36) The importance of cross-checking the cut

GB8 (eku37) How to cross-check and balance the cut

GB8 (eku39) The importance of applying the correct degree of tension to the hair when cutting

TUTOR SUPPORT

Discussion 5.2: Cutting problems and solutions

Finishing products for men

Product	Application	Purpose	Suitability
Dry wax 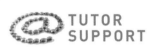	Applied in small amounts by the finger tips into pre-dried hair	A moderately firm hold providing a non-wet look or greasy finish. Ideal for men who really don't like the look of product on the hair, but need the benefits of the control it provides	Suited to short to medium length hair; the effects need to be created carefully and slowly by adding more as needed. It is very easy to add too much and overload the hair, particularly on finer hair types
Normal (grease-based) wax	Applied in small amounts by the finger tips into pre-dried hair	A firm hold that provides high definition and texture with a moist or slightly greasy effect. Ideal for most types of hair providing a groomed or sculpted look	Suited to short to medium length hair; the effects need to be created carefully and slowly by adding more as needed. It is very easy to add too much and overload the hair, particularly on finer hair types

Product	Application	Purpose	Suitability
Hair varnish WELLA	Applied in small amounts by the finger tips into pre-dried hair. Care needs to be taken in applying the product evenly, throughout the hair	A high-gloss look with a greasy texture. The styles created are moisture repelling. Ideal for men who do like product effects on their hair	Suits short hair with long-lasting, low maintenance looks, suitable for sports etc. Again the effect needs to be created slowly; it is easy to overload the hair and these types of product do produce a build up upon the hair
Hair gel L'ORÉAL PROFESSIONNEL	Applied with the finger tips or with a comb into wet or pre-dried hair. It is easy to see where it has been missed	A wet look effect with strong hold. Suitable for sculpted looks and ideal for men who do like product effects on their hair	You can't really overload the hair with gel as the look is based on 100 per cent coverage. The effects created are suited to short hair and are not moisture resistant and will start to drop if they get moist or wet
Styling glaze L'ORÉAL PROFESSIONNEL	Applied first to the hands and rubbed into wet or pre-dried hair all over. The hair is styled after and allowed to dry and fix into shape	A wet look effect with firm – strong hold. Suitable for controlled or groomed looks with a mild, wet look effect	Again like gel – you can't overload the hair as the look is based on 100 per cent coverage. The styles created are suited to short hair and are more resistant to moisture than gel but create less sculpted or high-hair effects than gel
Hair clay/putty L'ORÉAL PROFESSIONNEL	Applied in small amounts by the finger tips into pre-dried hair	A moderately firm hold providing a non-wet look or greasy finish with high definition, texture and control	Fairly easy to apply; these products are very versatile and create a wide range of effects on any hair texture generally on shorter hair lengths
Defining crème L'ORÉAL PROFESSIONNEL	Applied in small amounts by the finger tips into pre-dried hair.	A firm hold that doesn't dry on the hair providing an invent/reinvent option as the hair can be reworked throughout the day or night	Suits long-lasting low maintenance looks, on any hair length; suitable for sports, leisure, and work. The effect needs to be created slowly and it is easy to overload the hair, these types of product do produce a build up upon the hair

Product	Application	Purpose	Suitability
Hairspray	Applied to pre- dried hair by directional spraying from 30 cm away	Provides mild, moderate and firm hold, can be used as a final fixative or as a styling product when scrunched in	Easy to apply providing a long lasting effects on any hair length

Step-by-steps

Contemporary short

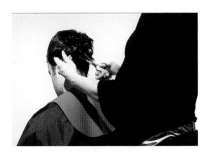

Step 1 Before

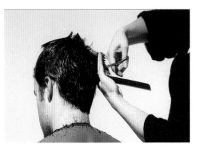

Step 2 Cut perimeter to length

Remember

Always use products sparingly. Most hair preparations are concentrated and can easily cause a product build-up as well as being an unnecessary waste.

Always follow the manufacturer's instructions and guidance for use when using any styling or finishing products.

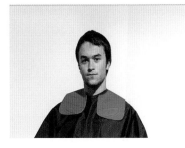

Step 3 Section off and fasten out of the way

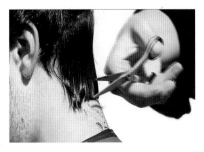

Step 4 Point cut layering to break up lines and create texture

@ LEARNER SUPPORT

Video: Short textured gents haircut

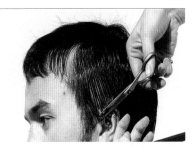

Step 5 Hold the ear whilst you cut around the perimeter shape

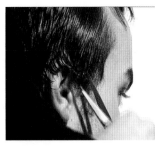

Step 6 Tidy up the side-burns as you progress

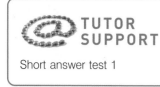

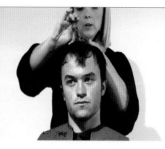

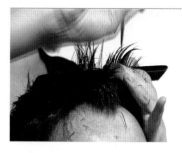

Step 7 Continue into the top layered length with pointing

Step 8 Break up the fringe area so that no lines are present

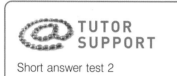

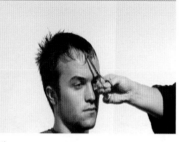

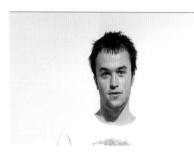

Step 9 Point cut to finish the profile

Step 10 Finished effect

GB8.3   Provide aftercare advice

Diversion The knowledge statements for level 3 in both the hairdressing and barbering standards are often repeated in different outcomes within units elsewhere.

EKU statement

GB8 (eku42) The recommended time interval between cuts

GB8 (eku43) How to use tools and styling products to maintain the look

GB8 (eku44) Products for home use that will benefit the client

GB8 (eku48) How to give effective advice and recommendations to clients

The aftercare advice that you should give your clients is comprehensively covered in Unit GH16 Creatively cut hair using a combination of techniques see pp. 100–101.

Home and aftercare checklist

✔	Talk through the style as you work; that way the client sees how you handle different aspects of the look.
✔	Show and recommend the products/equipment that you use so that the client gets the right things to enable them to get the same effects.
✔	Tell the client how long the style can be expected to last and when they need to return for reshaping.
✔	Demonstrate the techniques that you use so they can achieve that salon hair look too.

For more information on how to give advice to clients see Unit G18 Promote additional products and services to clients pp. 47–50.

Checkerboard

Checkerboard	I know my salon's requirements for client preparation, waste disposal, and expected service timings ☐	I know the safety considerations that I should make in respect to safe working practices ☐	I consult with the clients at all points during the cutting processes ☐
I always recognise style in limiting factors when I carry out consultation ☐	I can use a variety of cutting techniques and know what their benefits are ☐	I know how to negotiate, reaching a mutually beneficial conclusion ☐	I always carry out working practices according to the salon's policy ☐
I know how to maintain the cutting tools and equipment ☐	I always explain technical terms eliminating ambiguity and false beliefs ☐	I know when and who to refer clients to, in situations where external assistance is required ☐	I understand the necessity of personal hygiene and presentation ☐
I know how and when to advise or recommend other services and products to clients ☐	I know how to adapt cutting techniques to achieve a variety of different creative effects ☐	I can use a variety of cutting tools: scissors, thinning scissors, razors and clippers to achieve differing effects ☐	

Assessment of knowledge and understanding

Revision questions

Quick quiz: a selection of different types of questions to check your knowledge.

Q1	Accuracy is achieved by _____ and cutting the hair at the correct angle.	Fill in the blank
Q2	A razor should be used on dry hair.	True or false
Q3	Select the texturising techniques from the following list.	Multi selection

Club cutting	☐	1
Graduation	☐	2
Slice cutting	☐	3
Fading	☐	4
Point cutting	☐	5
Chipping	☐	6

Q4	Symmetrical styles produce outline shapes that are equally balanced.	True or false
Q5	Which of the following is not a cutting term?	Multi selection

Cross-checking	☐	a
Thinning	☐	b
Free hand	☐	c
Free style	☐	d

Q6	Disconnection is a term defining a continuous outline shape or layer patterning.	True or false
Q7	Which of the following hair growth patterns does not affect the way that hair lays after it is cut?	Multi selection

Nape whorl	☐	1
Double crown	☐	2
Widow's peak	☐	3
Low hairline	☐	4
Cowlick	☐	5
High hairline	☐	6

Q8	A graduated layer shape that tapers out on to the neck is referred to as _____.	Fill in the blank
Q9	Which of the following cuts would easily describe a disconnection?	Multi choice

Graduation in a long hairstyle	○	a
Reverse graduation in a long hairstyle	○	b
A fringe in a shoulder-length bob style	○	c
Texturising in a short cropped style	○	d

Q10	'Personalising' is the term that refers to any technique that is used to complete a style, tailoring it to the client's specific needs.	True or false

Chapter**six**
Styling beards and moustaches

LEE MORAN @ SANRIZZ

GB7

GB7.1

GB7.2

GB7.3

CREDIT VALUE
FOR UNIT GB7
4 Credits

More Information See units:

G21 Provide hairdressing consultation services

G22 Monitor procedures to safely control work operations

GB8 Creatively cut hair using a combination of barbering techniques

Diversion See appendices for Electricity at Work Regulations

EKU *statement*

GB7 (eku4) Your responsibilities under the Electricity at Work Regulations

EKU *statement*

GB7 (eku40) The meaning of avant-garde

Beards and moustaches: quick overview

Unit title

GB7 Design and create a range of facial hair shapes

This is a **mandatory** unit for barbering at level 3, it is made up of three main outcomes

Main outcomes

GB7.1 Maintain effective and safe methods of working when cutting facial hair

GB7.2 Create a range of facial hair shapes

GB7.3 Provide aftercare advice

What do I need to do for GB7.1?

● Make sure that the client is adequately covered and protected

● Make sure that your working position is comfortable and safe

● Keep the work area clean and tidy and that waste materials are disposed of properly

● Identify factors that influence the service prior to starting

● Work without causing risks to you or your client's health and safety

● Work efficiently and effectively

What do I need to do for GB7.2?

● Choose suitable visual aids to help with facial style selection for your client

● Prepare your client's facial hair before cutting

● Seek confirmation of the desired look before starting

● Cut your client's facial hair using a variety of creative cutting techniques

● Check that the final effect is accurate, that it has an even effect and that the client is satisfied with the results

129

Keywords

Keywords

Freehand

A method of cutting without holding the hair between the fingers or below or above a comb

Scissor over comb

A technique of cutting hair with scissors, using the back of the comb as a guide, especially when the hair is at a length that cannot be held between the fingers

Clipper over comb

A technique of cutting hair with electric clippers, using the back of the comb as a guide, especially on very short hair and hairline profiles

Avant garde

A genre of fashion that is considered progressive or exaggerated; it doesn't fit any of the usual modes such as classic and contemporary. The dramatic results of avant garde work are extrovert, individualistic and ultra-modern or futuristic in their design

Information covered in this chapter

- The tools and equipment used during cutting
- The preparations that you should make prior to cutting facial hair
- The factors that influence facial hair cutting decisions
- Cutting and styling facial hair techniques
- The aftercare advice that you should give clients

What do I need to do for GB7.3?

- Give the client accurate, constructive advice on how they can maintain the look themselves

What aspects do I need to cover for GB7.1, GB7.2 and GB7.3?

- A variety of cutting tools and equipment
- A range of factors that influence or limit the choice of styling
- Different types of cutting techniques that are used to create the effects

What aspects do I need to know for GB7.1, GB7.2 and GB7.3?

- Your salon's requirements for preparation, timings and standards of service
- How to work safely, effectively and hygienically when cutting facial hair
- Factors about the client that affect styling choice, suitability and durability
- The ways of methodically cutting facial hair to achieve the desired effects
- How to correct commonly occurring problems that can occur during cutting
- The aftercare advice and recommendations that you should give to clients

Introduction

There is nothing new in the shaping and lining of men's hair. Much of the current linear effects that can be seen etched over the scalps or around the faces of men today, have their roots in ancient tribal cultures. Many of the ancient civilisations used this as a form of body art to distinguish one unique culture from another.

This type of adornment, unlike jewellery or fine textiles, was achievable by many people because then, like now, its effects were short-lived and easily changed or modified to create something new.

Beards and moustaches have always been a feature of men's barbering and this chapter explores the different designs that can be created ranging from the traditional, professional to the progressive and avant garde.

Facial hair barbering

If you have already covered the men's cutting unit GB8 you will already be familiar with the techniques of freehand, scissor over comb and clipper over comb techniques. These techniques underpin nearly all of the skills needed to carry out this work; the only other things you need are care, control and creativity.

This chapter addresses all these things by covering:

- preparation and maintenance
- client consultation
- identifying the influencing factors that affect style choice
- cutting techniques and accuracy
- good customer care.

EKU *statement*

GB7 (eku9) The safety considerations which must be taken into account when cutting facial hair

GB7.1 Maintain effective and safe methods of working when cutting facial hair

Preparing the client

Your duty and responsibilities towards health and safety are reinforced throughout all hair-related services and each service has specific procedures that you should follow. This outcome addresses all of the health and safety issues that you need to consider when styling facial hair.

EKU *statement*

GB7 (eku1) Your salon's requirements for client preparation
GB7 (eku5) The range of protective clothing that should be available for clients

Gowning the client

Always use freshly clean, laundered protective equipment:

- Fasten a gown at the back, or secure the cutting square with a clip ensuring that the covering is close fitting around the neck and protects the client from any clippings or spillages.
- Place a towel around the front of the client so that the free edges are fastened at the back.
- Tuck a strip of neck wool (or neck tissue) in to the top edge of the towel to stop hair fragments from falling inside the client's clothes.
- (After consultation and just prior to starting) cover the client's eyes with a cotton wool pad to prevent snippings and clippings from entering their eyes.

EKU *statement*

GB7 (eku7) How the position of your client and yourself can affect the desired outcome and reduce fatigue and the risk of injury
GB7 (eku8) The importance of using the correct type of barber's chair

Positioning the client

Facial hair cutting requires the client to tilt their head back so that you can work at an angle that enables you to work safely and carefully. The barbering chair is designed for this with its inbuilt head rest and reclining ability. (If you need to recline the chair do it before the client is seated.)

Ensure that the client is sitting in the chair with their feet squarely on the foot rests. This posture stops them from twisting or 'hunching up' and allows the client to sit safely for long periods of time in a position that doesn't give them any discomfort, injury or fatigue and you the access and freedom to do your work properly and safely too.

Ask the client if they are comfortable and if you need to make any adjustments to working height or angle you can do this now.

Remember

Bad breath is offensive to clients too. Bad breath (halitosis) is the result of leaving particles to decay within the spaces between the teeth. You need to brush your teeth after every meal. Bad breath can also result from digestive troubles, stomach upsets, smoking and strong foods such as onions, garlic and some cheeses.

ISTOCKPHOTO.COM/GEORGE CAIRNS

 Diversion For more information on this topic see Unit GH16, pp. 75, 77 and 78

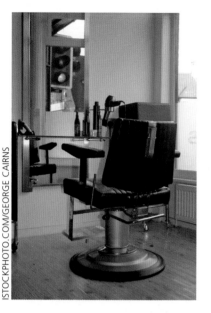

EKU *statement*

GB7 (eku15) The importance of personal hygiene

EKU *statement*

GB7 (eku12) Why it is important to position your tools and equipment for ease of use

GB7 (eku2) Your salon's expected service times for cutting facial hair to shape

GB7 (eku11) Why it is important to keep your work area clean and tidy

GB7 (eku14) Methods of working safely and hygienically and which minimise the risk of cross-infection and cross-infestation

 Diversion For more information on working efficiently, safely and effectively see Unit GH16, p. 77

 Diversion For more information on preventing infection see Unit GH16, p. 76

Your working position and posture

Barbering, as you already know, involves a lot of standing and because of this you need to be comfortable in your work. You should always adopt a comfortable but safe work position and sometimes comfortable and safe are not necessarily the same thing.

Your work position

The client's cutting position and height from the floor have a direct effect on your posture too. You must be able to work in a position where you do not have to bend 'doubled up' to do your work. Cutting involves a lot of arm and hand movements and you need to be able to get your hands and fingers into positions where you can cut the hair unencumbered without bad posture.

1 You should adjust the seated client's chair height to a position where you can work upright without having to over-reach on the top sections of their head.

2 You should clear trolleys or equipment out of the way so that you get good all-round access (300°) around the client.

3 Your equipment should be close enough at hand so that you can reach safely without putting you or the client at risk and the items should be clean, sterile and ready for use (having equipment at hand shows that you are organised and looks more professional).

Your personal hygiene

Personal hygiene can't be stressed enough; it is vitally important for anyone working in personal services. Your personal hygiene or lack of it, will be immediately noticeable to everyone you come into contact with. You may have overslept, but if you haven't showered it will be very uncomfortable for you, your colleagues and the clients as BO is unpleasant in any situation. Other strong smells are offensive too; the smells of nicotine and smoking are very offputting to the client, particularly if they are a non-smoker.

Working efficiently, safely and effectively

Working efficiently and maximising your time is essential so making the most of the resources available should occur naturally. One way of making the most of the salon's resources is being careful in the way that you handle the equipment and the products that you use. Always treat the salon's materials in the same way that you would look after your own equipment; always try to minimise waste, being careful how much product you use.

Prevent infection

Activity

Avoiding cross-infection

Answer the following questions in your portfolio.

1 Why is it important to avoid cross-infection/cross-infestation?

2 What things should you do to minimise the risk of cross-infection?

3 How does your work area affect hygiene and cross-infection?

Safe disposal of sharps

'Sharps' is the term describing any blades used in safety razors or shapers. When these items have been used and need to be replaced, they must be disposed of properly.

> **Activity**
> What is your salon policy for the use of razors and the disposal of sharp items?

EKU *statement*

GB7 (eku10) Why it is important to check for infestation and avoid cross-infection

GB7 (eku13) Methods of cleaning, disinfecting and sterilisation used in salons

EKU *statement*

GB7 (eku3) Your salon's and legal requirements for disposal of waste materials

Prepare the client's facial hair

Many men with longer beards never comb them out because they don't want to lose the shape they naturally take on, or they simply don't see the benefits of doing so. Obviously this is a mistake, as regular grooming keeps them free from debris and reduces the chance of infections or ingrowing hair. You should always make a point of giving the clients advice on this or at least tell them how they can manage their own facial hair between visits.

Moustaches and beards get matted as they get longer because the bristles tend to get curlier and lock together. So these tangles have to be removed so that the longer hair is revealed; this allows you to style *all* of the hair and not just part of it.

Cleansing is important too; a beard with debris or grease can not be styled until it has been cleaned. If you are shampooing the hair as part of another service, then the beard can be done at the same time or, alternatively, you can ask the client to wash their face and beard in the front wash basin, or cleanse with facial wipes.

> **Remember**
>
> **Disposal of sharp items**
> Used razor blades and similar items should be placed into a safe container ('sharps box'). When the container is full it can be discarded. This type of salon waste should be kept away from general salon waste as special disposal arrangements may be provided by your local authority.

Consultation

Check the client's requirements

The main aims of hairdressing and barbering are about delivering a continuing, repeated service that satisfies our clients. We can only satisfy the clients if we find out what they want and act upon those instructions. We demonstrate this by getting confirmation of the things we are doing throughout the service. This does a number of things:

- It ensures that we only do things that the clients want.
- It makes them more confident about what we are doing.
- It removes any ambiguity or confusion.
- It gives us more confidence in what we are doing for the client.
- It involves the client and helps to develop a professional relationship.

Effective communication is important in any hair service. Consultation is not just a process that takes place before a service; it is a continual process of reconfirming your intentions with those of the client. So, during your discussions, you must determine what the client wants and weigh this against the limiting factors that will influence what you need to do.

You need to understand your client fully and be able to negotiate and seek agreement with him throughout the service.

EKU *statement*

GB7 (eku23) How facial hair and skin should be prepared prior to cutting (e.g. cleansing, detangling)

EKU *statement*

GB7 (eku39) The importance of consulting with clients throughout the cutting process

GB7 (eku43) How to give effective advice and recommendations to clients

> **Diversion** For more information on effective communication see Unit G7 and G17.

EKU *statement*

GB7 (eku41) How to hold a discussion with a client and assist your client to come to an informed decision on a new look

GB7 (eku42) How to present information and recommendations on looks clearly to clients

EKU *statement*

GB7 (eku20) The factors that must be taken into consideration prior to cutting facial hair (e.g. suspected infections, suspected infestations, hair style, hair density, head and face shape, hair growth patterns, facial piercing, adverse skin conditions, facial contours

Diversion For more information see Unit G21 Provide hairdressing consultation services – Using visual aids in consultation p. 33.

EKU *statement*

GB7 (eku24) How the factors in the range can affect the way the facial hair is cut and shaped

GB7 (eku25) How to match beard shapes and styles to facial characteristics

Using visual aids

Visual aids such as men's styling magazines, internet downloads and trade publications are an excellent source for different effects. Pictures are a universal language and this is one simple way of collecting ideas and themes and working out what sorts of things work and those that don't. As a barber you are used to people bringing pictures of their ideas and you have probably spent a large amount of time trying to explain why some things work and others don't. Most clients have no self-visualisation; they need the reassurance of others to help them make their decisions. You are a professional and the aspects surrounding styling is your domain. Use your skills to find the most suitable images for your client and, more importantly, try to explain why your selections will work for them, taking in their physical features and personal image.

Activity
Develop a portfolio of effects
Finding examples of outline beard or moustache shapes is very difficult unless you have a pre-prepared selection of options.

Collect examples of different beard and moustache shapes so that you can use them as a visual aid with your clients.

When you have collected a suitable range you can mount them into a ring binder so that you can use them in the shop.

Identify factors that influence the service

Be sure to listen to your client's requests. Many mistakes can be avoided if you achieve a clear understanding of what the client is asking for.

The facial style that you choose with your client should take into account each of the following points about the client's:

- face and head shape/size
- facial physical features (including any scars or blemishes that need disguising)
- hair quality, abundance, growth and distribution
- age, lifestyle and suitability.

Aspects to consider

Facial features

Facial features	How best to work with it
Square and oblong facial shapes	Square and oblong are typically masculine and provide a perfect base for traditional classic well groomed looks. The angular features of the face can be augmented with closer, shorter beards or moustaches and would probably benefit from fewer curves and more angular, linear effects.
Round faces	The effect of a round face can be lessened or increased, it depends what the client wants. If the plan is to lessen the effects, then choose beard designs that lengthen the jaw line and incorporate lines and angles rather than curves. If the round features suit the personality and image of the client then work with it by cutting uniform-length shapes.

Facial features	How best to work with it
Square angular features, jaw, forehead etc.	Again these are traditionally accepted as a feature of masculinity. These can be handled in a similar way to that of the squarer features above. Squarer more angular features can also be easily softened with beards and moustaches.
Small faces	Smaller faces should be balanced with facial hair designs that don't overpower the overall effect. Keep your designs close cut and uniform in length.
Wider heads	These wide features will be increased with full–long beards. Create beard designs that are closer cut at the sides and extend to more length at the chin.
Scars, marks and blemishes	If the client has any scars or blemishes this may be the reason for growing a beard or moustache in the first place. You need to ask if there are any features that the client wants to disguise. *Always make a point of looking for these during your consultation.*
Facial piercing 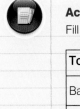 ISTOCKPHOTO.COM/FRANCK CAMHI	Facial piercings around the mouth and ears do need to be considered during your consultation. It is unlikely that the client will want to remove them/it so you have to be very careful in combing, detangling and the cutting, anywhere near to the area(s) of the piercing(s).

You need to find out how your client feels about his facial features. Sometimes these natural imperfections are not a concern; they are merely a characteristic of the client's personality. Don't forget to check on whether your client wears glasses or a hearing aid; take all of these factors into account.

Finally you and your client will be able to agree exactly what look is required, and you will then have a basis on which to decide how the work is to be carried out.

Activity
Fill in the table below with the missing information

Tools and equipment	What is it used for?	How is it used?
Barbicide™		
UV cabinet		
Autoclave		

EKU statement

GB7 (eku33) The importance of considering weight distribution and working with the natural growth patterns of the facial hair

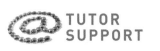

TUTOR SUPPORT

Project 6.1: Risk assessment for cutting facial hair services

Some men have a heavy, daily growth of facial hair and they find that they need to shave every day. This heavy growth can be obvious for a range of reasons.

1.	The growth appears heavy because of the contrast against the skin due to natural colour.
2.	The hair seems to grow particularly fast.
3.	The density of hair distributed on the face is particularly thick.
4.	Combinations of these factors put together.

Initially, men who are most likely to choose to grow beards and/or moustaches will have ticked two or more of the above. But they are not the only ones who choose to do this, as many others with a poorer growth or definition will grow facial hair for other reasons.

Head shape and size

As a general guide the facial hair should not outweigh the proportions of hair on the head. This may be fine for people with plenty of hair, as this would allow them to grow their beards to a longer length. But many men with male pattern baldness also like to grow a beard or moustache too. In these situations, closer cut effects seem to suit the wearer better than thick bushy ones.

Mouth and width of upper lip to base of nose

The size and width of the mouth forms the basis for any moustache. The distance between the upper lip and the base of the nose creates a sort of canvas for the moustache. If the distance between the two areas is quite deep, it will provide more outline shape options for the wearer rather than if it were narrow.

Similarly, the width of the face at the cheeks will also determine the best, suited effect. Someone with a wide face, will be able to wear a fuller moustache, whereas someone with a narrow face could be *swamped* by this much hair.

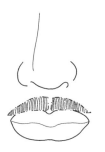
Thin moustache

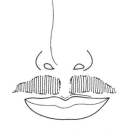
Thick narrow moustache

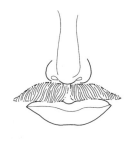
Wide thick moustache

Bone structure and facial contours

You should take particular care for clients who have a well-defined bone structure, i.e. cheekbones, jaws and facial contour. If they have a particularly linear aspect to their facial features then it would be wiser to retain that similar effect with the overall shapes and outlines. (That's unless they wanted to disguise themselves or have physical features they want to cover up.)

Conversely, the client who has a rounder, fuller face can benefit, aesthetically, from a shape that defines the face with a more structured effect. Remembering that these people can wear beards with fuller effects than those men with narrower facial features.

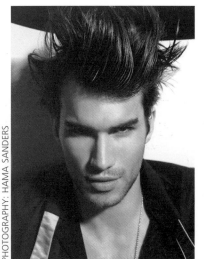

Width of chin and depth of jaw line

Facial hair growth forms a frame for the physical features of the face and it is the width of the chin and the depth down to the bottom of the jaw that become the focal point of any facial hair shaping. The outlines of the shapes created here are more noticeable than any others. Historically, beards were left relatively full; this meant that there was very little upkeep for the wearer, apart from keeping the beard from getting to bushy. Latterly, the fashion for wearing more chiselled effects has meant that not only thickness but an outline shape has to be maintained too.

Tools and equipment

The cutting tools are covered several times in this book so in order to prevent unnecessary duplication you are diverted elsewhere to find the relevant information.

However, there is a table which provides a quick reference guide to clipper grades/attachments and their effects when used on facial hair.

Scissors and cutting combs

> **Remember**
>
> Always take care when using any sharp items of equipment. Your safety and the safety of the client are in your hands; take care not to be distracted while you are working.

Clippers

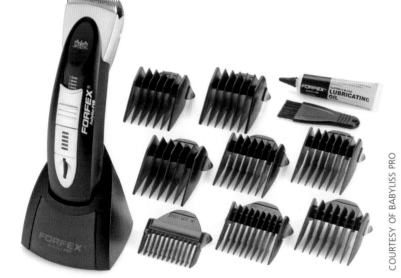

COURTESY OF BABYLISS PRO

EKU *statement*

GB7 (eku16) Methods of cleaning and maintaining all the tools and equipment in the range

GB7 (eku17) How to safely use the tools and equipment in the range

Diversion See Unit GH16 Creatively cut hair using a combination of techniques pp. 84–85 for information on scissors, cutting combs and clippers.

EKU *statement*

GB7 (eku19) The size of available clipper grades and the effects that these achieve

Diversion See Unit GB8 Creatively cut hair using barbering techniques pp. 117 and 118 for information on the use, handling and maintenance and cleaning of clippers.

TUTOR SUPPORT

Project 6.2: Cutting tools

Standard clipper grades/attachments

Clipper attachment size/ No. for attachment	Length of cut hair
Grade 1 = 3 mm ($\frac{1}{8}$ inch)	Very close to skin, almost as close as shaving.
	Very short, on darker hair it will only leave a stubbly shadowing effect.
Grade 2 = 6 mm ($\frac{1}{4}$ inch)	Close cut, will see some skin on finer hair types but short enough for the hair to appear straight even if it is naturally curly.
Grade 3 = 9 mm ($\frac{3}{8}$ inch)	Popular length grade for short groomed effects. Typically cuts to that of short scissor over comb lengths.
Grade 4 = 13 mm ($\frac{1}{2}$ inch)	Popular length which has a similar effect to longer scissor over comb type effects.
Grades 6–8 = 16 mm–25 mm ($\frac{1}{2}$–1 inch)	Popular longer length used for beard shaping.

Note: There are no set standard sizes for clipper attachment combs/grades; you will need to adapt the hair length required by your client in light of the make and model clippers that you have/or your salon provides.

EKU *statement*

GB7 (eku18) How to level and test the clippers

EKU *statement*

GB7 (eku16) Methods of cleaning and maintaining all the tools and equipment in the range

Cleaning the equipment

Diversion Levelling and checking clippers before use
For more information on levelling clippers and checking the cutting blades See Unit GB8 Creatively cut hair using barbering techniques on p. 117.

	Tools	Method of cleaning/sterilisation
DENMAN	Neck brush	Wash in hot soapy water and place in UV cabinet for 10 mins.
WAHL (UK) LTD	Sectioning clips	Wash in hot soapy water and immerse in Barbicide™ jar for 30 mins.
DENMAN	Cutting comb	Wash in hot soapy water and immerse in Barbicide™ jar for 30 mins.
www.gebetterton.co.uk	Scissors	Brush away hair fragments from pivot area and blades with a colouring brush. Carefully wipe the blades with sterile wipes and then place with open blades in the UV cabinet for 15 mins each side.

	Tools	Method of cleaning/sterilisation
www.gebetterton.co.uk	Thinning scissors	Brush away hair fragments from pivot area and blades with a colouring brush. Carefully wipe the blades with sterile wipes and then place with open blades in the UV cabinet for 15 mins each side.

@ TUTOR SUPPORT

Project 6.3: Facial hair shape for different face shapes

GB7.2   Create a range of facial hair shapes

Designing an outline shape

When a new look and outline shape is required, you will find it easier to draw the outlines first. This enables you to get an idea of balance and proportion in the mirror and it also enables the client to see a rough idea of where the new outlines will be in proportion to their face.

On fairer, lighter hair you can use an eyebrow pencil to mark the outlines and on darker hair you can use a white pencil. (Don't forget to remove any leftover marking when you complete the look.)

Facial hair cutting techniques

Many of the techniques used to cut men's facial hair are common to barbering practices. See Unit GB8 and Unit GH16 for more information on

- scissor cutting
- freehand cutting
- scissor over comb
- clipper over comb
- controlling the cut
- cross-checking the cut.

Every client is different; they all have differing needs, features and requirements. Therefore, they should always be handled with individual care and attention. Your consultation and analysis will need to reflect this and you will have to adapt to their requests. Normally, the process of trimming and shaping beards or moustaches will be the same in any event; that being:

- you remove the bulk from the interior of the feature first, then
- you tidy and shape the outline to finish the effect.

Facial hair is bristle; it is stiffer than hair on the head and this is due to the frequency that it is cut in relation to hairstyles. This makes the hair coarser and this creates its own problems, as it is more difficult to cut by 'scissor over comb' method. This leads stylists and barbers to choose 'clipper over comb', as the mechanical advantage makes the job far easier. But as you need to use one hand to steady and position the comb, you can only have one other holding the relatively heavy clippers. This technique is more complex than using clippers held with two hands and clipper grade attachments.

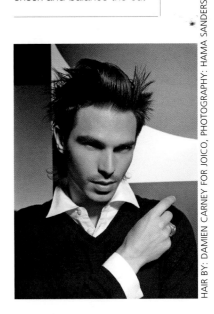

HAIR BY: DAMIEN CARNEY FOR JOICO, PHOTOGRAPHY: HAMA SANDERS

Remember

 Always look for any contra-indications before you start any facial hair shaping. Look carefully for any suspected infestations or viral or bacterial infections.

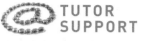 **TUTOR SUPPORT**

Discussion 6.1: Influencing factors as a result of the consultation

EKU *statement*

GB7 (eku6) Why it is important to protect clients from hair clippings

GB7 (eku34) The types of problems that can occur when cutting facial hair and ways in which they can be remedied, if possible

Clipper over comb

The clipper over comb technique should start by combing and lifting away the ends, then skimming over these to remove wispier bits first. The benefit of this will allow you to:

- see if any areas show less density in growth than others.
- make sure that you don't reduce these areas resulting in skin showing through in a patchy effect.

Bristles are strong and when they are cut into smaller fragments they can fly all over you and the client. This can be dangerous as bristles can stick in any areas of unprotected skin! Or worse, they can enter into the eye. To prevent this happening to the client, it would be safer get him to close his eyes while you trim or alternatively, place cotton wool pads over the eyes to protect them from the fragments.

Remember

Remember to check the clipper blade alignment before trimming the outline shape of beards and moustaches.

When the interior of the facial hair shape has been cut, you can then concentrate on defining the shape by creating the outside perimeter line. Hair growth can often be uneven across the head, let alone the face. Even if the client is a regular visitor to the salon you will need to check for balance throughout the shaping, to make sure that the growth doesn't occur thicker and deeper on one side than the other.

Although comfort is always a major concern, for beard trimming it may be easier to start your outlining with the clippers, centrally up the neck to the point below the chin to start the profile shape. By doing this, you can define the exact position where you stop and you will find that you can then work on either side of the client to create an even symmetrical finish. After this you can complete the shape behind or over the jaw and finally form the cheek area, down to the desired top profile of the beard.

On the other hand most moustaches are trimmed at or above the upper lip by scissors; this is easier to handle and stops the vibration of the clippers, tickling the client and causing them to pull back. The upper perimeter line can then be defined by the clippers to give a clean, finished profile shape.

Remember

Safety

Always take care when using sharp implements on the client's skin. Concentrate on the job in hand and ignore other distractions.

If you do cut the client:

1 Put on a pair of disposable vinyl gloves.
2 Use a medical sterilised wipe to clean the area and remove any hair or bristle.
3 Apply pressure to the cut to stem the flow of blood.
4 When the wound has stopped bleeding you can finish the service and give the client a clean, dry tissue for any minor seepage.

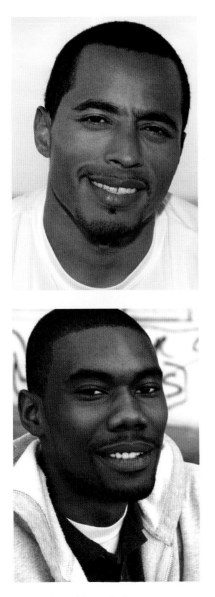
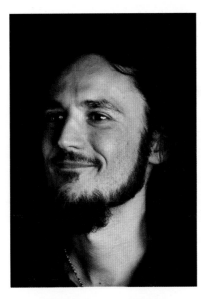
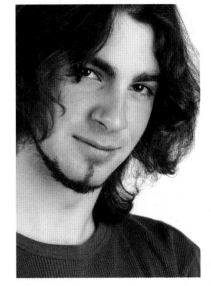
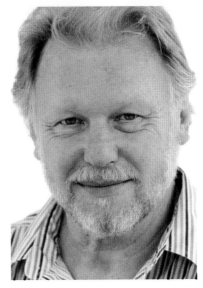

Examples of beard shapes

Removing unwanted hair outside the desired style line

Finishing and tidying is the last part of the service; you need to clean-up any hair or stubble that lies outside the desired style line. After you have agreed with the client that the overall shape and design is OK, you take the electric clippers and turn them so that the fixed blade works away from the design line. You may find that you need to stretch the skin around the neck and face to get a cleaner, straighter cut close to the skin. Then working back from the design line; draw the clippers away over the neck/cheek or jaw to create a clean finish. Take a neck brush and carefully brush away any fragments. Then finally re-cut any areas still with signs of uncut bristle. A final brush and the cutting part is over.

EKU *statement*

GB7 (eku26) The range of traditional and current facial hair shapes

Step-by-step

Maintenance–based trim

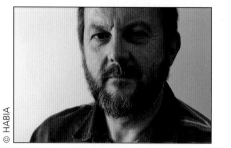

Step 1 Before

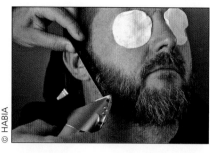

Step 2 Remove excess hair using the clippers-over-comb technique. Note the pads to protect the eyes from clippings

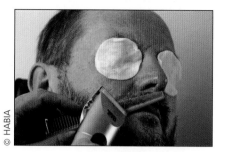

Step 3 Remove excess hair from the moustache using the clippers-over-comb technique

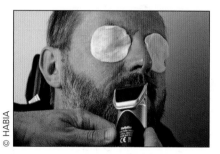

Step 4 Use the clippers carefully to produce a tidy edge above the top lip

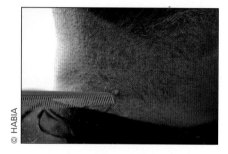

Step 5 Be aware of critical influencing factors such as moles, scars, infected spots etc

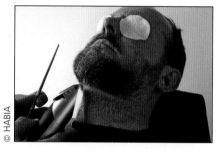

Step 6 Mark out and create an edge using the clippers

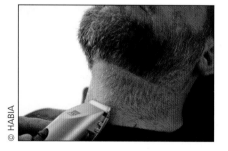

Step 7 Remove unwanted hair up to the edge

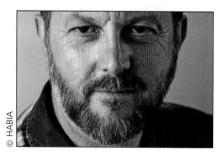

Step 8 The finished result

GB7.3   Provide aftercare advice

No service is complete unless the client leaves in the knowledge that he can achieve the same result as that done in the salon. If he can't achieve a similar effect he is unlikely to return. You can make sure that he does and the real sign of client satisfaction is the rebooking of his next visit before he leaves the salon.

You can help to achieve this by making sure you tell him:

- how long the effect will last and when he needs to come back
- which products and equipment you have used and how they might benefit the client at home
- how changes in hairstyle may affect the overall look.

How long will it last?

Hair grows at an average 1.25 cm per month so a shorter, closer styled beard or moustache will have grown out within a month whereas longer facial designs will last longer. (Or, rather, the growth won't be quite as noticeable and therefore the client tends to go longer in-between visits.) Remember, if the effect incorporates a moustache too; then that will need trimming anyway, as that will over-fall the upper lip fairly quickly.

> **Remember**
> Whatever the length or effect created you need to tell your client from the outset how long they can expect it to last, so that they don't have any unrealistic expectations.

Products and skin care

Explain to the client how they can manage the effect themselves. You need to provide advice on cleansing – what to use, in relation to their hair and skin types, how often to use it and what products wouldn't suit them and therefore should be avoided and your reasons why.

Exfoliation is beneficial to the client; it removes dead skin cells from the epidermis and stimulates blood circulation, which will generally improve the skin's condition. There are many different products now available for men and these can be bought as grains that are mixed with water and applied as a paste or, alternatively, a wide range of ready-to-use products with a variety of bases such as fruit acids or herbal with essential oils.

> **Remember**
> **Avoid ingrowing hairs**
> Ingrowing hairs are an uncomfortable aspect of closely cut wavy or curly hair. When hair is razored or clippered close to the skin, say at the neckline, the action of the cutting implement tends to slightly pull the hair within the follicle. After the hair is cut, the hairshaft tends to retract back into the follicle giving a very close, smooth finish to the touch. Unfortunately, if the area isn't kept thoroughly clean the open area of the follicle can become partially blocked with dead skin cells or dirt. This will change the growing direction of the hair within the follicle, often allowing it to find a new position within the skin. Bearing in mind that the average rate of hair growth is about 10–12 mm per month, if this is allowed to continue, an ingrowing hair will result. The physical effects of this will not be noticed until:
>
> - it starts to create a raised area often accompanied with a mild infected spot
> - it begins to itch as it causes irritation beneath the skin.
>
> If the ingrowing hair is not brought to the surface or removed from the skin a longer-term, more serious condition/infection will result.

Diversion Much of the advice relating to homecare advice is covered in Unit GH16 pp. 100–101.

EKU *statement*

GB7 (eku35) The recommended time interval between cuts and why they need to have their facial hair cut regularly

GB7 (eku21) The average rate of hair growth

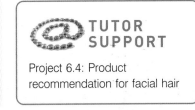

TUTOR SUPPORT

Project 6.4: Product recommendation for facial hair

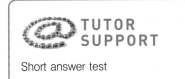

TUTOR SUPPORT

Short answer test

EKU *statement*

GB7 (eku37) Suitable products and equipment for home use that will benefit the client and those to avoid and why

EKU *statement*

GB7 (eku22) The potential risk of in growing hair resulting from continual cutting of curly hair

EKU *statement*

GB7 (eku38) The personal factors which could affect the client's potential for style change (e.g. hair length, hair growth patterns, hair density etc.).

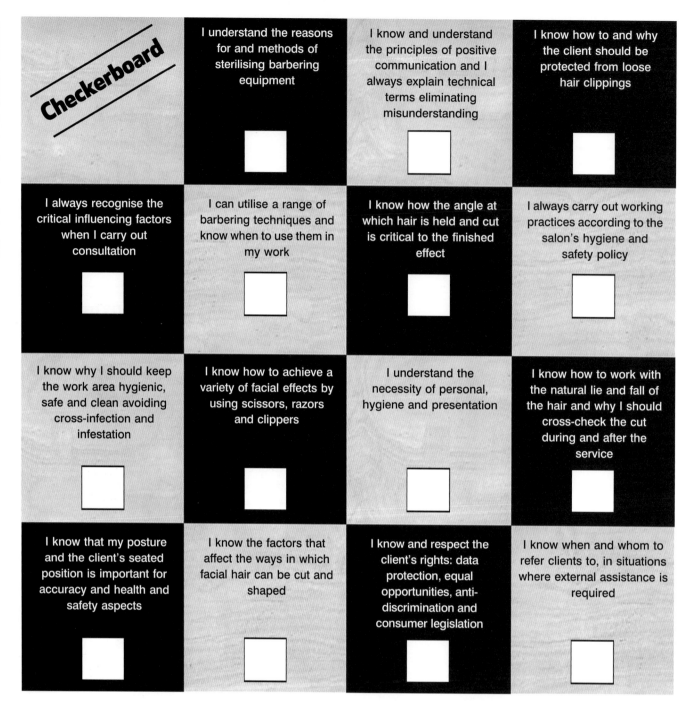

Checkerboard

I understand the reasons for and methods of sterilising barbering equipment

I know and understand the principles of positive communication and I always explain technical terms eliminating misunderstanding

I know how to and why the client should be protected from loose hair clippings

I always recognise the critical influencing factors when I carry out consultation

I can utilise a range of barbering techniques and know when to use them in my work

I know how the angle at which hair is held and cut is critical to the finished effect

I always carry out working practices according to the salon's hygiene and safety policy

I know why I should keep the work area hygienic, safe and clean avoiding cross-infection and infestation

I know how to achieve a variety of facial effects by using scissors, razors and clippers

I understand the necessity of personal, hygiene and presentation

I know how to work with the natural lie and fall of the hair and why I should cross-check the cut during and after the service

I know that my posture and the client's seated position is important for accuracy and health and safety aspects

I know the factors that affect the ways in which facial hair can be cut and shaped

I know and respect the client's rights: data protection, equal opportunities, anti-discrimination and consumer legislation

I know when and whom to refer clients to, in situations where external assistance is required

Revision questions

Quick quiz: a selection of different types of questions to check your knowledge.

Q1   Barbicide™ is a form of chemical ....   Fill in the blank

Q2   UV radiation is suitable for hygienic preparation of scissors?   True or false

Q3   Which of the following is suitable for immersing into Barbicide?   Multi selection

Scissors	☐	1
Combs	☐	2
Thinning scissors	☐	3
Clipper blades	☐	4
Plastic brushes	☐	5
Open razor	☐	6

Q4   Grade 1 is shorter than grade 2.   True or false

Q5   You are going to use all of the following clipper grades in a gent's clippered graduation. Which clipper grade would you start with?   Multi selection

1	☐	1
2	☐	2
3	☐	3
4	☐	4

Q6   Facial hair is stiffer than scalp hair.   True or false

Q7   Which of the following factors would influence the choice of shape of a beard?   Multi selection

Facial features	☐	1
Hair length	☐	2
Parting position	☐	3
Facial hair density	☐	4
Height	☐	5
Weight	☐	6

Q8   Quality combs are strong but ....   Fill in the blank

Q9   Which of the following will cause ingrowing hairs?   Multi choice

Leaving a beard too long	○	1
Repeated close cutting with a razor	○	2
Fading out to a hairline	○	3
Blunt clipper blades	○	4

Q10   Alopecia does not affect facial hair.   True or false

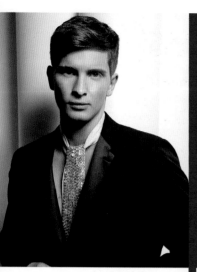

Chapter**seven**
Shaving

LEONARDO RIZZO @ SANRIZZ

GB6

GB6.1

GB6.2

GB6.3

GB6.4

**CREDIT VALUE
FOR UNIT GB6**

4 Credits

 More information See Unit G21 Provide hairdressing consultation services for information of adverse hair and skin conditions

 Diversion See Unit GB7 Design and create a range of facial hair shapes for information on client preparation, hygiene and work efficiency

See appendices for Electricity at Work Regulations

EKU *statement*

GB6 (eku4) Your responsibilities under the Electricity at Work Regulations

Shaving: quick overview

Unit title

GB6 Provide shaving services

This is a **optional** unit for barbering at level 3, it is made up of four main outcomes

Main outcomes

GB6.1 Maintain effective and safe methods of working when shaving

GB6.2 Prepare the hair and skin for shaving

GB6.3 Shave hair

GB6.4 Provide aftercare advice

What do I need to do for GB6.1?

- Make sure that the client is adequately covered and protected
- Make sure that your working position is comfortable and safe
- Keep the work area clean and tidy and that waste materials are disposed of properly
- Identify factors that influence the service prior to starting
- Work without causing risks to you or your client's health and safety
- Work efficiently and effectively

What do I need to do for GB6.2?

- Choose suitable tools and equipment based on your consultation
- Prepare and apply hot towels
- Pre-cut unwanted facial hair prior to shaving
- Prepare and apply appropriate lathering products

What do I need to do for GB6.3?

- Confirm the look required prior to shaving
- Maintain or replace cutting edges throughout the process
- Take appropriate remedial action as and when problems arise
- Remove lather and moisture after the service
- Cool the client's skin and apply appropriate finishing products

What do I need to do for GB6.4?

- Give the client accurate, constructive advice on aftercare treatment

What aspects do I need to cover for GB6.1, GB6.2, GB6.3 and GB6.4?

- A variety of cutting tools and equipment
- A range of factors that influence shaving
- A range of products and techniques applicable to the service

What aspects do I need to know for GB6.1, GB6.2, GB6.3 and GB6.4?

- Your salon's requirements for preparation, timings and standards of service
- How to work safely, effectively and hygienically when shaving
- Factors about the client that affect shaving
- How to handle, use and maintain the shaving equipment
- The ways of using tools and products to suit the needs of the client
- Aspects of facial hair and skin and how this influences the provision of shaving services
- The aftercare advice and recommendations that you should give to clients

Introduction

The recent popularity of contemporary facial shapes has helped to promote the need for careful and skilled shaving. The intricate shapes that are popular with the modern man along with the needs of busy professionals have helped to drive forward a service that is luxuriant, soothing and something that men find as yet another intrusion upon the little time that they have in the mornings.

Keywords

Forehand razoring
A method of razoring where the cutting action occurs with a forehand technique

Backhand razoring
A method of razoring where the cutting action occurs with a backhand technique

Astringent
A substance applied after shaving to close the pores

Exfoliating
The removal or shedding of a thin outer layer of skin from the epidermis

Moisturising balms
Cooling, soothing and moisture replenishing lotions applied after shaving to counteract the abrasive effects of the process

Information covered in this chapter

- The tools and equipment used during shaving
- The preparations that you should make prior to shaving
- The factors that influence shaving
- Shaving techniques
- The aftercare advice that you should give clients

TUTOR SUPPORT

Project 7.1: Hazards and risks associated with shaving

The barber's shave

The everyday bind of shaving for men is a tedious necessity; it takes up extra time on an already busy morning which could be used in other ways. The barber's shave is considered to be a luxury, but still a valuable service. This chapter addresses the various aspects and considerations of the service by covering:

- tool preparation and maintenance
- client preparation
- client consultation
- identifying the influencing factors that affect the service
- shaving techniques, problems and accuracy
- good customer care.

GB6.1 Maintain effective and safe methods of working when shaving

EKU statement

GB6 (eku1) Your salon's requirements for client preparation

GB6 (eku2) Your salon's expected service times for shaving facial hair

GB6 (eku6) The range of protective clothing that should be available for clients and yourself

GB6 (eku10) The safety considerations which must be taken into account when shaving

GB6 (eku12) Why it is important to keep your work area clean and tidy

GB6 (eku13) The importance of positioning tools and equipment for ease of use

GB6 (eku18) The importance of personal hygiene

Remember

 Safety first
Open cut-throat razors are extremely sharp and must always be handled with care and respect

Tool preparation and maintenance

The tools that you use must always be sterilised and ready for use; the razors need to be kept close at hand, but well out of the way of clients and children. If you use razors that use disposable blades, make sure that any used blades are disposed of properly in the 'sharps' box. Alternatively, if you use a fixed blade razor it must be hygienic and sharp ready for use.

Your main concern during shaving is damage to the skin and this can be avoided by careful, shaving techniques and the use of sterile and sharp tools.

Remember

 A new blade needs to be used on every client to prevent cross-infection.

Remember

 Facial hair cutting requires the client to tilt their head back so that you can work at an angle that enables you to work safely and carefully. The barber's chair is specifically designed for this with both its inbuilt head rest and reclining ability, this ensures both the client's comfort and safety.

Shaving tools and equipment

You will be using a variety of equipment, some of which you may already be familiar with whilst others may be a completely new experience. If you want more information on clippers and clipper maintenance or razors see Chapter 5, Unit GB8 Creatively cut hair using a combination of barbering techniques pp. 116–120.

Diversion For more information on client preparation, working efficiently and sterilising equipment, see Chapter 6, Unit GB7 Design and create a range of facial hair shapes pp. 129–145.

Remember

Local bye-laws
Different local authorities have different local bye-laws. Some areas do not allow the use of fixed blade open razors and only permit the use of disposable bladed types.
Find out what the policy is in your area.

EKU *statement*

GB6 (eku14) The importance of using the correct type of barber's chair for shaving services

GB6 (eku15) Methods of cleaning disinfecting and/or sterilisation used in salons

Clippers

Clippers can be used as a pre-shaving procedure for men who have longer facial hair. Dense, heavy growth needs to be removed before shaving so that only short, stubbly growth remains. This is particularly beneficial as it not only saves time during the shaving process, it enables you to see the client's skin and their facial hair growth patterns more clearly.

EKU *statement*

GB6 (eku17) The correct use and maintenance of shaving tools and equipment

EKU *statement*

GB6 (eku34) When and why it is necessary to reduce beard length prior to shaving

Remember

Bristles are strong and when they are cut into smaller fragments they can fly all over you and the client. This can be dangerous as bristles are stiff and sharp and can pierce areas of unprotected skin! Or worse, they can enter into the eye. To prevent this happening to the client, it would be safer get him to close his eyes while you trim or, alternatively, place cotton wool pads over the eyes to protect them from the fragments.

EKU *statement*

GB6 (eku8) Why it is important to protect clients from hair clippings

Open blade razor

There are two types of razor that are used for shaving: the safety razor, which has a disposable blade and the fixed blade razor that has a blade that is kept sharp by honing and stropping.

If you use a safety razor you would always replace the disposable blade with a new blade for every client. This hygienic practice prevents the risk of cross-infection and eliminates the need for any sharpening processes.

The fixed blade razor can have two types of blade:

- *The hollow ground* – the more popular, lighter and durable type that is made out of tempered steel. It has a narrower, waist-like profile that is more sensitive during use, which discloses resistance to cutting when in need of sharpening.

- *The solid blade* – which are made of a softer metal that 'dulls' more easily and therefore needs sharpening more frequently.

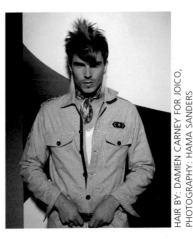

HAIR BY: DAMIEN CARNEY FOR JOICO, PHOTOGRAPHY: HAMA SANDERS

WWW.GEBETTERTON.CO.UK

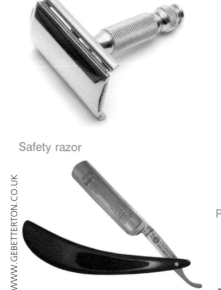

Safety razor

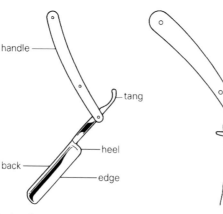

Parts of a razor

handle

tang

heel

back

edge

How to hold an open blade razor

Fixed blade razor

Remember

 A fixed blade razor must always be sterilised between clients and therefore, for handiness, a barber may own a couple, so that one can be cleaned, prepared and always ready for use.

Diversion For more information on preventing infection see Unit GB7, Design and create a range of facial hair shapes p. 132 and Unit GH16, Creative cutting p. 76.

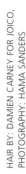

HAIR BY: DAMIEN CARNEY FOR JOICO,
PHOTOGRAPHY: HAMA SANDERS

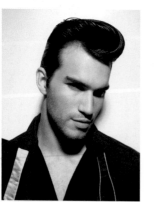

EKU *statement*

GB6 (eku29) The types of open blade razors with disposable blades available for professional use

Honing (setting) fixed blade razors

If you looked at the cutting edge of a razor through a powerful magnifying glass, you would see that it has very fine teeth like a saw. During routine use, this cutting edge is 'dulled' and must be re-sharpened by the barber; this is done by honing and stropping.

There are three different types of hone: natural, synthetic and combination.

A natural hone is a rectangular block of stone and the most popular of these originate from Belgium and Germany.

A synthetic hone is made from a material called carborundum. It produces a sharp edge to a razor more quickly than that of natural stone. Care should be taken to not over-hone as this will damage the edge of the blade.

The third type of hone is double sided and is a combination of the natural on one side and synthetic on the other. So if a razor has a badly damaged edge then the synthetic side of the hone is used to quickly bring back its keenness.

Alternatively, if a razor only needs a slight re-sharpening than the natural stone side is used.

Honing technique

A fixed blade razor is sharpened by a technique of drawing the edges over the lubricated surface on the stone in a particular way.

- Wipe over the surface of the hone to remove any oil or debris.
- Drop a little lubricating oil on to the surface of the hone.
- With the edge of the blade pointing left, start at the upper right area of the hone with the heal of the blade.
- Draw down diagonally towards the lower left area of the hone, keeping the blade flat and parallel to the abrasive so that it sharpens the edge up the blade towards the point.
- Turn the blade over and slide it upwards towards the upper left area of the hone.
- Then repeat the diagonal movement again from upper left to the lower right.
- The complete movement is like a figure of '8' on its side.

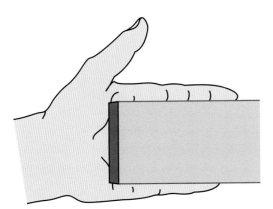

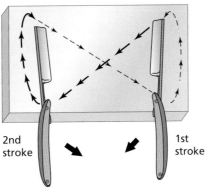

2nd stroke

1st stroke

Correct way to hold a hone

Proper method to hone a razor

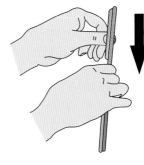

Test the sharpness of the razor on moistened thumbnail

Testing the razor's edge

During honing the edge of the razor's blade needs to be tested to prevent over honing. This is done by lightly drawing the razor over a moistened thumbnail to feel for any signs of roughness or snagging.

- A sharp razor will dig in to the nail with a smooth, continual draw.
- A blunt razor will glide over the surface of the nail without digging in.
- Any nicks or damaged parts of the blade will feel rough and uneven.

Stropping

A fixed blade razor is stropped to produce what is known as a 'whetted' edge. Stropping cleans (but does not sterilise) a razor's edge and re-aligns the microscopic serrations or teeth, to provide an extremely sharp blade. There are two types of strop:

1 *Hanging strop* – this is the most popular type of strop which is flexible and has a canvas and leather side.
2 *Solid (French or German) strop* – these strops are used for solid blade razors and are made of a combination of materials.

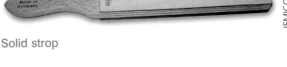

Solid strop

JEMICO

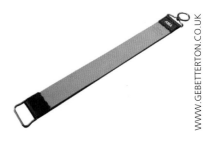

Hanging strop

WWW.GEBETTERTON.CO.UK

EKU statement

GB6 (eku30) How to prepare an open blade razor with disposal blade for use

EKU statement

GB6 (eku11) Why it is important to avoid cross-infection

GB6 (eku16) Methods of work-ing safely and hygienically and which minimise the risk of cross-infection and cross-infestation

Activity

Answer the following questions in your portfolio.

1 Why is it important to avoid cross-infection/cross-infestation?
2 What is meant by setting a razor's blade?
3 When would you do a sponge shave?
4 How would you dispose of the waste items produced during shaving?
5 How do you test a razor's edge?

Remember

Never try to strop a razor with the cutting edge facing towards the direction of sharpening. This will damage the razor's edge and also the surface of the strop.

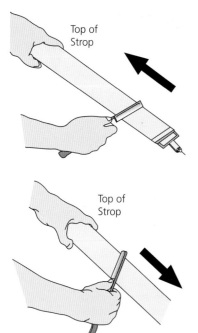

Top of
Strop

Top of
Strop

Stropping a hollow ground razor

1 Hang the strop at one end by its hook.

2 Then, holding the other end, pull it out horizontally so that the strop is flat.

3 Position the razor near the hook end with the heel of the blade pointing towards you and holding it by its metal shank between the thumb and forefinger.

4 Draw the razor down the strop towards you; then as it reaches ¾ of the way down, carefully turn the blade over.

5 Repeat the stroke in the opposite direction.

6 Repeat this for about 10 strokes and the blade should be ready for use.

Correct stropping will extend the useable life of the razor and will reduce the risk of damaging the client's skin. You should always sterilise the razor after stropping and honing to prevent the risk of cross-infection to the client.

Stropping a solid razor

The movement or technique is similar to that used for the hanging strop, except the strop is placed on a flat, solid surface rather than hung from a hook.

EKU statement

GB6 (eku9) How the position of your client and yourself can affect the desired outcome and reduce fatigue and the risk of injury

EKU statement

GB6 (eku7) Why it is important to wear gloves when shaving

Activity

This activity relates to the variety of products that are used during shaving. Complete this activity by filling in the missing information.

Product	What does it do?	When is it used?
An astringent		
An exfoliating crème		
A moisturising balm		
A solid hone		
A hanging strop		

GB6.2 Prepare the hair and skin for shaving

Client preparation

Remember

If you do need to remove excess beard length first, place a couple of cotton wool swabs over the eye sockets as this will stop bristle clippings from entering the eyes.

After making sure that your hands and nails are scrupulously clean, make sure that your client is comfortable and correctly positioned, seated in the barber's chair. Find out what the client wants and agree your course of action. Now check to see that the client's beard is clean, free from debris and short enough to work on. (If the beard is long the excess length can be removed by clippering first.) After looking for contra-indications to shaving as well as checking the beard's hair growth directions, you can make your adjustments to the position of the headrest to suit the client's neck and head.

Place a towel across the client's chest covering the gown and tuck the edges into the neckline.

Diversion For more information on working position, safety and efficiency see Unit GB7, Design and create a range of facial hair shapes p. 132.

Remember

If you want to apply the lather with your hands rather than a brush make sure that you wear vinyl disposable gloves as this is more hygienic and prevents cross-infection.

Remember

If, during the process of shaving, the lather dries out then re-apply it as you may cause damage to the client's skin.

Contra-indications to shaving

There are a variety of situations when shaving is not suitable for the client at that time. Look for signs to see if the service *can* be provided and *ask* the client if they have any reasons that they know of that would *not permit* the service to be conducted.

Possible contra-indications could be due to:

- infections or infestations that you see during your examination
- cuts or abrasions within the facial hair areas
- uneven skin due to acne, eczema or other conditions
- skin sensitivity.

EKU *statement*

GB6 (eku19) The importance of questioning clients to establish any contraindications to the shaving service

GB6 (eku24) The factors that must be taken into consideration prior to and during the shaving service (e.g. suspected infections, infestations, hair growth patterns, facial piercing, skin disorders, unusual facial features)

GB6 (eku33) When not to carry out shaving

Lathering

Before applying the lather, the skin and beard need to be prepared; this is done by applying hot towels to the face. Hot towels can be prepared by pre-soaking them in a basin of hot water; then, after wringing out the excess water, they are placed around the facial area (but not covering the nose) to:

- soften the bristly hair
- open up the follicles and
- prepare the skin for lathering.

Always make sure that the towels are not dripping wet and they are not too hot for the client.

Hot lather is generally applied to the beard area of the face using a brush and bowl, it needs to be done quickly and take care not to cover the mouth, nose or go anywhere near the client's eyes. Begin lathering by placing the brush on the point of the chin and by making small circulatory movements, extend the area of lather to cover all of the beard area. Keep the brush and lather hot by dipping it in hot water; as a hot lather produces a better, closer shave.

Diversion To see more information about the types of questions that you should ask clients and the different adverse conditions that exist and the skin's physical structure, see Unit G21 Provide hairdressing consultation services pp. 4–43.

Remember

If you have any doubts about symptoms and contra-indications, always ask a more experienced member of staff for their assistance. You may be putting the salon at risk from legal action or pursuance if you don't follow this process properly. If you do offer shaving services and have covered the above contra-indications, make sure that you keep a record of your consultation and the responses made by the client after the service, for future reference.

EKU statement

GB6 (eku20) Why it is important to record client responses to questioning

GB6 (eku21) The legal significance of client questioning and of recording the client's responses

GB6 (eku22) The importance of keeping and maintaining client records

GB6 (eku26) The importance of lathering and the function it performs on the skin and the hair

GB6 (eku27) The effect of heat on the hair and skin

GB6 (eku31) How to prepare and use lathering products correctly

GB6 (eku38) When and why to use brush and massage techniques to apply lathering products

EKU statement

GB6 (eku23) The structure of the skin

GB6 (eku25) The scalp and facial skin disorders commonly affecting men and how to recognise them

Activity

Shaving problems

Review this chapter then complete this table by filling in the missing information.

After you have completed this; keep a copy for future reference within your portfolio.

Problem	Possible cause	Remedy
	1 Poor skin tensioning 2 Blunt razor	1 Administer first aid – continue after bleeding stops 2 Re-hone the blade and test for sharpness; then shave again with the correct tension
Skin rashes		1 Re-hone the blade and test for sharpness; 2 Let the skin rest 3 Check heat and allow to cool first 4 Incorrect cutting angle – change
	1 Shaving curly hair too close 2 Blocked pores/ follicle	
Uneven skin		
Folliculitis	1 Inflamed follicles 2 Ingrowing hairs	
		1 Re-hone the blade and test for sharpness, then re-shave with an even tension

GB6.3 Shave hair

EKU statement

GB6 (eku35) How to carry out the shaving techniques listed in the range

EKU statement

GB6 (eku36) Why skin needs to be tensioned during shaving

There are two main movements to shaving; the forehand and backhand techniques.

First time over

The first time shave is always done in the same direction as the client's natural hair growth. If you are right handed stand on the right-hand side of the client (left-handed stand on left) begin with the outer cheek area nearest to you.

Tension the skin with your free hand so that it is taut; keeping it free from lather so that you don't slip and allow the skin to relax. (This would be dangerous as it would allow the skin to cut easily.) With the skin taut the razor will be able to glide easily over the skin and cut the hair cleanly and smoothly.

1 Holding the razor loosely with your thumb on the blade.

2 Begin the shave on the nearest sideburn area to you.

3 Move the razor in steady sweeping movement starting at the top of the stroke, moving downwards.

4 Follow the sequence shown in the diagram.

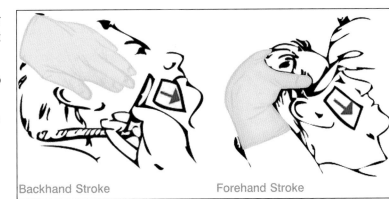

Backhand Stroke   Forehand Stroke

Shaving techniques

Second time over

The second time shave is done against the natural growth direction; this ensures that the shave is as close as possible. This will be the last shave unless the client has a particularly coarse, stubborn growth which will then require a sponge shave.

1 Re-lather the face and start the shave at the neck area.

2 Work upwards towards the chin, then upwards again on each side of the face.

3 Clean the face with a damp, warm towel then pat dry, without rubbing.

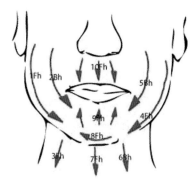

Shaving procedure

Finishing

1 Apply a little talcum powder to remove any moisture.

2 Then apply an astringent to close the pores of the skin and a moisturising balm to cool and replenish the skin with moisture.

3 Sit the client back-up to an upright position and get him to check the result.

EKU *statement*

GB6 (eku37) The importance of adapting shaving techniques in relation to the direction of hair growth

Remember

Hot and cool towels

Hot towels should not be used on a client with sensitive skin as this will irritate the skin further and prevent you from carrying out the service.

Cool towels are used to sooth the face after shaving and to close the pores to finish the service.

Cool towels should not be used on a client who is going to have a facial massage as this will close the pores prematurely and prevent the client from gaining the full benefit of the massage service.

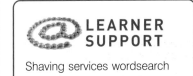

LEARNER SUPPORT

Shaving services wordsearch

Sponge shaving

If the client has particularly heavy, coarse or thick growth, it may be necessary to do a sponge shave after the second time over.

● Dip a sterilised sponge into hot water and wipe it over the skin directly before shaving.

Remember

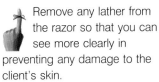 Remove any lather from the razor so that you can see more clearly in preventing any damage to the client's skin.

EKU *statement*

GB6 (eku39) The reasons for and effects of using cool towels after shaving

GB6 (eku40) Why cold towels should not be used if the face is to be massaged

EKU *statement*

GB6 (eku41) When and why to use sponge shaving

GB6 (eku42) The importance of working in a way which maintains the right skin temperature throughout the shaving process

EKU *statement*

GB6 (eku43) Problems which may arise during the shaving process (e.g. shaving hair too close, damage to your client's and your own skin) and ways of resolving such problems

EKU *statement*

GB6 (eku3) Your salon's and legal requirements for disposal of sharps, hazardous and waste materials

GB6 (eku5) Typical limitations placed on the use of fixed blade razors by local bye-laws and legislation

EKU *statement*

GB6 (eku48) How to give effective advice and recommendations to clients

Diversion For more information see preventing infection Unit GB7 Design and create a range of facial shapes p. 133.

- This opens the hair follicle and lifts the hair/bristle enabling the closest of shaves.
- Take particular care as you can damage the skin or cause ingrowing hairs.
- Don't do this type of shave unless absolutely necessary.

Shaving problems

Problem	Possible cause	Remedy
Facial cuts	1 Poor skin tensioning 2 Blunt razor	1 Administer first aid – continue after bleeding stops (wear PPE) 2 Re-hone the blade and test for sharpness; then shave again with the correct tension
Skin rashes	1 Blade is dull and is pulling the hair before cutting 2 Shaving too close 3 Towels too hot 4 Dragging the razor	1 Re-hone the blade and test for sharpness 2 Let the skin rest 3 Check heat and allow to cool first 4 Incorrect cutting angle – change
Ingrowing hairs	1 Shaving curly hair too close 2 Blocked pores/ follicle	1 Avoid cutting that close 2 Face not deep cleansed enough– provide advice for exfoliation
Uneven skin	1 Acne, moles	1 Take extra care in uneven skin areas
Folliculitis	1 Inflamed follicles 2 Ingrowing hairs	1 and **2:** Refer client to pharmacist for remedial treatment, do not carry out shaving
Patchy shaving results	1 Blunt dull razor	1 Re-hone the blade and test for sharpness, then re-shave with an even tension

Disposal of waste materials

There will always be some waste materials at the end of a shave and 'sharps' must be disposed of in line with local authority bye-laws and regulations. All used razor blades are disposed of in a sharps bin, this must be clearly labelled and the top always re-tightened after disposal.

Any unused lather should be washed away down the sink; it cannot be used again on another client as this may cause cross-infection.

Any used towels need to be laundered and should be removed from the work area or temporarily placed into a covered towel bin prior to washing.

GB6.4 Provide aftercare advice

Recommended re-shaving intervals

Hair growth on men differs greatly, some men have less dense facial hair that is fine in texture, and others have heavy, coarse growth that seems to show as a shadow within hours. So the advice and recommendations that you give to clients is individual to them and their needs. Some men don't mind showing a small amount of regrowth whereas others need to be clean shaven all the time.

A lot depends on what they do professionally; a busy executive meeting people or business clients' throughout the day needs to be seen as a smart professional. Stubble or several days' growth may be OK in certain circles, but not in others. Your advice needs to reflect their individual lifestyle and personal needs.

Aftercare advice

You need to provide advice to the client on suitable shaving equipment and skin care and cleansing – they need to know what products they should be using, in relation to their facial hair and skin types. They need to know how often to use the items and, particularly, the products that won't suit them and the reasons why they should be avoided.

Skin care for men is now a very popular and growing business area. It is important to men as it is for women; the only difference is the ranges of products that are available. Men who shave regularly will already know that blunt razors and close shaving are a contributing factor for causing minor skin infections or blocking pores and follicles and starting ingrowing hairs. When this occurs, a spot forms on the surface of the skin and the bacteria will have started a small infection. This, like ingrowing hairs, is uncomfortable and itchy and can easily be avoided if you give the client the correct advice.

Exfoliation is beneficial to the client; it removes dead skin cells from the epidermis and stimulates blood circulation, which will generally improve the skin's condition. There are many different products now available for men and these can be bought as grains that are mixed with water and applied as a paste or, alternatively, a wide range of ready-to-use products with a variety of bases such as fruit acids or herbal with essential oils.

EKU *statement*

GB6 (eku32) The types of finishing products available for use and their effects on skin

GB6 (eku44) Suitable shaving equipment and products for home use that will benefit the client and those to avoid and why

GB6 (eku45) How to shave effectively and when to do so to maintain the desired lock

GB6 (eku47) How lifestyle can influence their choice and possible change of style

EKU *statement*

GB6 (eku28) The potential risk of ingrowing hair resulting from continual close shaving

EKU *statement*

GB6 (eku46) When and how to cleanse, exfoliate and moisturise

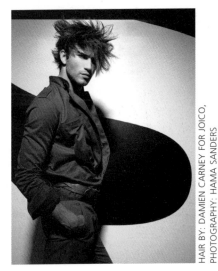

HAIR BY: DAMIEN CARNEY FOR JOICO,
PHOTOGRAPHY: HAMA SANDERS

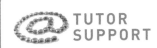

TUTOR SUPPORT

Project 7.2: Product recommendation for shaving

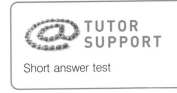

TUTOR SUPPORT

Short answer test

Checkerboard

I understand the reasons for and methods of sterilising barbering equipment	I know and understand the principles of effective sterilisation of tools and equipment	I know how to and why the client should be protected from loose hair clippings
I know what to ask clients and recognise contra-indications to shaving	I know the variety of protective clothing available for clients prior to shaving	I know how the angle at which facial hair is cut is critical to the shaving result	I always carry out working practices according to the salon's hygiene and safety policy
I know why I should keep the work area hygienic, safe and clean avoiding cross-infection and infestation	I know the structure of the skin	I know how to apply lather prior to shaving	I understand the necessity of personal, hygiene and presentation
I know how and why to work with the natural growth directions of the hair	I know that my posture and the client's seated position is important for accuracy and health and safety aspects	I know the factors that affect the ways in which facial hair can be cut and shaped	I know how to advise clients on a range of shaving products and equipment that suits different hair and skin types

Assessment of knowledge and understanding

Revision questions

Quick quiz: a selection of different types of questions to check your knowledge.

Q1 An _____ produces sterilisation by heat.   Fill in the blank

Q2 Honing is also known as 'setting' a blade.   True or false

Q3 A hollow ground blade has the following features: Multi selection

It is not as sharp as a solid blade razor	☐ 1
It is more sensitive during use	☐ 2
It is less sensitive during use	☐ 3
It is narrower than a solid blade razor	☐ 4
It is heavier than a solid blade razor	☐ 5
It needs sharpening more often	☐ 6

Q4 Natural hones originate from Germany and Belgium.   True or false

Q5 Which of the following is not a contra-indication to shaving?   Multi selection

Infections	☐ 1
Infestations	☐ 2
Uneven skin	☐ 3
Alopecia	☐ 4

Q6 A solid strop is suitable for solid razors.   True or false

Q7 Which of the following are the main contributors to skin rashes?   Multi selection

Dull razor blade	☐ 1
Sharp razor blade	☐ 2
Shaving too closely	☐ 3
Towels too hot	☐ 4
Towels too cold	☐ 5
Poor skin tensioning	☐ 6

Q8 A _____ shave is suitable for particularly heavy,   Fill in the blank
coarse thick growth.

Q9 A 'first time over' shave: Multi choice

Should be done in the same direction of the client's natural growth	○ 1
Should be done in the opposite direction to the client's natural growth	○ 2
Should be done very quickly	○ 3
Should be done with a blunt razor	○ 4

Q10 Alopecia does not affect facial hair   True or false

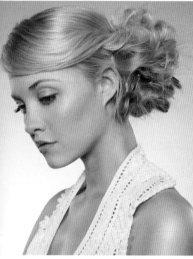

ADAM HARRIS @ MG MARTIN GOLD, STANMORE

GH19

GH19.1

GH19.2

GH19.3

CREDIT VALUE FOR UNIT GH19
4 Credits

 More Information See Unit G22 Monitor procedures to safely control work operations

- Personal hygiene GH19 (eku15)
- Contact dermatitis GH19 (eku6)
- General salon hygiene

See also appendices for following relevant legislation:

- COSHH GH19 (eku3)
- Electricity at Work Regulations GH19 (eku4)

Chapter**eight**
Creatively style and dress hair

Style and dress Hair: quick overview

Unit title

GH19 Creatively style and dress hair

This is a **optional** unit for students taking hairdressing level 3, it is made up of three main outcomes

Main outcomes

GH19.1 Maintain effective and safe methods of working when styling hair

GH19.2 Creatively style and dress hair

GH19.3 Provide aftercare advice

What do I need to do for GH19.1?

- Take adequate precautions in preparing yourself and the client before any setting or styling procedure
- Work tidily, safely and effectively at all times
- Maintain standards of personal health and hygiene
- Use a range of tools and equipment suitable for styling and dressing
- Work to your salon's expectations for service and image

What do I need to do for GH19.2?

- Confirm and agree the techniques and style requirements with the client
- Prepare the hair suitably for the styling requirements
- Work in a controlled and methodical way when setting
- Apply added hair to achieve the desired effect
- Adapt your styling techniques with non-conventional materials to achieve the desired effect
- Take into account a variety of factors that influence the way that the style is created

What do I need to do for GH19.3?

- Give the client recommendations and advice for maintaining their own hair

What aspects do I need to cover for GH19.1, GH19.2 and GH19.3?

- A range of styling and winding techniques suitable for creating the effect

- A variety of tools and non-conventional materials suitable for creating the effect

What do I need to know for GH19.1, GH19.2 and GH19.3?

- Your salons requirements in relation to salon policies and current legislation

- How to work safely and hygienically when styling or dressing hair

- The science that affects styling and dressing

- How to use a range of non-conventional styling and dressing materials and when they are applicable for your client's needs

- The current fashion trends

- The ways of handling and applying added hair

- How different techniques achieve different results and effects

- How to recommend or provide advice to the client on hair maintenance at home

Introduction

Creative styling is so far removed from what you learnt at level 2. In setting hair you worked with heated, Velcro and general wet setting rollers. You learnt how to backbrush and tease the roller marks out; to create a finished look that didn't quite look as natural as it could.

The task of producing really creative work is achieved by two things:

1 You need to think of your experiences as a sort of 'toolbox' and the tools within it are the little tips, techniques and methods that you use and experiment with, ones that you will always keep building upon.

2 You need to think creatively and that means *laterally*; you need to use those tools in different ways, sometimes in a different order, so that you can create a variety of finished effects on different hair types.

- The science of the physical changes that take place during styling as well as the effect that heat and humidity have on the hair
- The advice you should give to clients in order to maintain their own hair

This chapter takes you beyond the routine to explore other ways of doing things and that is what level 3 is about.

Remember

Always look after your brushes, combs and other tools. Make sure they are washed, dried and hygienically clean before you start your work.

GH19.1 Maintain effective and safe methods of working when styling hair

Although Unit G22 covers much of the general aspects that you need to know about health, safety and hygiene within the salon environment, such as preventing cross-infection, methods for sterilising equipment and personal hygiene etc. Each technical procedure you carry out has particular things that are relevant to health and safety.

Styling and dressing hair are always carried out at the styling units and therefore the main health and safety concerns should relate to the client's comfort, positioning and protection as well as your posture, accessibility and care.

As much of the essential information surrounding client preparation, health and safety and working effectively are common throughout the standards, the following essential knowledge and understanding statements can be referenced in Unit GH16 Creatively cut hair using a combination of techniques (see pp. 72–103).

Preparing, protecting and positioning the client

GH19 (eku1) Your salon's requirements for client preparation

GH19 (eku7) The range of protective clothing that should be available for clients

GH19 (eku8) Why it is important to use personal protective equipment,

GH19 (eku9) The type of personal protective equipment available

GH19 (eku10) How the position of your client and yourself can affect the desired outcome and reduce fatigue and the risk of injury

Preparing and positioning the equipment ready for use

GH19 (eku12) The importance of positioning equipment for ease of use

GH19 (eku13) Why it is important to keep your work area clean and tidy

Working safely and preventing infections

This area of work is covered in Chapter 15, Unit G22 Monitor procedures to safely control work operations, pp. 374–396.

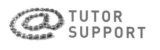

TUTOR SUPPORT

Project 8.1: Risk assessment for styling and dressing services

REDUCING RISKS – GOOD SALON SAFETY and SALON EQUIPMENT (pp. 389–395)

GH19 (eku11) The safety considerations which must be taken into account when setting and dressing hair

GH19 (eku14) Methods of working safely and hygienically and which minimise the risk of cross-infection and cross-infestation

GH19 (eku16) Why it is important to check electrical equipment used to aid the styling and finishing processes

GH19 (eku17) Methods of cleaning, disinfecting and or sterilisation used in salons

Your personal health and hygiene

PERSONAL HEALTH and HYGIENE (pp. 388 and 394)

GH19 (eku15) The importance of personal hygiene

REDUCING RISKS – PREVENTING DERMATITIS (p. 393)

GH19 (eku6) What is contact dermatitis and how to avoid developing it whilst carrying out styling and finishing services

REDUCING RISKS – HANDLING CHEMICALS (pp. 391 and 394)

GH19 (eku3) Your own responsibilities under the current Control of Substances Hazardous to Health Regulations in relation to the use of styling and finishing products

Working with electricity

REDUCING RISKS – WORKING WITH ELECTRICITY (p. 394)

GH19 (eku4) your responsibilities under the current Electricity at Work Regulations

> **Remember**
>
> **Lateral thinking**
>
>
> Non-conventional styling equipment can be things like highlighting foils, rags or pre-formed plastic containers cut to shape. It's up to you to think about applying materials in different ways; that's what creative thinking is.

> **Remember**
>
> Always make sure that your choice of non-conventional styling equipment is safe and hygienic to use.

Preparing the tools and equipment for setting and dressing hair

Make sure that you have prepared the area. Get everything that you need together beforehand and this includes the equipment that you need, as well as the products. You should have your trolley prepared with all the materials you will need. Styling materials should have been previously prepared by thorough washing/sterilising and combs, brushes, sectioning clips etc. should be all cleaned, sterilised and made ready for use.

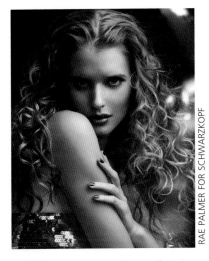

RAE PALMER FOR SCHWARZKOPF

> **Diversion** For more information on cleaning, sterilisation and general hygiene, see Chapter 15, Unit G22 monitor procedures to safely control work operations.

EKU *statement*

GH19 (eku29) The suitability of specific products and equipment for use with different hair types and for achieving different effects

GH19 (eku30) The types of non-conventional items that may be used when setting hair and the effects they can create (e.g. rags, chopsticks, straws, rik-rak etc.)

GH19 (eku19) The health and safety factors to consider when making a choice of non-conventional items

Remember

Make sure that you always

✔ Follow your salon's policy in respect to standards and public image

✔ Prepare yourself in a professional manner ready for work

✔ Wear the minimum of jewellery that can dangle or tangle in the client' hair

✔ Wear appropriate footwear

✔ Be aware of your personal hygiene

✔ Minimise the risk of cross-infection to your colleagues and clients

✔ Work responsibly and respectfully within the salon's service timescales

Styling materials and tools

Equipment	Effects achieved	Precautions	Cleaning
Highlight foil (concertina folded)	Produces zig zag set effects that can have uniform or tapering effects on wet or dry hair	If you use a hood dryer to help set the hair, remember that foil retains heat, so it could burn the client!	It is unlikely that you would keep used foils, as these can be disposed with in a sealed bin
Rags	Creates twisted spiralled curl effects on wet hair	No obvious problems, as rags tend to be kinder on hair than any other setting equipment	Machine (hot) wash (if they are to be retained)
Chopsticks	Hair wound in a figure of '8' around two chopsticks produces a softer zig zag effect than foil with wet hair	Be careful not to buckle the ends of the hair, it will produce fish hooks (like perming can). Use end papers or foil	Washed with hot soapy water and scrubbed clean, then dried and put in UV cabinet and finally back in trolleys/trays
Straws	Single long straws can be bent in half to create two legs; on which the hair can be wound in figure of 8 (similar to chopsticks)	Be careful not to buckle the ends of the hair, it will produce fish hooks (like perming can). Use end papers or foil	It is unlikely that you would keep used straws, as these can be disposed with in a sealed bin.
Pre-formed plastic items (e.g. conical vase shape)	Plastic formers can be used to create the bases for all sorts of avant garde effects. Wet hair is wrapped or styled onto bases and fixed in place	The initial fixing of the former to the head is important to the durability of the effect. Spend more time thinking how it can be pierced and gripped to secure it	Make sure that any item is thoroughly washed before it is used! – It is unlikely that you would keep used formers after; so, disposed with safely.

Equipment	Effects achieved	Precautions	Cleaning
Bendy foam covered rollers	These can be used to create spiral curls on wet or dry longer hair, or used more conventionally to produce loose, set results like rollers	Damaged rollers should be thrown away	Washed with hot soapy water and scrubbed clean, then dried and put in UV cabinet and finally back in trolleys/trays in sized order ready for future use
Velcro rollers	On dry hair they produce a softer (and not as durable) curl effect as wet setting rollers	Self-clinging rollers tend to lock onto finer hair types. Be careful when removing as they will not only pull the hair but damage it too	Washed with hot soapy water and scrubbed clean, then dried and put in UV cabinet and finally back in trolleys/trays in sized order ready for future use
Heated rollers	On dry hair they produce a soft but longer-lasting, more durable effect than velcro rollers	These are very hot when they are first put into the client's hair. Use cotton neck-wool as a insulating base between the bottom of the curler and the client's scalp	Washed with hot soapy water and scrubbed clean, then dried and put in UV cabinet and finally back on to their appropriate heating stems ready for future use
Heated tongs/rik-rak stylers	Provides long lasting waves or spiralled curls on dry hair	Electrical item: remember to check the condition of the lead before use. Very hot when in use, be careful not to burn the client or yourself.	Spray cleaner and dried thoroughly after. Remove hairstyling product build up from the curling surfaces
Heated straighteners	Can produce super flat effects on dry hair that is unruly, or curly hair. Can also be used to create spiral curls on longer hair	Electrical item: remember to check the condition of the lead before use. Very hot when in use (up to 200°C) be careful not to burn the client or yourself	Spray cleaner and dried thoroughly after. Remove hairstyling product build up from the styling surfaces
Grips and hair pins	Hair ups, partial hair up/back effects	Grips and pins are metal with sharp points; care should be used when putting them in and when removing them to avoid tugging snatching the hair	Washed and dried and put into trolleys or trays
Pin clips	On wet hair, they provide a narrow curl stem that can be positioned either flat against the skin or standing away	Pin clips tend to have fairly strong durable springs. These can pull the hair if not careful	Washed with hot soapy water and scrubbed clean, then dried and put back in trolleys/trays

Note: Information from level 2

The following information about styling tools is also required at NVQ level 2. If you have recently covered this or you remember the facts, you can skip this information and go on to GH19.2 Creatively style and dress hair.

	Uses	Description	Technique	Cleaning and maintenance
Denman Classic Styling brush DENMAN	General brushing, detangling hair before: shampooing, styling and blow-drying straight hair of any length	A parallel, flat brush with removable cushioned bristles. Available in small (5), medium (7), and large (9) rows of plastic bristles	Blow-drying is achieved by placing the leading edge of the bristles against the mesh of hair then turning the brush to engage the hair across all of the width. The brush is used from roots to points with the dryer blowing across the cushioned surface	Denman brushes can be dismantled by removing the rubber cushioned head from the brush handle and the bristle rows can be removed and washed in hot soapy water, then dried and replaced. Rows of bristles can be replaced if damaged or overheated. Brushes can be placed in a UV cabinet for 15 mins to complete the cleaning sterilisation/sterilisation process
Vented brush DENMAN	For blow-drying straight short and mid-length hair	A parallel, flat brush with a double row of rigid plastic bristles (short and long) affixed to a brush head that is not solid. Allowing air to pass between the bristles	Blow-drying is achieved by placing the leading edge of the bristles against the mesh of hair then turning the brush to engage the hair across all of the width. The brush is used from roots to points with the drier blowing across the cushioned surface	Vented brushes can be cleaned by raking out any loose or tangled hair from the bristles, then washing in hot soapy water. The brush is then dried before use. Brushes can be placed in a UV cabinet for 15 mins to complete the cleaning/sterilisation process
Bristle (curved head) brush COURTESY OF BABYLISS PRO	General brushing detangling hair and pre-dressing hair	A brush with a wide, curved head usually with a cushioned head with finer, closer teeth than a Denman. Sometimes the bristles are natural in composition, but generally plastic	Flatter, curved bristle brushes are not generally used for blow-drying, unlike their radial counterparts. They are more associated with general brushing and brushing out	Bristle brushes can be cleaned by raking out any loose or tangled hair from the bristles, then washing in hot soapy water. The brush is then dried before use. Brushes can be placed in a UV cabinet for 15 mins to complete the cleaning/sterilisation process

	Uses	Description	Technique	Cleaning and maintenance
Radial brushes DENMAN	Blow-drying with volume, lift, wave and curl on shorter or longer length hair	Radial brushes are completely round in section and come in a wide variety of sizes. The bristles are usually made of plastic although pure bristle brushes are still available. The inner body of radial brushes are often made of metal allowing the brush to heat up; improving the drying speeds of the underneath hair within a section.	Blow-drying volume and movement is achieved by placing meshes of damp hair around the brush and drying the hair in position from both sides. When dry, the curl or movement can be affixed or set into position by applying a cool shot to increase the durability of the set	Radial brushes can be cleaned by raking out any loose or tangled hair from the bristles, then washing in hot soapy water. The brush is then dried before use. Brushes can be placed in a UV cabinet for 15 mins to complete the cleaning/ sterilisation process
Diffuser (although not a brush it is a piece of equipment used to style the hair) 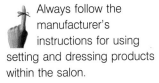 COURTESY OF BABYLISS PRO	Scrunch-drying and finger-drying hair to optimise the natural or permed movement within the hair	A diffuser is an attachment for a blow-dryer that suppresses the blast of hot air and turning it into a multidirectional diffused heat	The hair is styled with the fingers by either pressing into the cupped diffuser to dry or by working through the hair with the fingers until the hair is dried with the required amount of texture or definition	Diffusers are cleaned by spraying with an antibacterial spray then wiped with paper towels

Remember

Scrunch-drying is a way of drying hair more naturally with a diffuser. It uses the natural body or movement within the hair to create tousled and casual effects.

Remember

Root direction will determine hair flow within a style.

Remember

Portable appliance testing (PAT)
All items of electrical equipment have to be annually tested and certified fit for use by a competent person. The items are tested, labelled and recorded and a compiled list is made available for inspection.

Remember

Always follow the manufacturer's instructions for using setting and dressing products within the salon.

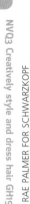

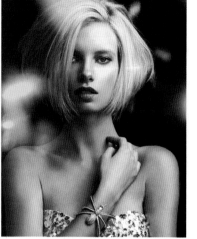

RAE PALMER FOR SCHWARZKOPF

The classic dressing out brush has a cushioned, pure bristle head. This brush is an essential part of the dressing out collection as it is designed to fit into the hand often with a shaped handle that fits the fingers and provides good control for applying backbrushing. The bristled end of the brush can be 'spoon' shaped or be, narrow and parallel in section. This allows the user to take sections between their fingers and applying back-brushing across the whole section in one movement without missing areas. This is particularly useful because back-brushing is softer and less tangling to the hair than back-combing and an even amount needs to be applied throughout the voluminous parts of the hairstyle.

EKU statement

GH19 (eku31) The manufacturers' instructions on the use of the specific setting and dressing products in your salon

Activity
Ionic styling equipment
The term *ionic* crops up a lot with modern styling tools and equipment. It is used to describe new types of blow-drier, heated styling tools and brushes and combs.

Q. What are the claims of ionic equipment technology and in what ways do they benefit the hair?

Tip. You could find more information about these products on the internet. Write your answer in your portfolio.

EKU statement

GH19 (eku30) The types of non-conventional items that may be used when setting hair and the effects they can create (eg rags, chopsticks, straws, rik-rak etc.)

Activity
Styling materials
For each of the items listed below; write down how these items could be used for styling hair and what sort of effects it will produce.

Styling item:	What effects will it produce?	How could the item be used?
Bendy foam rollers		
Highlighting foil		
Rik-rak waving irons		
Rags		
Chopsticks		
Straws		

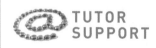 **TUTOR SUPPORT**

Project 8.2: Tools and equipment to style and dress hair

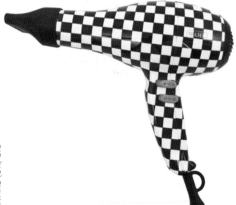

WAHL (UK) LTD

Blow-dryers

The blow-dryer is one of the most commonly used items of equipment in the salon. There is a huge range of models available; with a variety of power outputs, speeds and heat settings. The latest ionic dryers can even reduce the 'flyaway' effect that is produced by static electricity when hair is heated in a colder environment.

Well-designed professional dryer needs to have a number of special features and you should bear this in mind if you buy one.

A good professional hair blow-dryer should:

- have at least two speeds and two heat settings
- have different shaped nozzles to channel the heat onto the brush or comb.
- have a lead long enough not to tangle around the chair or client
- be powerful enough to dry damp hair quickly (1300w–1500w)
- have a 'cool shot' button – to enable hot, dried hair to be quickly cooled and fixed (set) into shape around a brush
- be not too long so that it is balanced in the hand and can be held away from the client's hair during drying
- be light enough so that it can be manipulated easily and used for long periods without fatigue
- be quiet enough so that it allows natural conversation with the client.

Styling products

There is an ever-growing range of styling and finishing products available to the profession. As this has been the major growth area, careful market research and product development have ensured that each one is specifically designed to do a particular job. As a result the huge range is confusing and is driven by successful advertising and brand awareness. If you look closely at each manufacturer's range you will find that the brand leaders all have similar and competing products. The more these numbers of similar products increase, the more confused the purchaser becomes. At this stage the only factor that can help someone to make a choice between one product and another is a reputable and recognisable name.

Styling products contain plasticisers as a fixative to hold and support the hair in its shape. Apart from hold, they often have other agents and additives within the products that can repel moisture, provide protective sunscreens, add shine and lustre or add definition and shape.

Setting lotions Such as mousses protect the hair from excessive heat. They increase the time that the hair is held in shape and the volume and/or movement created, all whilst being exposed to the blast from the dryer's nozzle. They can be in a variety of different strengths for differing hair types and holds.

Finishing products Are products that enhance the hair by giving hold, adding shine or gloss and improve handling and control by removing static, fluffiness or frizziness from the hair. Certain finishing products like waxes will define the movement in hair, giving texture or spikiness that could not otherwise be achieved.

Heat protection Many products provide protection from heat styling. Regular use of straightening irons could damage the hair so there are a number of products that can be applied to eliminate any long-term effects. Other products provide protection from harsh UVA in sunlight in a variety of 'leave-in' treatments that can be used at any time. They are put on before exposure to harsh sunlight and can be removed after by washing. This is particularly useful for clients who have coloured hair, as the bleaching effects of sunlight will quickly remove colour. Other products have the ability to resist or remove the effects of minerals on the hair such as chlorine from swimming pools. This is particularly useful as blonde hair that is regularly subjected to chlorine tends to look green!

EKU *statement*

GH19 (eku18) The importance of using products economically

GH19 (eku23) The physical effects of styling and finishing products on the hair and how they work to maintain the style

Remember

Always use products sparingly and economically within the salon and avoid over loading the hair during styling.

Make a point of explaining the benefits of using professional products to your clients so that they can achieve similar effects themselves at home.

Remember

Moisture is the enemy of any finished set. It weakens the hold and therefore how long the overall effect will last.

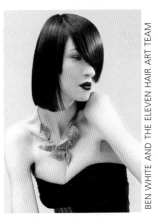

BEN WHITE AND THE ELEVEN HAIR ART TEAM

EKU *statement*

GH19 (eku21) The effects of humidity on hair

GH19 (eku22) The physical effects of styling on the hair structure

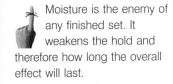

Pros and cons for products

Properties → Product ↓	Positives	Negatives	Advice for clients
WELLA — Mousse (styling product)	Good for general styling use; Can be used in blow-drying or as a setting agent	None really, although mousses between manufacturers vary a great deal	Explain that not all products are the same. Professional products are very different from that available in high street shops
IMAGE COURTESY OF GOLDWELL — Setting lotion (styling product)	Good for setting, easy to apply and distribution throughout the hair is very good	Limited uses: not really suitable for any brush dried styling, tends to 'bind' to easily	If the client needs to get support from setting rather than blow-drying this could be a better option than mousse
WELLA — Styling gel/glaze (styling product)	Produces a firm hold that will provide long lasting textured effects	Takes a while to dry so any 'high-hair' effects need to be held in place until dry. Absorbs moisture from the air readily; so tends to collapse quickly	Match the client's needs with the product. If the client has an outdoor lifestyle the product will not hold height or volume in humid conditions
IMAGE COURTESY OF GOLDWELL — Dressing cream (finishing product)	Good for applying texture into any texture hair as a finishing product. Easy to apply, lasts well	Be careful in the application of finishing products. If you over apply you might find yourself starting over!	Match the client's needs with the product. Very easy to use and essential for quick invent-reinvent hairstyling
WELLA — Serum (setting/ blow-drying finishing product)	Good for achieving a smooth controlled finish on straighter hair	Be careful in the application of finishing products. If you over apply you might find yourself starting over!	Match the client's needs with the product. Great for improving the handling of dry, or unruly hair. Adds lustre and shine
IMAGE COURTESY OF GOLDWELL — Wax (setting/ blow-drying finishing product)	Good for applying texture into any texture hair as a finishing product. Easy to apply, lasts well repels moisture	Be careful in the application of finishing products. If you over apply you might find yourself starting over!	Match the client's needs with the product. Choose the right wet or dry type wax to suit the client and tell them why you recommend one rather than another

Properties → Product ↓	Positives	Negatives	Advice for clients
Hairspray (setting/blow-drying finishing product)	There are hairsprays for every type of hold and for producing all sorts of finishes. Still a great favourite with easy application	None: ensure that you use the right product for the right finish	Match the client's needs with the product. Recommendation is essential for the client to maximise the benefits of hairsprays
Heat protection	Essential products for straightening irons or crimpers. Protects and helps to set the hair all in one	None	Essential recommendation for anyone using very hot styling equipment on a regular basis

WELLA

IMAGE COURTESY OF GOLDWELL

TUTOR SUPPORT

Project 8.3: Benefits of styling products

Activity
Equipment and their uses
From the following list of equipment indicate which ones are suitable for the lengths of hair indicated in the three columns.

For those that you have marked as suitable now describe what sorts of effects they will achieve.

	Short hair	Medium length	Long hair
Denman brush			
Vented brush			
Rags			
Chopsticks			
Heated straighteners			
Heated rollers			

Hair science

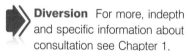

The physical changes that take place during setting

Hair is both flexible and elastic. As alpha keratin, or unstretched hair, is curled or waved, it is bent under tension into curved shapes. The hair is stretched on the outer side of the curve and compressed on the inner side. If it is dried in this new position, the beta keratin, or stretched hair curl will be retained. This happens because when hair is set the hydrogen bonds and salt bonds between the keratin chains of the hair are broken. The linking system is moved into a new temporary position. (The stronger disulphide links remain unbroken.)

Hair, however, is hygroscopic – it is able to absorb and retain moisture. It does so by capillary action: water spreads through minute spaces in the hair structure, like ink spreading in blotting paper. Wet hair expands and contracts more than dry hair does, because water acts as a lubricant and allows the link structure to be repositioned more easily. So the amount of moisture in hair affects the curl's durability. As the hair picks up moisture the rearranged keratin chains loosen or relax into their previous shape and position. This is why the humidity – the moisture content of air – determines how long the curled shape is retained, so moisture causes a set to drop.

The condition and the porosity of hair affect its elasticity. if the cuticle is damaged, or open, the hair will retain little moisture, because of normal evaporation. The hair will therefore have poor elasticity. If too much tension is applied when curling hair of this type it may become limp, overstretched and lacking in spring. Very dry hair is likely to break.

GH19.2 Creatively style and dress hair

Consultation

Diversion For more, indepth and specific information about consultation see Chapter 1, Unit G21 Provide hairdressing consultation services p. 6.

Consultation is an essential part of every hairdressing process; you will always need to find out a variety of information before you start.

If you have already reviewed this information or covered it previously within your training, here is a quick checklist to cover the applicable aspects for setting and dressing hair.

Consultation checklist before setting hair

✔	What is the texture, type, tendency and condition of the hair like?
✔	How much hair is there, how long is the hair?
✔	Are there any limiting factors or adverse hair or scalp conditions?
✔	What type of effect does the client want?
✔	Does the hair type/texture/tendency/amount and length support the client's ideas?
✔	What tools and equipment do you need?
✔	What lifestyle limitations are there?
✔	How much time will it take?
✔	How much will it cost?
✔	Do you need to use any products to achieve the effect?
✔	Will the client benefit from using these products too?
✔	Agree and confirm desired effects with the client prior to starting the service.

EKU *statement*

GH19 (eku24) How the incorrect application of heat can affect the hair and scalp

GH19 (eku25) Why hair should be allowed to cool prior to dressing

The principles of heat styling

Both setting and blow-drying are methods of forming wet or damp hair into shape and then fixing it with the aid of heat to create a finished look. These methods of styling and dressing hair are temporary and the looks can be either classic or fashionable. You can make hair straighter, curlier, fuller, flatter or wavier.

The styling involves placing and positioning wet hair in to selected positions, and fixing the movement in to it, while it is dried into shape. You may roll the hair round curlers, or around a brush. Once dry, you complete the process by dressing the hair with brushes and combs.

The hair should never be excessively heated otherwise permanent damage will result, so always keep an eye on the:

- time the client is seated under the dryer, so that they don't get too hot and longer-term hair damage doesn't occur
- direction of heat and the time it is focused on the hair from the hand dryer.

Before removing rollers or formers from the hair; allow them to cool down in position after taking out of the dryer. The cooling allows the hair set to fix into position as hot hair can 'relax' back to its previous state. In Blow-drying this principle is assisted by a cool shot, this helps to fix the curl in after using a round or curved brushes.

The dressing part involves the manipulation of the hair in a planned and controlled way. It starts with the removal of the setting marks by brushing and then continues as the hair is combed out. The level of finish achieved during the comb out relies upon the dexterity and skill of the stylist.

Activity
Using electrical equipment
A lot of the equipment safety issues are more to do with common sense.

What things come to your mind when you handle salon electrical equipment?

List down at least six safety precautions that should be considered when handling electrical equipment.

1

2

3

4

5

6

Checklist:

Before styling:

✔	Prepare the client by carefully gowning them and making sure that they are comfortable
✔	Find out what the client wants, the type of occasion/event
✔	Look for factors that will influence your styling options: i.e. physical features, style suitability, growth patterns or density for example
✔	Use visual aids to agree on the effect
✔	Get your materials, products and equipment ready
✔	Check the condition of the electrical tools
✔	Pre-wash, condition and detangle (if working on wet hair)

During styling:

✔	Check the heat from the dryer: is the client comfortable?
✔	Check the style's construction: is the shape and proportions correct?
✔	Do you need additional movement from heated styling equipment?
✔	Does the hairstyle need additions: added hair, ornamentation, grips pins etc?
✔	Is the finished hairstyle OK; if not, what aspect needs to be changed?

EKU *statement*

GH19 (eku21) The effects of humidity on hair

Hair science

The effects of humidity on the hair

As with other techniques, setting/blowdrying produces only a temporary change in hair structure (and this is covered below). The fixed or set effect is soon lost if/when moisture is absorbed or introduced to the hair. You have probably already discovered this yourself: if, after having your hair done, you take a bath in a steamy bathroom, what happens to the hairstyle?

Moisture is all around us though and, in more extremes of **humidity**, it is seen as mist and fog. To help prevent style deterioration from happening, a wide variety of setting aids are available to slow down the 'collapsing' process and therefore hold the shape longer.

Different effects can be produced by different techniques:

- *increasing volume* – adding height, width and fullness, by lifting and positioning 'on base' when rollering or curling
- *decreasing volume* – producing a close, smooth, contained or flat style by pin-curl stem direction, or by dragged or angled rollering 'off base'
- *movement* – variation of line waves and curls, produced by using differently sized rollers, pincurls or finger waving.

Relaxed hair effects can be produced by wrapping hair or by using large rollers. Different techniques are used for hair of different lengths:

- Longer hair (below the shoulders) requires large rollers, or alternating large and small rollers, depending on the amount of movement required.
- Shorter hair (above the shoulders) requires smaller rollers to achieve movement for full or sleek effects.

- Hair of one length is ideal for smooth, bob effects.
- Hair of layered lengths is ideal for full, bouncy, curly effects achieved by, say, barrel or clockspring curls.

Different techniques can also be used to improve the appearance of hair of different textures:

- Fine, lifeless hair can be given increased body and movement. Lank hair can be given increased volume and movement.
- Coarse thick hair requires firmer control.
- Very curly hair can be made smoother and its direction changed.

Setting techniques

Curls and curling

Curls are series of shapes or movements in the hair. They may occur naturally, or be created by hairdressing – this could be chemically by perming or physically by setting. Curls add 'bounce' or lift to the hair, and determine the direction in which the hair lies.

With styled curls, each has a root, a stem, a body and a point. The curl base – the foundation shape produced between parted sections of hair – may be oblong, square, triangular and so on. The shape depends on the size of the curl, the stem direction and the curl type. Different curl types produce different movements.

You can choose the shape, size and direction of the individual curls: your choice will affect how satisfying the finished effect is and how long it lasts. The type of curl you choose depends on the style you're aiming for – a high, lifted movement needs a raised curl stem; a low, smooth shape needs a flat curl. You may need to use a combination of curl types and curling methods to achieve the desired style – for example, you might lift the hair on top of the head using large rollers, but keep the sides flatter using pincurls.

Winding root to point

Root to point winding is normally carried out on longer-length hair to produce spiralling type curls that can be formed on bendy foam wavers, chopsticks, spiral wavers as a setting method or, alternatively, with heated tongs or spiral tongs. These tend to produce curl formations that have a uniform curl diameter throughout the length.

Winding point to root

On the other hand, conventional (croquignole) winding, which is used in normal setting, produces a curl formation that has a larger curl size at the root that tapers to tighter near the points.

Rollering hair

There are various sizes and shapes of roller. In using rollers or non-conventional formers, you need to decide on the size and shape, how you will curl the hair on to them and the position in which you will attach them to the base.

- Small rollers produce tight curls, giving hair more movement. Large rollers produce loose curls making hair wavy as opposed to curly.

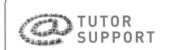

TUTOR SUPPORT

Project 8.4: Materials and items that could be used to 'set' hair

EKU *statement*

GH19 (eku36) Why and how to use point to root and root to point winding techniques

EKU *statement*

GH19 (eku32) Current fashion styling and dressing looks

GH19 (eku34) How the factors in the range affect the setting and dressing processes and finished look

GH19 (eku35) How the angle of winding on and off base influences the volume and direction of the hair movement

GH19 (eku38) The variety of styling techniques available and why and when they are used

GH19 (eku39) Current techniques for creatively styling, dressing and finishing hair

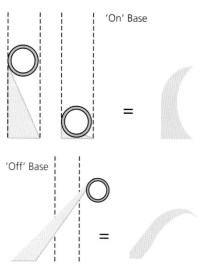

'On' Base

'Off' Base

=

=

On and off base diagrams

- Rollers pinned on or above their bases so that the roots are upright, produce more volume than rollers placed below their bases.
- The direction of the hair wound on the roller will affect the final style.

Pincurling

Pincurling is the technique of winding hair into a series of curls or flat waves which are pinned in place with pin clips while drying. The two most common types curl produced in this way are the barrel curl and the clockspring.

- The *barrel spring curl* has an open centre and produces an even effect. When formed, each loop is the same size as the previous one. It produces an even wave shape and may be used for *reverse curling*, which forms waves in modern hairstyles. In this, one row of pincurls lies in one direction, the next in the opposite direction. When dry and dressed, this produces a wave shape. When used in just the perimeter outline of a short hairstyle they can control the shape and stop the ends (that could be otherwise be set on rollers) from buckling.

- The *clockspring curl* has a closed centre and produces a tight, springy effect. When formed each loop is slightly smaller than the previous one. It produces an uneven wave shape throughout its length. It can be suitable for hair that is difficult to hold in place.

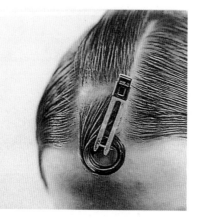

Barrel curl

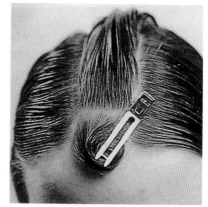

Clockspring curl

Step-by-step: Pincurling

1 Neatly section the hair and comb through any setting lotion – the size of the section will relate to the degree of movement achieved.

2 Hold the hair in the direction it will lie after drying.

3 Hold the hair at the midpoint in one hand using the thumb and first finger, with the thumb uppermost. Using the thumb and first finger of your other hand and thumb underneath, hold the hair a little way down from the hair points.

4 Turn the second hand to form the first curl loop. The hand should turn right round at the wrist.

5 On completion of the first loop, transfer the hair to the finger and thumb of the other hand.

6 Form a series of loops until the curl base is reached. The last loop is formed by turning the curl body into the curl base. The rounded curl body should fit into the curl base.

7 Secure the curl with a clip without disturbing the curl formed in the process.

Curl body directions

A flat curl may turn either clockwise or anti-clockwise. The clockwise curl has a body that moves around to the right and the anti-clockwise a body that moves around to the left. Reverse curls are rows of alternating clockwise and anti-clockwise pincurls; these will produce a finish that has continuous 's' waves, similar to the effect of finger waves throughout the style. Stand-up pincurls produce a waved movement the same as barrel spring curls but with raised crests and deep troughs

Step-by-step: Finger waving

Finger waving is a technique of moulding wet hair into 'S'-shaped movements using the hands, the fingers and a comb. It is sometimes called water waving or water setting. The technique is often used as part of an overall finished style. To form the wave:

1 Use one finger of one hand to control the hair and to determine the position of the wave. Comb the hair into the first part of the crest, and continue along the head.

2 Place the second finger immediately below the crest formed, and comb the hair in the opposite direction.

3 Form the second crest similarly, to complete the final wave shape.

Remember

Common pincurl faults

✔ Tangled hair is difficult to control. Comb well before starting.

✔ If the base is too large curling will be difficult.

✔ If you hold the curl stem in one direction but place it in another the curl will be misshaped.

✔ If you don't turn your hand far enough it will be difficult to form concentric loops.

Remember

✔ Never place grips or pins in your mouth – this is unhygienic and could cross-infect.

✔ Never place tailcombs in your pocket – you could injure yourself and pierce your body.

✔ Never work on wet slippery floors and always clear up loose clippings of hair.

✔ Never use any items of personal equipment that have not been cleaned or sterilised.

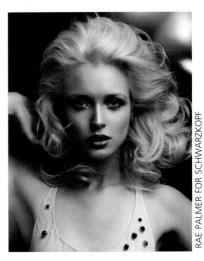

RAE PALMER FOR SCHWARZKOPF

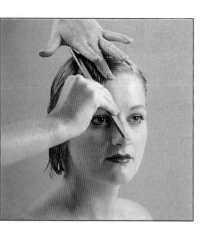

Step 1

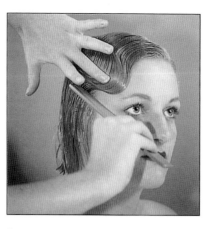

Step 2

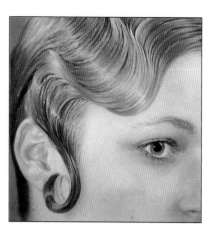

Step 3

> **Remember**
>
> **Finger waves**
>
> - Finger waving is most successful on medium or fine hair that is about 10 cm long. Coarse or lank hair can be difficult.
> - Setting lotion, gel, mousse or emulsion will be needed to hold the waves.
> - Keep your forearm level with or slightly higher than the wrist, to control the hair and your hand during waving. Hold the comb upright and don't use too much pressure when combing, to avoid tearing the scalp.
> - Keep the waves the same size and depth. About 3 cm (the tips of two fingers) between crests is usually best.
> - Pinching or forcing the crests will distort the waves. Correct control and angling will produce the best waves.
> - Positioning is important. Comb the hair to make it lie evenly, and return it to this position after each wave movement is complete.
> - Keep the hair wet (but not dripping) during waving. If you find that it is drying out, dampen it while you work and apply more setting lotion if necessary.
> - Dry the completed shape under a hood dryer, preventing movement or slip.
> - Dressing out should not disturb the waves. The hair is not normally brushed.

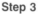

Remember

Clean the gauze filters out on the back of the hand dryer regularly. This will prolong the dryer's life and enable it to work more efficiently too.

Blow-drying hair

Prior to blow-drying hair a hand dryer is fitted with a heat and air focusing nozzle; this stops the dryer from randomly blasting the hair (and anything else) in a haphazard way. As a style is progressed, the nozzle can be moved around so that the client's scalp can be shielded from the potentially damaging, very hot blast and other sections of hair (awaiting styling) are not disturbed by the jet stream.

When the client's hair is ready for styling the excess water must be removed so that:

- only damp and not saturated sections are worked upon
- that the benefits of any styling products are not lost and diluted by excess water

- the client's hair is not unduly or excessively overheated
- the client remains comfortable and dry throughout the process rather than getting wet and cold.

Drying the hair – roots to points

Blow-drying from root to point ensures that the cuticle lays flat therefore reducing fly away frizz and smoothing the overall result.

Water moisture will naturally fall down the hairshaft with gravity, so by starting near the root area will always quicken the drying process. After a couple of passes through the hair the section will be dry If you are using a radial type brush you will find that you need to take a section (like that of rollering) and wind the hair around the brush. Again, focus the jet stream over the curved surfaces of the brush, but this time from both sides. This will enable the hair to dry around the brush forming part of the wave. Then after drying and while still warm, use a **cool shot** from the dryer (or use blast only without heat settings) to quickly cool and fix the wave into place. (This fixes the style with more durability like in setting; when rollers are allowed to cool down before removal and final brushing and dressing out.) If you do not allow the meshes of hair to cool it will result in a less firm result and will not last as long.

EKU *statement*

GH19 (eku20) The reasons why tools and heated styling equipment should be kept free from product build up

GH19 (eku24) How the incorrect application of heat can affect the hair and scalp

Step-by-step: Blow-drying hair

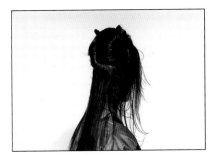

Step 1 Section off the hair and secure out of the way

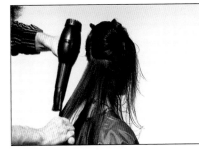

Step 2 Keep an even tension and the heat blast parallel to the hair

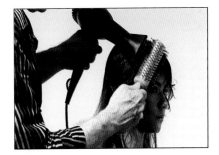

Step 3 Dry the hair in different ways to ease out the movement

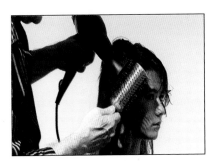

Step 4 Turn the nozzle to keep the air blast parallel to the brush surface

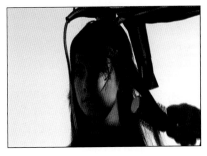

Step 5 Continue on the other side

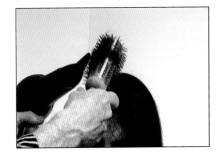

Step 6 Finish off the drying by styling the fringe

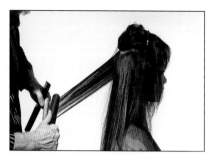

Step 7 Retrace your steps by working through with the straightening irons

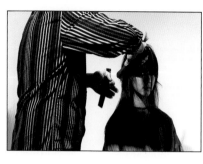

Step 8 Take care not to burn the client

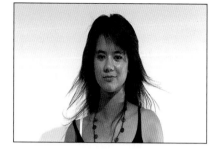

Step 9 Finished effect

Remember

If too much heat is applied to the hair it will sustain permanent, unrepairable damage.

Excessive heat will damage cuticle, remove essential moisture from the hair and make hair very difficult to manage.

Remember

Alpha and beta keratin
The keratin bonds of unstretched hair are in alpha keratin state and the keratin bonds of stretched hair are in beta keratin state. This is the basis of cohesive or temporary setting.

Remember

The temporary bonds (beta keratin state) within the hair are only reformed when the hair is completely dry.

However, they will revert to their former (alpha keratin state) if moisture or water is introduced to the hair.

Remember

Always let the hair cool before removing all the rollers. Hot hair may seem dry when you first check it, but when it cools it may actually be damp.

Dressing hair

Dressing is the process of achieving finish to previously set or styled hair. Dressing uses brushing and combing techniques, and dressing aids such as hairspray to keep the hair in place. If you have constructed the set carefully and accurately only the minimum of dressing will be required. The initial part of any dressing out requires a partial removal of the roller or styling marks so that the final dressing can begin. The hair is then finished with backbrushing and smoothing or the use of heated styling equipment such as tongs, straighteners or crimpers etc.

Backbrushing

Backbrushing is a technique used to give more height and volume to hair. By brushing backwards from the points to the roots, you roughen the cuticle of the hair. Hairs will now tangle slightly and bind together to hold a fuller shape. The amount of hair backbrushed determines the fullness of the finished style.

Tapered hair, with shorter lengths distributed throughout, is more easily pushed back by brushing. Most textures of hair can be backbrushed because it adds bulk, the technique is especially useful with fine hair.

Step-by-step: Backbrushing

1 Hold a section of hair out from the head; for maximum lift, hold the section straight out from the head and apply the backbrushing close to the roots.

2 Place the brush on the top of the held section at an angle slightly dipping in to the held section of hair.

3 Now, with a slight turn outwards with the wrist, turn and push down a small amount of hair towards the scalp.

4 Repeat this in a few adjacent sections of hair.

5 Smooth out the longer lengths in the direction required, covering the tangled backbrushed hair beneath.

Note: **The more the hair is backbrushed the greater the volume and support will be.**

Backcombing

This technique is similar to backbrushing above; however, in this situation a comb is used rather than a brush to turn back the shorter hairs within a section to provide greater support and volume. Backcombing is applied deeper toward the scalp than back-brushing and therefore provides a stronger result.

> **Activity**
>
> This activity is designed to satisfy the essential knowledge statement above. You will need to gather information from a variety of sources. Collect together photographs, digital images and magazine clippings about different creative styling, blow-drying, setting and dressing techniques.
> Make sure that you include styles for long hair as well as short; for weddings, special occasions and casual wear.
> Then in your portfolio describe:
>
> 1 How the styles were achieved.
>
> 2 Why each is suitable for its purpose.
>
> 3 The equipment (with examples) that was used to create the effects.
>
> 4 The products (with examples) used to help hold or define the effects.

Added hair

Hair pieces, wefts and extensions have been around for many years and they are a popular option for providing temporary, alternative, styling effects. The main reasons why people want to use them is because they are a relatively quick and cost effective way of achieving:

- more volume, for people who have finer or lank hair or
- additional length for people that want their hair to appear longer.

There are many types of hair piece or extension available. People can choose between:

- added hair pieces that match their own hair – therefore disguising the fact that hair has been added in the first place
- added hair pieces that contrast against their hair to quickly achieve highlighted or partial block colour effects – a way of achieving colour for those people who may otherwise not be able to have colour
- added hair pieces that provide strong fashion statements as an extension of their personality and personal image, e.g. Amy Winehouse.

EKU *statement*

GH19 (eku26) The effects of backcombing and back brushing on the hair structure

Remember

Backcombing is applied to the underside of the hair section. Don't let the comb penetrate too deeply otherwise the final dressing and smoothing out will remove the support you have put in.

EKU *statement*

GH19 (eku37) Methods of handling and securing added hair and accessories

GH19 (eku43) How to remove pins, accessories, any added hair and any backcombing and/or back brushing

GH19 (eku27) The potential effects on the hair structure of using and securing added hair and accessories

GH19 (eku33) Sources of creative information and inspiration (e.g. historical, cultural and fashion)

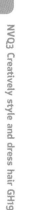

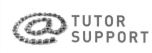

TUTOR SUPPORT

Project 8.5: Types of added hair

▶ **Diversion** For more information about hair pieces, wigs etc., see Banbury Postiche www. banburypostiche.co.uk.

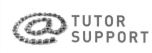

TUTOR SUPPORT

Discussion 8.1: Situations in which extra hair could be used on clients

EKU *statement*

GH19 (eku40) The type of checks needed during styling and dressing services to ensure the intended shape, direction, balance and volume is achieved.

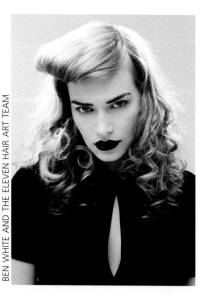

BEN WHITE AND THE ELEVEN HAIR ART TEAM

Generally speaking, the base or fixing of the hair must be well hidden and secure. Your client must feel confident that the hair will stay in place for the duration it is worn. You can make sure that the fixing is secure by interlocking two kirby grips into (backcombed hair if necessary) the hair and placing the comb or clip behind them.

Most hair pieces/extensions are artificial. They are made of a form of acrylic or nylon which is more difficult to manage than real hair itself. Make sure that you tell your client this during the styling as they can not be heat styled after they have been placed. Show them how to remove them and any hair ornaments from the hair without putting any tension on the rest of the hair as this may cause damage.

Acrylic pieces can only be cleaned in cold water using specialist products suitable for extensions and avoid using hairspray or other styling products as this tends to bind them making them difficult to separate or manage.

Not all hair pieces are artificial; interest is growing and there are more natural hair type pieces available. These are more expensive, but if they are looked after properly they do pay back in the longer term as they can be coloured, styled, permed, washed and dried just like normal hair.

Activity

Answer these questions in your portfolio:

1 What difference would there be from setting with rollers on base as opposed to off base?

2 What type of effect do you get from clockspring pin curls?

3 What type of effect do you get from barrel spring curls?

4 Why do you need to brush the hair first when combing out?

5 What is the difference between backcombing and backbrushing?

Use the styling mirror to check your progress

As you work keep using the mirror to check the shape that you are creating. If you find that the outer contour is mishaped or lacking volume, don't be afraid to go back to resection and backbrush/comb again or even take down the area of hair that lacks shape and support.

Heated styling equipment

Tongs, brushes and straightening irons

Electrical accessories health and safety checklist

✔	Never get too close to the client's head with hot styling equipment
✔	Never leave the styling equipment on one area of hair for more than a few moments
✔	Always replace the styling tools into their holder at the workstation when not in use
✔	Always check the filters on the back of hand dryers to make sure that they are not blocked (this will cause the dryer to overheat and possibly ignite)

✔	Look out for trailing flexes across the floor or around the back of styling chairs
✔	Let tools cool down before putting them back into storage
✔	Always check for deterioration in flexes or equipment damages
✔	Never use damaged equipment under any circumstances

Activity

In your portfolio explain each of the following:

1 alpha keratin

2 beta keratin

3 why hair should be allowed to cool before it is brushed out

4 the effects of humidity on hair

5 the effects of excessive heat upon the hair

6 what advice on hair maintenance you could give to the client.

Remember

Heated equipment – advice for the client
Heated styling equipment such as straightening irons and tongs work at very high temperatures. When you are ready to use them, tell your client to keep their head still as any sudden movement or twisting could draw the hot surfaces closer to the scalp or even burn them.

Straightening irons, heated brushes and tongs

Electric curling tongs, heated brushes and straightening irons are a popular way of applying finish to a hairstyle. They are particularly useful in situations where:

- setting or blow-drying will not achieve the desired look
- the hair is not in a suitable condition to be dried into shape.

Professional heated tongs (and many hair straighteners) usually have a thermostatic temperature control, this is particularly useful so that you can *dial up* the heat setting required to achieve the desired effect for a particular hair type. This eliminates the chance of damage to the hair caused by excess heat.

Straightening irons and particularly ceramic straightening irons have been a very popular way of calming unruly hair. They work by electrically heating two parallel plates so that the hair can be run between them in one movement from roots to ends, smoothing out the unwanted wave or frizz in the process.

Ceramic straighteners have been particularly successful as they heat up in just a few moments and have a higher operating temperature than metal irons (170°C). This alarmingly high temperature would initially be considered as damaging to hair but, because they have the ability to transfer heat quickly and smoothly to the hair without *grabbing*, they are very effective in creating smoother effects. But because of their temperature you must check them before you introduce them to the hair so that you don't permanently damage the client's hair.

When straightening is needed to complement the look on longer hair, it is often better to straighten each section as the blow-dry proceeds. If you start underneath, each section is completely finished before you move on up the head. The hair will stay flatter from the outset and each section is totally dry, stopping the hair from reverting to its previous state (i.e. reverting to alpha keratin).

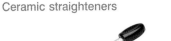

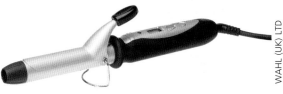

Ceramic straighteners

WAHL (UK) LTD

Curling tongs

WAHL (UK) LTD

Remember

Very hot styling tools without a non-slip coating or ceramic surface can often tend to stick when they are introduced to hair that has styling products on it.

This grabbing effect can cause damage as the hair will bond to the edges of the equipment until it is removed. Always check the temperature settings before you use heated equipment and where possible start at a lower temperatures. Remember you can always turn the temperature up.

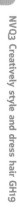

TUTOR SUPPORT

Short answer test 1

EKU *statement*

GH19 (eku41) Products for home use that will benefit the client and those to avoid and why

GH19 (eku42) How to maintain their style

GH19 (eku44) How to give effective advice and recommendations to clients.

The use of crimping irons tends to go through phases of popularity at least once every decade or so. They too have parallel fixed plates but these are wavy and produce flat 'S' waves on longer hair. They are a great styling accessory for competition and stage work as crimped effects are visually striking and very unusual. In staged hairdressing shows models with crimped hair will often accompany the look with strong fashion colours.

Unlike tongs and straightening irons, crimpers are not turned, twisted or drawn through the hair.

1 Each mesh of hair is started near the head and works down to the points of the hair.

2 The meshes should be no wider than the crimping irons and are crimped across the width of the plates.

3 After a few moments of heating each section of the mesh the crimpers are moved to the last wave crest created and pressed again.

4 This is repeated down the lengths of the hair until all of the hair is crimped.

5 The final look is not combed out or brushed, but allowed to fall in waved sections.

Crimping is not advisable on shorter, layered hair unless a frizzy, fluffy look is wanted. The most successful results are on longer, one-length hair.

GH19.3 Provide aftercare advice

Remember

Styling is only part of the formula; clients need the advice on what things they should be using themselves and the products and bad practice that they should be avoiding. Most of the advisory things that you should cover are within this chapter; although others can be found within Chapter 1, Unit G21 Provide hairdressing consultations services.

A good professional service is supported through sound advice and recommendation. The client appreciates what you do and you can tell that by the way that they keep coming back on a regular basis. But unless you tell them how to achieve and maintain the same effects at home, it is unlikely that anyone else will get to see the endeavours of your work.

The checklist below outlines a summary of the things that you should cover.

Home- and aftercare checklist

✔	Talk through the style as you work; that way the client sees how you handle different aspects of the look.
✔	Show and recommend the products/equipment that you use so that the client gets the right things to enable them to get the same effects.
✔	Tell them what products or styling practices that they need to avoid and why.
✔	Explain how routine styling with heated equipment such as tongs or straighteners can have detrimental effects.
✔	Demonstrate the techniques that you use so they can achieve that salon hair look too.
✔	If you have put the client's hair up, or added a hair piece or extensions; give them advice on how to take the style down/remove the hair pieces.

TUTOR SUPPORT

Short answer test 2

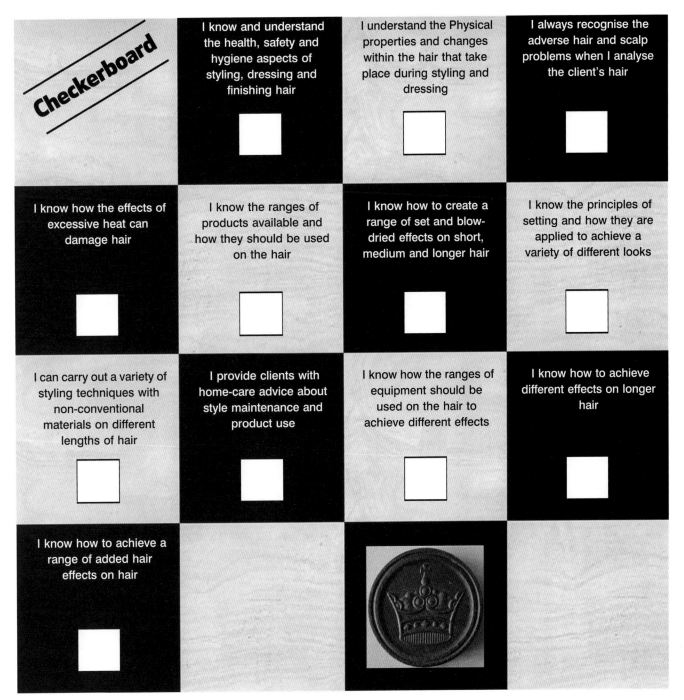

Checkerboard

I know and understand the health, safety and hygiene aspects of styling, dressing and finishing hair ☐	I understand the Physical properties and changes within the hair that take place during styling and dressing ☐	I always recognise the adverse hair and scalp problems when I analyse the client's hair ☐
I know how the effects of excessive heat can damage hair ☐	I know the ranges of products available and how they should be used on the hair ☐	I know how to create a range of set and blow-dried effects on short, medium and longer hair ☐	I know the principles of setting and how they are applied to achieve a variety of different looks ☐
I can carry out a variety of styling techniques with non-conventional materials on different lengths of hair ☐	I provide clients with home-care advice about style maintenance and product use ☐	I know how the ranges of equipment should be used on the hair to achieve different effects ☐	I know how to achieve different effects on longer hair ☐
I know how to achieve a range of added hair effects on hair ☐		

Assessment of knowledge and understanding

Revision questions

Quick quiz: A selection of different types of questions to check your knowledge.

Q1 Self-cling rollers are commonly known as _____ rollers.   Fill in the blank

Q2 Humidity in the atmosphere will help to retain set hairstyles.   True or false

Q3 Which of the following are pincurling techniques?   Multi selection

Rik-rak winding	☐ 1
Off-base rollering	☐ 2
Barrel curls	☐ 3
Clockspring curls	☐ 4
Tonged curls	☐ 5
Chopstick winding	☐ 6

Q4 The keratin bonds of stretched hair are said to be in the beta state.   True or false

Q5 Which chemical bonds within the hair are not affected during setting?   Multi choice

Hydrogen bonds	◯ a
Disulphide bonds	◯ b
Salt bonds	◯ c
Oxygen bonds	◯ d

Q6 Heated rollers are a quick way of setting wet hair in to style.   True or false

Q7 Hair set with rollers on-base, produces which of the following results and effects?   Multi selection

Increased body at the roots	☐ 1
No body at the roots	☐ 2
No movement at the ends	☐ 3
Straighter effects	☐ 4
Wavy effects	☐ 5
Same as blow-dried effects	☐ 6

Q8 Rik-rak stylers produce a _____ waved effect.   Fill in the blank

Q9 Which item of equipment would smooth and flatten frizzy, unruly hair best?   Multi choice

Curling tongs	◯ a
Ceramic straighteners	◯ b
Crimping irons	◯ c
Blow-dryer	◯ d

Q10 Hair should be brushed out with a radial brush before dressing.   True or false

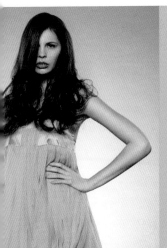

Chapter**nine**
Creatively dress long hair

ADAM HARRIS @ MG MARTIN GOLD, STANMORE

GH20

GH20.1

GH20.2

GH20.3

CREDIT VALUE FOR UNIT GH20

5 Credits

More information

See Unit G22 Monitor procedures to safely control work operations

- Personal hygiene GH20 (eku15)
- General salon hygiene

See also appendices for following relevant legislation:

- COSHH GH20 (eku3)
- Electricity at Work Regulations GH20 (eku4)

Dressing long hair: quick overview

Unit title

GH20   Creatively dress long hair

This is a **optional** unit for students taking hairdressing level 3, it is made up of three main outcomes

Main outcomes

GH20.1   Maintain effective and safe methods of working when dressing long hair

GH20.2   Creatively dress long hair

GH20.3   Provide aftercare advice

What do I need to do for GH20.1?

- Take adequate precautions in preparing yourself and the client before any long hair dressing procedure
- Work tidily, safely and effectively at all times
- Maintain standards of personal health and hygiene
- Use a range of tools and equipment suitable for dressing hair
- Work to your salon's expectations for service and image

What do I need to do for GH20.2?

- Confirm and agree the techniques and style requirements with the client
- Prepare the hair suitably for the styling requirements
- Work in a controlled and methodical way when adding hair or ornamentation
- Produce creative effects in an innovative way
- Conceal any grips, clips, pins or supporting materials

Keywords

Pleats

A finished long hair effect which resembles a vertically folded pleat; more often that not it is centrally positioned at the back of the head to create the style known as a 'French' pleat

Rolls

A roll produces a folded, pleat-like effect in the lateral (horizontal plane) around or at the sides of the head

Knot

When long hair is wound, positioned and secured to take on a tied or knotted rope-like effect

Twist

A technique of styling hair (or multiple stems of hair) by twisting it together to produce head hugging styles or free hanging lengths; they have a similar effect to that produced by fine plaits (corn rows)

Added hair

A general term that covers the addition of hair pieces, wefts and extensions

Traction alopecia

A condition that is caused by the excessive pulling of hair at the root, it is often associated with longer hair worn in plaits, twists and hair ups

Information covered in this chapter

- The materials and tools used for dressing long hair and what they can achieve

- Make sure that your creative shaping, balance, proportions and effects suit the client and meet their expectations
- Apply finishing products to complete the effect

What do I need to do for GH20.3?

- Give the client recommendations and advice for maintaining their own hair

What aspects do I need to cover for GH20.1, GH20.2 and GH20.3?

- A range of long hair dressing techniques e.g. rolls, pleats, knots, twists and plaits
- The factors that influence style suitability

What do I need to know for GH20.1, GH20.2 and GH20.3?

- Your salon's requirements in relation to salon policies and current legislation
- How to work safely and hygienically when dressing hair
- The science that affects dressing long hair
- How to apply added hair and hair ornaments
- The current fashion trends
- How different techniques achieve different results and effects
- How to recommend or provide advice to the client on hair maintenance at home

Remember

Long hair is easier to work with the day after it is washed and that is because clean, well-conditioned, just-washed hair, is often too 'slippy' to work with when it has been dried.

So if you book a long 'hair-up' get your client to wash their hair the night before.

Introduction

Long hair can be daunting, particularly if you are not used to working with it on a regular basis. It's like anything else: if you don't keep the skills up then, when you want to recall how you would tackle something you did ages ago, your confidence lets you down.

'Hair ups' needn't be too difficult, especially if you keep the basics elements firmly in your mind and that is:

- having a clear idea of what you are trying to achieve
- building enough structure and support in to the look to ensure that the finished effect is comfortable and durable.

Other than that, the most important things to remember are:

- choosing a style suitable for the occasion
- assessing whether a particular look or effect is going to suit the client
- giving the client enough visual information to help her get an idea of what can be achieved.

- How to dress long hair creatively into a style
- A variety of dressing techniques that you can use
- The science aspects that impact the dressing of long hair
- The advice you should give to clients in order to maintain their own hair

GH20.1 Maintain effective and safe methods of working when dressing long hair

Long hair dressings are always carried out on dry hair at the styling units and because of this, the main health and safety issues relate to work positioning and client comfort.

Preparing, protecting and positioning the client

GH20 (eku1) Your salon's requirements for client preparation

GH20 (eku6) The range of protective clothing that should be available for clients

GH20 (eku7) How the position of your client and yourself can affect the desired outcome and reduce fatigue and the risk of injury

Preparing and positioning the equipment ready for use

GH20 (eku9) The importance of positioning equipment for ease of use

GH20 (eku10) Why it is important to keep your work area clean and tidy

Working safely and preventing infections

REDUCING RISKS – GOOD SALON SAFETY AND SALON EQUIPMENT (pp. 389–395)

GH20 (eku8) The safety considerations which must be taken into account when setting and dressing hair

GH20 (eku11) Methods of working safely and hygienically and which minimise the risk of cross-infection and cross-infestation

GH20 (eku13) Why it is important to check electrical equipment used to aid the dressing process

GH20 (eku14) Methods of cleaning, disinfecting and or sterilisation used in salons

Your personal health and hygiene

PERSONAL HEALTH AND HYGIENE (pp. 388 and 394)

GH20 (eku12) The importance of personal hygiene

Diversion Much of the other essential information addressing client preparation, health and safety and working effectively and efficiently are a common thread that appears throughout the NVQ level 3 standards, so for your information the following essential knowledge and understanding statements can be found in: Chapter 4, GH16 Creatively cut hair using a combination of techniques (see pp. 72–103).

Diversion This area of work is covered in Chapter 15, Unit G22 Monitor procedures to safely control work operations pp. 374–396.

Remember

Always make sure that your choice of non-conventional hair accessories are safe and hygienic to use.

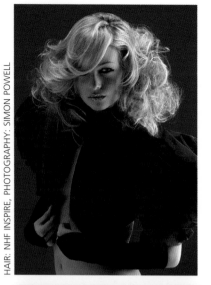

HAIR: NHF INSPIRE, PHOTOGRAPHY: SIMON POWELL

HAIR: MARK WOOLLEY, PHOTOGRAPHY BY PETE WEBB

EKU statement

GH20 (eku14) Methods of cleaning, disinfecting and or sterilisation used in salons

GH20 (eku26) The range of products, tools and equipment available for dressing long hair and how to use them

GH20 (eku5) Your salon's image and expected standards of service

 Diversion For more information on cleaning, sterilisation and general hygiene see Chapter 15, Unit G22 monitor procedures to safely control work operations.

Working with electricity

REDUCING RISKS – WORKING WITH ELECTRICITY (p. 394)

GH20 (eku4) Your responsibilities under the current Electricity at Work Regulations

GH20 (eku13) Why it is important to check electrical equipment used to aid the dressing process

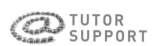 **TUTOR SUPPORT**

Project 9.1: Risk assessment for dressing long hair

Remember

☞ **Think laterally when it comes to ornamentation**
Non-conventional hair accessories can be anything from flowers and foliage to crystals and sequins. It's up to you to think about applying hair ornaments in different ways; that's what creative thinking is.

Activity
Styling materials
For each of the items listed below; write down how these items could be used for styling hair and what sort of effects it will produce.

Styling item:	How could the item be used?	What effects will it produce?	How should this item be hygienically maintained?
Heated rollers			
Heated tongs			
Heated straightening irons			
Crimping irons			

Preparing the tools and equipment for setting and dressing hair

Make sure that you have prepared the area. Get everything that you need together beforehand and this includes the equipment that you need, as well as the products. You should have your trolley prepared with all the materials you will need. Styling materials should have been previously prepared by thorough washing/sterilising and combs, brushes, sectioning clips etc. should be all cleaned, sterilised and made ready for use.

Service timings

Different services take differing lengths of time; you need to be clear in your own mind how long these services take. For example, a French pleat is going to take less time than a full bridal look. So therefore the cost implications in relation to materials used, cost of labour and profit margin required by the salon will all vary considerably. You need to be aware of how much your salon charges for each type of service so that you can inform clients about the range of options available to them.

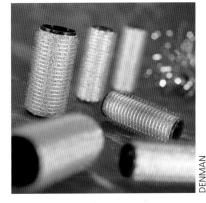

DENMAN

Remember

Make sure that you always:

✔ Follow your salon's policy with respect to standards and public image

✔ Prepare yourself and your materials in a professional manner ready for work

✔ Wear the minimum of jewellery that can dangle or tangle in the client's hair

✔ Be aware of your personal hygiene

✔ Minimise the risk of cross-infection to your colleagues and clients

✔ Work responsibly and respectfully within the salon's service timescales

EKU *statement*

GH20 (eku27) The suitability of specific products and equipment for use with different hair types and for achieving different effects

GH20 (eku28) The types of non-conventional items that may be used as accessories when dressing long hair

GH20 (eku17) The reasons why tools and heated styling equipment should be kept free from product build up

Styling materials and tools

Equipment	Used for	Benefits	Precautions	Cleaning
Heated rollers	Adding more wave/curl to dry hair prior to dressing out.	Makes hair easier to style, improves handling, gripping and pinning into place	These are very hot when they are first put into the client's hair. Use cotton neck-wool as a insulating base between the bottom of the curler and the client's scalp	Washed with hot soapy water and scrubbed clean, then dried and put back on to their appropriate heating stems ready for future use
Heated tongs	Dry curling only. Used for adding more movement.	Provides quick, added support for hair that lacks movement prior to dressing the hair. Or, alternatively, a quick, simple option for styling tendrils, of hair as a way of finishing a 'hair up'	Electrical item: remember to check the condition of the lead before use. Very hot when in use be careful not to burn the client or yourself	Spray cleaner and dried thoroughly after. Remove hairstyling product build-up from the curling surfaces NOTE* Look out for product build-up on heated styling equipment. Clean before use to avoid 'grabbing'

Equipment	Used for	Benefits	Precautions	Cleaning
Heated straightening irons	For use on dry hair; makes hair straighter or adds curls/movement.	Provides a fail-safe way of improving the look and smoothness of the hair before dressing. Provides quick, added support for hair that lacks movement prior to dressing the hair. Or, alternatively, a quick, simple option for styling tendrils, of hair as a way of finishing a 'hair up'	Electrical item: remember to check the condition of the lead before use. Very hot when in use be careful not to burn the client or yourself	Spray cleaner and dried thoroughly after. Remove hairstyling product build up from the curling surfaces

NOTE* Look out for product build-up on heated styling equipment. Clean before use to avoid 'grabbing' |
Tail or pin comb	Sectioning hair into workable sizes dependant on the setting, plaiting or twisting technique used.	They will provide tension when combing through sections and help to manage the hair	The point ends of tail combs can be metal or plastic, but both types are sharp. Be careful in sectioning or combing that you don't scratch the client's scalp	Washed in hot soapy water then kept in Barbicide™ until needed. When needed for setting they should be rinsed and dried first
Straight combs	Dressing out hair; enabling the hair to be backcombed and smoothed	They will provide tension when combing through sections and help to manage the hair	Be careful during combing or backcombing that you don't scratch the client's scalp	Washed in hot soapy water then kept in Barbicide™ until needed. When needed for setting they should be rinsed and dried first
Flat bristle brushes	Flat, bristle brushes when used on wet hair can work setting agents through distributing the product more evenly	Used during dressing to remove roller/setting marks, smooth or shape the hair or introduce backbrushing into the hair	Be careful not to brush to vigorously as it can make hair static or be painful to the client	Washed in hot soapy water and scrubbed clean to remove hair and particles. They should be dried thoroughly and put in a UV cabinet for sterilisation
Ornamental grips and hair pins	Fixing hair into position as part of the finished hairstyle	Provides simple ways of accessorising hair to create, decorative or themed effects	Most metal ornaments have sharp edges; care should be used when putting them in and when removing them to avoid tugging snatching the hair	Handwash carefully in warm soapy water. Can be put into a UV cabinet for storage purposes
Pin clips	Wet or dry setting hair	Provides a narrow curl stem that can be positioned either flat against the skin or standing away	Pin clips tend to have fairly strong durable springs. These can pull the hair if not careful	Washed with hot soapy water and scrubbed clean, then dried and put back in trolleys/trays
Hair grips	Fixing hair into position as part of the finished hairstyle	Choose kirby grips or similar with crimped leg for better grip. Hair ups, partial hair up/back effects	Grips and pins are metal with sharp points; care should be used when putting them in and when removing them to avoid tugging snatching the hair	Washed and dried and put into trolleys or trays

Equipment	Used for	Benefits	Precautions	Cleaning
Hair 'doughnut' rings (see step-by-step 8 later in the chapter for an example)	Used for providing a base for chignons	Great for adding more bulk to hair that lacks density or volume. Makes knots and chignons an easy option for anyone with long enough hair	Take care when removing as hair grips tend to bond on very well	Washed in hot soapy water. Put into washing machine

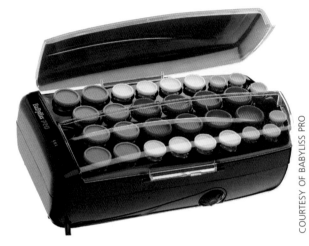

Heated rollers

COURTESY OF BABYLISS PRO

EKU statement

GH20 (eku23) The potential effects on the hair structure of using and securing added hair and accessories

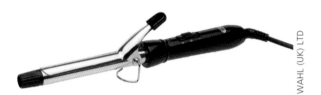

Heated tongs

WAHL (UK) LTD

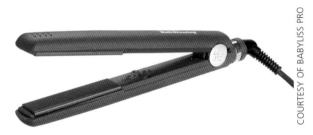

Heated straightening irons

COURTESY OF BABYLISS PRO

Tail or pin comb

DENMAN

Added hair and hair pieces

Added hair type	Advantages	Disadvantages
Synthetic artificial wefts with clip on or comb attachments 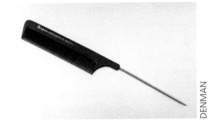 CONNECT-2-HAIR LTD	Very easy and relatively quick to apply Colours don't fade; they are pre-coloured in a variety of single or multi-toned effects Can be shaped and cut easily (not with best hairdressing scissors) to suit or achieve the desired effect Bulks up fine hair, or hair that lacks volume Can provide a quick cost effective solution to people who want longer hair They can be removed at home with care providing the right advice has been given	Needs careful handling, tends to get matted very easily Needs to be brushed regularly when applied to avoid tangling Avoid heat styling as all synthetic extensions are very susceptible to becoming mis-shaped or damaged when excess heat is applied Can cause traction alopecia if incorrectly applied

Added hair type	Advantages	Disadvantages
Natural hair pieces with stitched bases	Lasts for a long time with care and attention Can be shampooed conditioned, styled and shaped with heated equipment just like natural hair Provides a cost effective solution for repeated long term use Fairly easy to apply for the client as well as the professional Colours can be changed just like natural hair. (i.e. decoloured or lightened, toned and coloured) Can be shaped and cut easily to suit or achieve the desired effect Bulks up fine hair or hair that lacks volume	Need some care and attention with handling needs to be shampooed, conditioned and detangled now and again Needs to be gripped into place to secure the added hair base against the rest of the hair Can cause traction alopecia if incorrectly applied
Synthetic – artificial full-head (wigs)	A wide range of price options, providing choice to suit many budgets Lots of choices in natural, fashion and multi-toned effects Pre-styled with little maintenance, can be shampooed and reshaped back into style with little effort (not with best hairdressing scissors) Easy option for those who want to look different or would like 'instant' hair length change Good-quality synthetic wigs are long-lasting, can take daily wear with care for anything up to one year. (Ideal for clients who have lost hair through ill health, radiology or chemotherapy)	Need some care and attention with handling needs to be shampooed, conditioned and detangled now and again
Natural full head hair pieces (wigs)	Can be pre-made or made to order; provides options for any length depending upon needs. Beautifully crafted to suit the wearer Can be shampooed, conditioned, shaped and styled just like normal hair Easy option for those who want to look different or would like 'instant' hair length change Capable of daily wear (with care) for several years. (Ideal for clients who have lost hair through ill health, radiology or chemotherapy)	Expensive

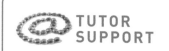

TUTOR SUPPORT

Project 9.2: Added hair that can be used in long hair dressings

---

EKU *statement*

GH20 (eku29) The manufacturers' instructions on the use of the specific finishing products in your salon

Remember

Traction alopecia

The tension on the hair is increased with the use of added hair; this can exert exceptional pressure on the hair follicle particularly on scraped back hair styles or on free hanging effects.

In extreme cases hair loss may be caused by this continued pulling action; areas of hair become thin and even baldness may be result!

Brushes

The variety of brushes available for combing out and hair dressings has been comprehensively covered elsewhere in this book.

Activity

Styling materials

For each of the items listed below; write down how these items could be used for dressing hair and how it should be maintained.

Styling item:	How could the item be used?	How should it be maintained?
Artificial hair wefts		
Natural hair piece		
Full head hair piece (wig)		
Hair 'doughnut' ring		

Remember

Control is the secret when handling long hair; when you have hold of the hair whilst brushing don't let go or lose your grip. You need to keep an even tension upon the hair until it is fixed/pinned into position.

Styling products

There is a wide variety of products available for dressing and adding hair. As a rule of thumb, you should always try to use the minimum amount of product whilst you are dressing the hair as it is very easy to overload the hair and this will:

- make the hair harder to manage as the hair starts to lock together whilst you work with it
- make the hair look greasy as you will not really be able to much about it short of starting again
- look unprofessional – in providing a very average, amateur result
- look unnatural – which most people want to avoid.

Most hairdressers who do use lots of product during the dressing out phase do so because they:

- do not have control of the hair they are trying to manage
- are taking sections that are too large
- have not applied sufficient backbrushing or interlocked grips
- lack the confidence to create the result in the first place or
- have had very little experience in this type of work.

Diversion For more information on added hair/hair pieces see Chapter 8, Creatively Style and dress hair, pp. 181–182.

Diversion To review brushes information again see Chapter 8, GH19 Creatively style and dress hair pp. 166–167.

Remember

Always follow the manufacturer's instructions for using dressing and finishing products within the salon

EKU statement

GH20 (eku24) The potential consequences of excessive tension on the hair and scalp

GH20 (eku25) How to identify the first signs of traction alopecia

EKU statement

GH20 (eku15) The importance of using products economically

GH20 (eku22) The physical effects of finishing products on the hair and how they work to maintain the style

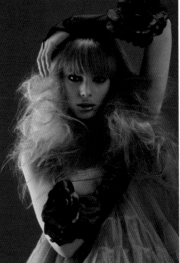

HAIR: NHF INSPIRE, PHOTOGRAPHY: SIMON POWELL

Specific styling products for hair-ups

There are products that are extremely useful in helping you to create the right sorts of results and they fall into the following ranges:

Product	Do use...	Avoid...
Hairspray	Finer atomised, dry hairsprays. They are particularly useful when used during the dressing out as a way of smoothing out unwanted frizzies Hairsprays that repel/resist moisture	Slow drying, hand-pump type hairsprays as these tend to 'clog' up or spray globules onto the hairstyle making it impossible to get a satisfactory finish on the hair Applying too much hairspray as a finish, it's too easy to spoil the effect right at the end when you can do little else about it
Heat protection	Heat protection sprays on the hair if you are going to use heated styling equipment and particularly, straighteners as these operate at very high temperatures	Using these as well as other finishing products. It is easy to overload the hair and spoil the result
Serums	A little initially, as you work and brush the hair when you start Or as a finishing product by applying a small amount on any free hanging tendrils, but not on any part of the fixed hairstyle	Applying too much at any point during the dressing as it will make the hair VERY oily very quickly
Wax	Some dry wax as a *finishing* product to bind 'spiky' or sculpted areas	Using them at any other point of the dressing

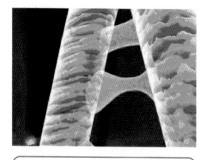

Remember

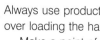 Always use products sparingly and economically within the salon and avoid over loading the hair during styling.

Make a point of explaining the benefits of using professional products to your clients so that they can achieve similar effects themselves at home.

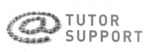 **TUTOR SUPPORT**

Project 9.3: Styling products features and benefits

How styling products bond the hair together

Styling products contain plasticisers as a fixative to hold and support the hair in its shape. Apart from hold, they often have other agents and additives within the products that can retain or repel moisture, provide protective sunscreens, add shine and lustre or add definition and shape.

Remember

 Moisture is the enemy of any finished hairstyle; It weakens the hold and therefore how long the overall effect will last. This can be improved with some moisture-repelling products such as hair spray for example, L'Oréal's AirFix in the Techni-Art range.

Make sure that you point this out to your client, so that they can make the most of their hairstyle.

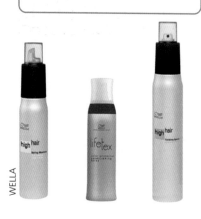

WELLA

Creatively dress long hair

Consultation

The things that you need to find out during consultation change with the type of service that you are going to do. General information for this such as dealing with:

- different hair textures
- different hair types
- different densities of hair
- contra-indications to styling
- client communications
- recording client information.

Can be found in Chapter 1, Unit G21 Provide hairdressing consultation services pp. 4–43.

Other information that specifically relates to dressing long hair can be found below.

Have clear ideas of what you are trying to achieve

Without clear ideas you could be wasting both your time and the client's. Hair ups can be fun, as they tend to be non-routine work and individual in the design. But overrunning the allotted appointment time is both unproductive and stressful, make sure that you keep to time and you will keep calm too.

If the work is for a forthcoming wedding, the bride will often try to get a package price deal that includes a series of trials too. You need to make sure that from the very first consultation (or before that, if at all possible) you ask the bride-to-be to start collecting images of the sorts of things that she would feel happy with. Remember your creation is part of her total look, so ask her to bring in pictures of the dress and also the theme of the wedding that she is trying to create.

Assessing the suitability

This is the first aspect that you should consider. In most cases, hair up is a special situation. It's not a quick, casual throw up that the client does to get her hair out of the way. Clients come to the salon for the things that they can't achieve themselves – that's what hair for special occasions is.

The problem from a suitability point of view is how will the client know if she is going to like her hair up if she seldom has it styled that way? For people that don't normally wear their hair up there are always underlying reasons and these could be:

- their hair is too thick
- they don't like the shape of their ears
- it makes their nose appear bigger
- they prefer their hair to have volume so they don't like it scraped back
- their hair isn't really long enough in the first place.

Don't cut corners! Make sure you look from all different angles too. True, the client only sees what they look at in the mirror, but don't forget that everyone else sees the rest!

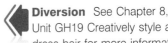

Diversion See Chapter 8, Unit GH19 Creatively style and dress hair for more information on:

- hair styling on the hair structure
- the effects of humidity on hair and hairstyles
- products in general.

EKU *statement*

GH20 (eku18) The effects of humidity on hair

GH20 (eku22) The physical effects of finishing products on the hair structure

EKU *statement*

GH20 (eku2) Your salon's expected service times for dressing hair

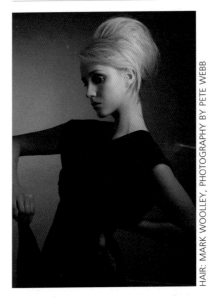

HAIR: MARK WOOLLEY, PHOTOGRAPHY BY PETE WEBB

EKU *statement*

GH20 (eku38) The type of checks needed during long hair dressing services to ensure the intended shape, direction, balance and volume is achieved

EKU *statement*

GH20 (eku35) How the factors in the range affect the dressing process and the finished look

EKU *statement*

GH20 (eku30) The importance of preparing the hair correctly prior to dressing

GH20 (eku39) The importance of maintaining correct tension when dressing up long hair

@ TUTOR SUPPORT

Project 9.4: Current fashion in long hair styling

Take your time If you ignore part of the main construct of the hairstyle it will have a detrimental effect on the overall finished effect. Check and re-check it's worth it in the long run.

Agree the effect before you start

When you have selected a suitable look and you have shown the client examples of how this would look you will need to help with her self-visualisation. Self-visualisation from the client's point of view is very difficult but you can help very easily. You need to try to rearrange the hair loosely, so that she can get an idea of the balance, proportions and weight distribution.

Simple, quick placement can eliminate problems or unwanted effects right from the start such as:

- added height
- extra width
- revealed physical features – forehead, ears or jaw lines.

If you can convey to your client what it will look like roughly, when her face is exposed, and she likes what she sees, you are halfway there. It will save lots of time later and avoid you having to unpick everything that you have done.

General rules for style suitability

Physical features			Facial shapes			Protruding ears	Prominent nose	Short neck
Hairstyle	Oval ○	Round ○	Heart ♥	Triangular ▽	Square □			
Vertical roll/pleat	✔	With height to compensate	✔	With height to compensate	With height and width to compensate	Volume at the sides to cover	Volume at the sides	Needs to be sleek
Barrel spring curls	✔	✔	✔	✔	✔	Volume at the sides to cover (not triangular)	Volume at the sides	Needs to be sleek
Low knot or chignon	✔	With height	✔	✗	With height	Volume at sides except triangular	✗	✗
High knot	✔	✔	✔	✔	✔	Volume at sides except triangular	✗	Needs to be sleek
Plaits	✔	With height	✔	✔	✗	Volume at sides except triangular	✔	Needs to be sleek
Twists	✔	With height	✔	✔	✔ Use designs that involve curves and not straight lines/ linear effects	Volume at sides except triangular	✔	Needs to be sleek

Building enough structure and support in to the look

The simplest mistake that stylists make with 'hair ups', is not making sure that there is enough secure support from the very beginning. This is usually caused by:

- Not putting enough backcombing into the hair initially, because the client isn't used to that type of technique.
- Not creating a comfortable, secure base from which to position and fix the hair into style.
- Not maintaining an even tension on the hair during manipulation; allowing lengths or ends to fall out during the dressing.

The style needs support; it cannot be durable without it. It needs to be secure as well as creative in its effect. It can only be secure if you use things like backcombing, grips or bands.

Reassure your client first; then don't be afraid to backcomb the hair. It may look as if the whole thing is getting too big, but don't forget you can take out as much as you like within the dressing. Backcombing provides you with a solid base that you can grip to without the fear of the grips dropping out.

Maintain your grip and an even tension on the hair as you work; not too tight or rough, but firm enough to gain a grip on all the hair that you are trying to fold, pin or fix into place.

As you become more experienced in handling long hair, you will find that you won't need to use much spray in the styling stage, but only later in the finishing off.

 Diversion For more information on backbrushing, backcombing and other dressing techniques see Chapter 8, Unit GH19 Creatively style and dress hair pp. 160–186.

> **Remember**
>
> Backcombing is applied to the underside of the hair section. Don't let the comb penetrate too deeply otherwise the final dressing and smoothing out will remove the support you have put in.

 Remember

Don't put grips in your mouth: it's unhygienic and could cross-infect your client.

The other main tool for giving structure and support is grips. Kirby grips have one leg with a serrated profile; this helps them to interlock together to stay in the hair much better or to comfortably hold large amounts of hair together without pulling or tugging.

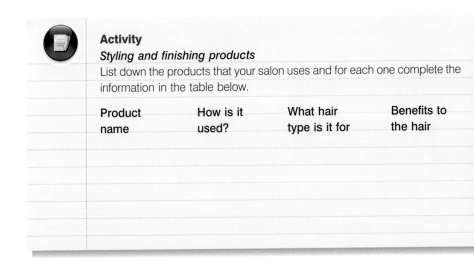

Activity
Styling and finishing products
List down the products that your salon uses and for each one complete the information in the table below.

Product name	How is it used?	What hair type is it for	Benefits to the hair

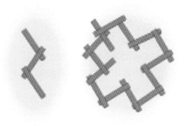

Interlocking grips

Consultation checklist before dressing hair

✔	What is the purpose for the dressing/hair up?
✔	What is the texture, type, tendency and condition of the hair like?
✔	How much hair is there, how long is the hair is there enough to achieve the result?
✔	Are there any limiting factors or adverse hair or scalp conditions?
✔	What type of effect does the client want?
✔	Does the hair type/texture/tendency/amount and length support the client's ideas?
✔	What tools and equipment do you need?
✔	How much time will it take?
✔	How much will it cost?
✔	Do you need to use any products to achieve the effect?
✔	Will the client benefit from using these products too?
✔	Agree and confirm desired effects with the client prior to starting the service.

EKU statement

GH20 (eku19) How the incorrect application of heat can affect the hair and scalp

GH20 (eku20) Why hair should be allowed to cool prior to dressing

Diversion For more information about the effects of heat upon the hair see Chapter 8, Creatively style and dress hair EKU GH19.21, 24 and 25.

Remember

✔ Never place grips or pins in your mouth – this is unhygienic and could cross-infect.

✔ Never place tail combs in your pocket – you could injure yourself and pierce your body.

✔ Never use any items of personal equipment that have not been cleaned or sterilised.

Activity
How are the following items made safe and hygienic and prepared for salon use: Write down your answers in your portfolio.

1 Heated curling tongs

2 Crimpers

3 Ceramic straighteners

4 Hot brushes

5 Heated rollers

6 Hand driers

Remember

Because longer hair takes longer to dry, it is far easier to apply too much heat during the drying. If you have set the hair prior to adding hair or dressing the hair, make sure that you don't burn the client's hair or head.

Activity

Knowing which sort of hair shape will suit which facial shape is part of thinking creatively. In this activity use a simple tick to identify which type of hairstyle is suitable for type of facial shape.

Hair style	Facial shapes				
	Oval ○	Round ○	Heart ♥	Triangular ▽	Square □
Vertical roll/pleat					
Barrel curls					
Low knot or chignon					
High knot					
Plaits					
Twists					

EKU *statement*

GH20 (eku31) The preparation procedures required for the different dressing techniques in the range

TUTOR SUPPORT

Project 9.5: Designing a style for an event

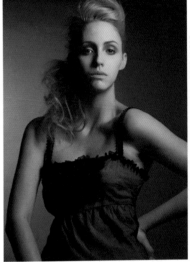

HAIR: MARK WOOLLEY, PHOTOGRAPHY BY PETE WEBB

Vertical roll (French pleat)

The vertical roll is a formal classic dressing that suits many special occasions. The hair can be enhanced further by the additions of accessories or fresh flowers. If you review the planning stages for putting hair up you will see under building the support, that backcombing is an essential aspect for creating a solid foundation. This should be your starting point for the step-by-step procedure.

Step-by-step: Vertical roll (French pleat)

1 Apply a little backbrushing to the back and the sides.
2 Smooth the hair over to cover any visible tangles.
3 While holding the hair across, interlock a row of grips down from the lower crown to the nape.
4 Take the remaining hair back over smoothly to cover the grips.
5 Fold the ends in and secure into place.
6 Finally, arrange any showing ends into place.

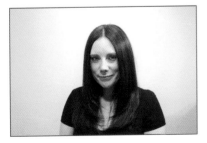

Step 1 Before

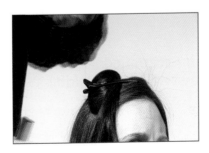

Step 2 Clip hair to be styled later out of the way

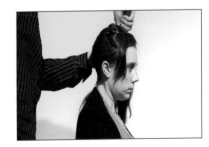

Step 3 Now taking a bristle brush, smooth the hair and hold over to the left

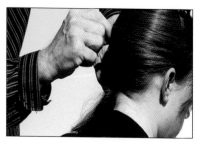

Step 4 Starting at the bottom, create a row of interlocking grips vertically from the left of center

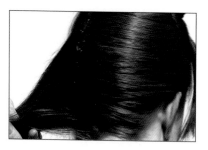

Step 5 Grip base in place

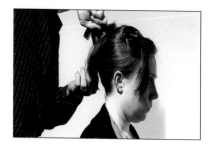

Step 6 Now smooth the hair from the left over to the right and turn inwards to form the fold

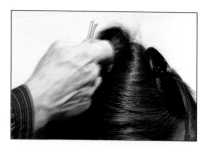

Step 7 Grip down the sides to secure the pleat and tuck in any loose ends

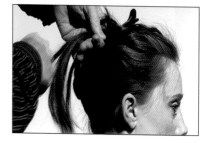

Step 8 Arrange the hair from the front as a decoration for the style

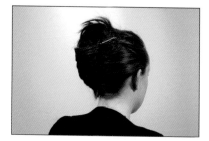

Step 9 The finished pleat

Plaiting hair

Plaiting is a method of intertwining three or more strands of hair to create a variety of woven hairstyles. When this work is done for specific occasions, it is often accompanied by ornamentation: fresh flowers, glass or plastic beads, coloured silks and added hair are also popular.

The numerous options for plaited effects are determined by the following factors:

- number of plaits or twists used
- positioning of the plait or twist across the scalp or around the head
- the way in which the plaits are made (under or over)
- any ornamentation/decoration or added hair applied.

'Plaits' usually refers to a free-hanging stem(s) of hair that is left to show hair length. This length can be natural or can be extended by adding hair during the plaiting process; an example is the 'French' or 'Fish tail' plait.

Step-by-step: Loose plaiting (three-stem (loose) plait)

The three-stem plait is easily achieved and demonstrates the basic principle of plaiting hair.

1 Divide the hair to be plaited into three equal sections.
2 Hold the hair with both hands, using your fingers to separate the sections.

3 Starting from either the left or the right; place the outside section over the centre one. Repeat this from the other side.

4 Continue placing the outside sections of hair over the centre ones until you reach the ends of the stems.

5 Secure the free ends with ribbon thread or a covered band.

Step-by-step: Three-stem 'French' plaiting

1 Brush the hair to remove all tangles.

2 With the hair tilted backwards, divide the foremost hair into three equal sections.

3 Starting from either the left or the right, cross an outside stem over the centre stem. Repeat this action with the opposite outer stem.

4 Section a fourth stem (smaller in thickness than the initial three stems) and incorporate this with the next outside stem you are going to cross.

5 Cross this thickened stem over the centre, and repeat this step with the opposite outer stem.

6 Continue this sequence of adding hair to the outer stem before crossing it over the centre.

7 When there is no more hair to be added, continue plaiting down to the ends and secure them.

Weaving

Hair weaving is a process of interlacing strands of hair to produce a wide variety of effects. A small area of woven hair can be very effective by itself, or used to highlight a particular part of a style. Hair weaving is also used to place and hold lengths of hair. At its simplest, hair weaving may be used to hold long hair back from the face. This may be done by taking strands of hair from each side, sweeping them over the hair lengths, and intertwining them at the back. More intricate is the *basket weave,* which uses a combination of plaiting, twisting and placing to form many shapes and patterns. It is important to wet or gel the hair before starting to weave. Weave tightly or loosely according to the effect you are aiming for. The hair may be woven as follows:

1 Use six meshes of hair, three in the left hand and three in the right.

2 Start with the furthest right-hand mesh. Pass this *over* the inner two meshes.

3 From the left, pass the outside mesh *under* the next two and *over* one.

4 Continue to the ends of the hair.

5 Tuck in the hair ends and secure them in position.

Remember

The tension used in plaiting can exert exceptional pressure on the hair follicle and scalp-type plaits/corn rows create more vulnerability than free-hanging plaits. In extreme cases hair loss may be caused by this continued pulling action; areas of hair become thin and even baldness may be result!

This condition is called 'traction alopecia' and is particularly obvious at the temples of younger girls with long hair who regularly wear their hair up for school, sport or dancing.

EKU statement

GH20 (eku33) Sources of creative information and inspiration (e.g. historical, cultural and fashion)

Remember

Practise on colleagues or models and experiment with different woven shapes before you attempt to weave hair for clients.

EKU *statement*

GH20 (eku32) Current fashion long hair looks

GH20 (eku34) When, why and how to use the different types of – securing equipment – accessories – added hair

GH20 (eku36) The sequence of working necessary to create the dressing techniques and effects listed in the range (i. e. rolls, pleats, knots, twists, plaits, curls, woven effects)

GH20 (eku37) Methods of handling, controlling and securing long hair during the dressing process

GH20 (eku28) The types of non-conventional items that may be used as accessories when dressing long hair

Activity

This activity is designed to satisfy the essential knowledge statement above. You will need to gather information from a variety of sources.

Collect together photographs, digital images and magazine clippings about different types of creative dressings. Look for styles covering a range of themes *and* for different occasions.

Make sure that you include styles for adding hair to short hair as well as long hair.

Then in your portfolio describe:

1   How the styles were achieved

2   Why each is suitable for its purpose

3   The equipment (with examples) that was used to create the effects

4   The products (with examples) used to help hold or define the effects

Step-by-steps

Barrel curls with cross-branding

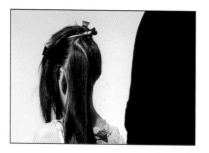

Step 1 Before

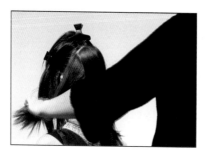

Step 2 Brush and separate the hair

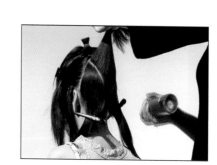

Step 3 Divide into blocks and temporarily secure

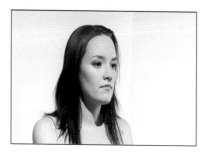

Step 4 The left section will start the cross-banded effect

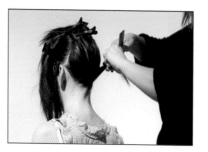

Step 5 Take a neat small section across to the right and secure with a grip

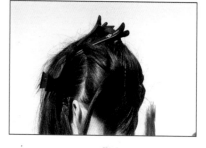

Step 6 Do the same on the right back over to the left

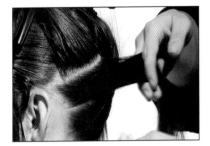

Step 7 Close-up of section

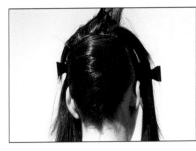

Step 8 The back effect

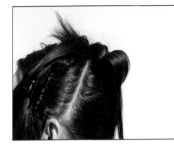

Step 9 Form a barrel curl high up just beneath the crown

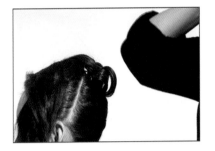

Step 10 Check your profile shape

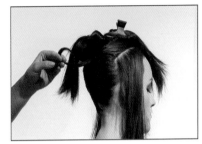

Step 11 Form the second barrel curl

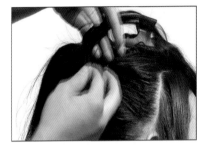

Step 12 Continue shaping to form a nest of curls

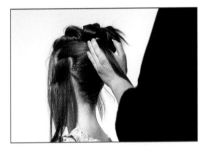

Step 13 Take the side lengths back and fix into place beneath the curls

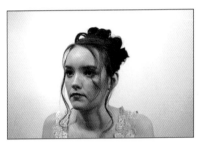

Step 14 Finished effect

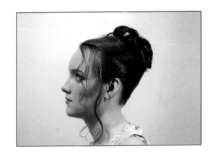

Step 15 Finished effect from the side

Contemporary knots

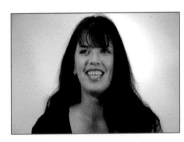

Step 1 Before

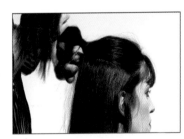

Step 2 Take a horse-shoe section and secure with a band

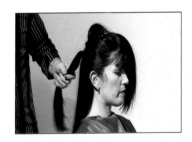

Step 3 Take a second horse-shoe section

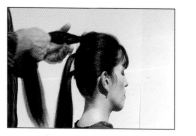

Step 4 And a third, leaving the tails to hang freely

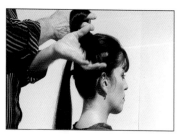

Step 5 Take the top pony and tie in a loose knot, temporarily secure the free ends out of the way

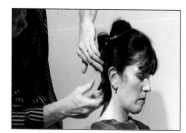

Step 6 Do the same with the second

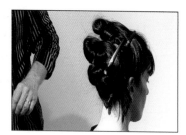

Step 7 And again with the third

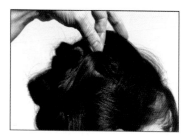

Step 8 Now take the bottom ends up to the top knot and secure the ends out of sight

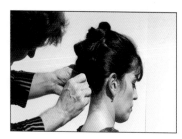

Step 9 Fold in the ends from the other loose pony tails in a 'figure of eight'

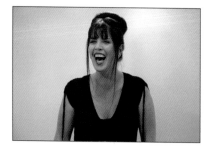

Step 10 Finished effect

Contemporary beehive

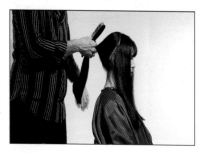

Step 1 Divide off the back hair away from the front

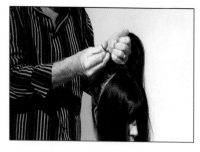

Step 2 Secure in a high position above the crown

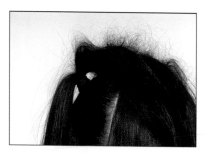

Step 3 Backcomb the hair to add extra body

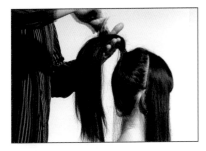

Step 4 Smooth the hair to cover the backcombing

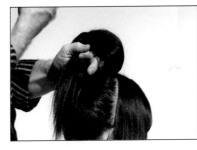

Step 5 Form a shell shape and apply a little spray

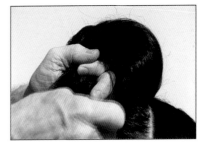

Step 6 Secure the shell shape

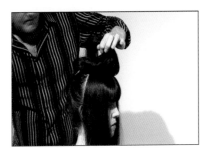

Step 7 Check the balance in the mirror

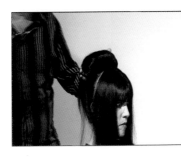

Step 8 Grip into position

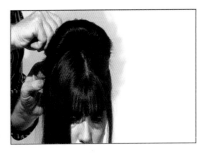

Step 9 Apply the decoration and cover the grips

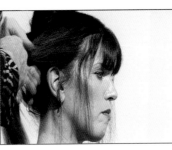

Step 10 Take the sides back and secure into place

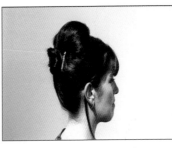

Step 11 Finished effect

Contemporary effect with a twist

Finding hair ups that are not too formal or too casual can be very difficult. So where do you draw the line? What is the difference between fun and formal?

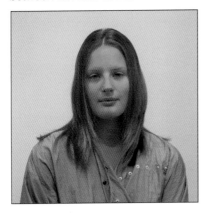

Step 1 Before

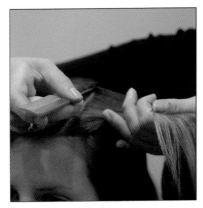

Step 2 After brushing the hair to remove any tangles, start the style at the front by dividing the hair with a tail-comb

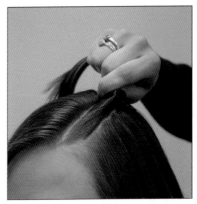

Step 3 Twist the section of hair firmly but not too tightly back towards the crown area

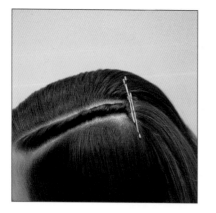

Step 4 Grip the twisted section into place before starting the next channel

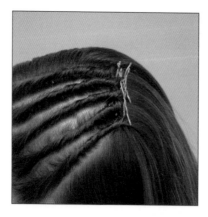

Step 5 Continue with the same technique on each of the channels

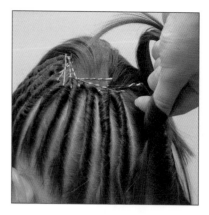

Step 6 Twist the sections at the back from the nape up to the crown in the same way

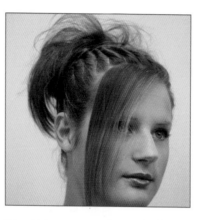

Step 7 Leave a section at the front to soften the hairline profile. Lightly backcomb the remaining hair to finish effect

Party look 1

There are classic, traditional looks and avant garde dramatic effects. This is an example of a romantic effect for special occasions.

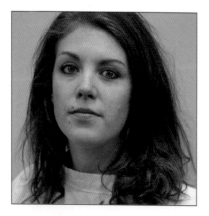

Step 1 Before: clients with this type of look 'shout out' for soft, romantic effects. In this hair up the hair is prepared by curling it first

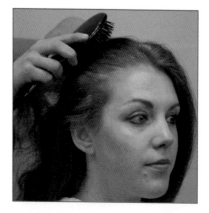

Step 2 Brush the hair to remove tangles

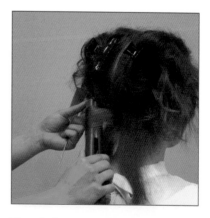

Step 3 Start at the lower nape, so that each curl placed does not disturb those done previously

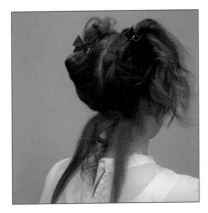

Step 4 Use ceramic straighteners to produce curls by drawing them quickly down the section of hair in one continuous movement

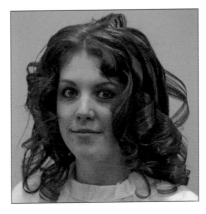

Step 5 The hair after curling, ready for positioning

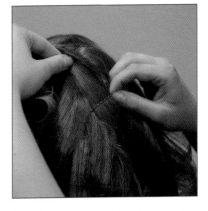

Step 6 Lift and grip into place sections of curls

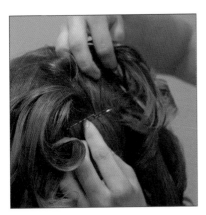

Step 6 *Continued*

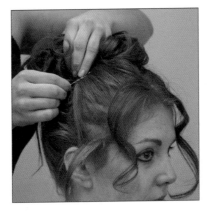

Step 7 Work up and around to the final placements at the front

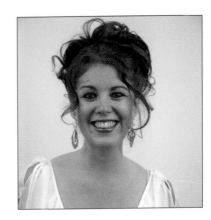

Step 8 The final effect

Party look 2

Cross-banded to produce an interwoven effect, this style incorporates a low asymmetric chignon to complete the look.

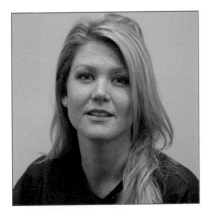

Step 1 Before: Kim suits classic effects such as chignons, pleats and soft folded hair

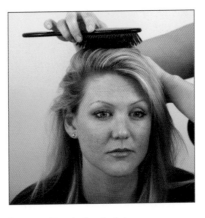

Step 2 Brush the hair to remove tangles

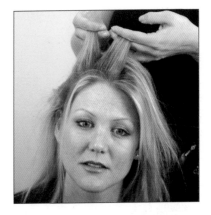

Step 3 Then, starting at the front, take two sections of hair

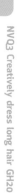

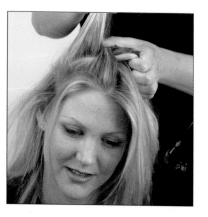

Step 4 Holding the two sections in one hand, take a third

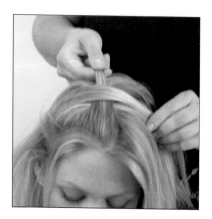

Step 5 Interlock the sections by weaving them together

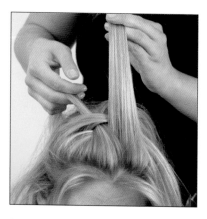

Step 6 Introduce another section of hair

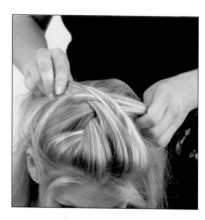

Step 7 Continue the technique through the top

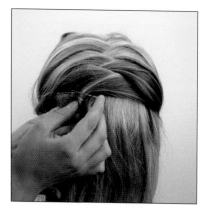

Step 8 Now fix these sections into place with grips

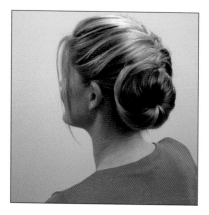

Step 9 A low, asymmetrical chignon finishes the effect to create a simple, classic look suitable for any event

Simple chignon (with the aid of a 'hair doughnut')

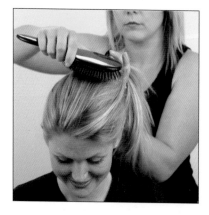

Step 1 Brush the hair through to remove any tangles

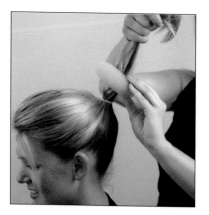

Step 2 Apply 'doughnut' former around a pony tail at the position where you want the chignon to be

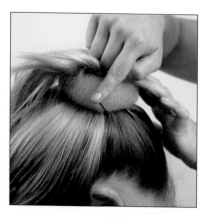

Step 3 Position and grip the former into place

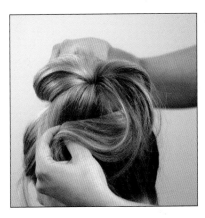

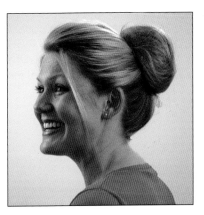

Step 4 Separate the hair and place it around the former. Grip the hair to the base underneath

Step 5 A light mist with spray and the effect is complete

GH20.3 | Provide aftercare advice

A good professional service is supported through sound advice and recommendation. The client appreciates what you do and you can tell that by the way that they keep coming back on a regular basis. But unless you tell them how to achieve and maintain the same effects at home, it is unlikely that anyone else will get to see the endeavors of your work.

Before the client leaves the salon, you need to give advice on what things they should be using themselves and the products and bad practice that they should be avoiding.

In your summing up you should at least cover the following:

Aspect to cover	What to say
The effects of humidity on the hairstyle	Tell the client what will happen if they take a bath before going out. If they are in a steamy environment for a long period the style could drop. Perhaps showering would be a better option.
How traction alopecia can occur	Tell the client to avoid putting their own hair up with too much tension on their hair. Explain the signs of traction alopecia and long-term effects.
Products for home use	Explain the benefits of buying the products that you use with the salon, as opposed to buying from the supermarket without professional recommendation or knowledge.
How to take down the style – remove the grips and pins	Tell the client how they can remove the pins without tension or pulling, tell them where to start and what to avoid.
What sorts of materials and ornaments they should avoid	Tell them about the benefits of using covered bands and fabric covered 'bungees'. Tell them what sorts of ornaments would be suitable and how they can be positioned/fixed without excess weight or damage to the hair.

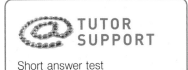

TUTOR SUPPORT

Short answer test

EKU *statement*

GH20 (eku16) The health and safety factors to consider when making choices of ornamentation

GH20 (eku23) The potential effects on the hair structure of using and securing added hair and accessories

GH20 (eku40) Products for home use that will benefit the client and those to avoid and why

GH20 (eku41) How to maintain their style

GH20 (eku42) How to remove pins, accessories, any added hair and any backcombing and or back brushing

GH20 (eku43) How to give effective advice and recommendations to clients.

Aspect to cover	What to say
What sorts of tools and equipment they should avoid	Explain how the use of heated styling equipment can damage hair if temperature settings are too high. Tell them about the benefits of heat protecting sprays.
Hair condition	Explain how the hair can be maintained in good condition, what products to use, how they should brush their hair to avoid tangling or damage.

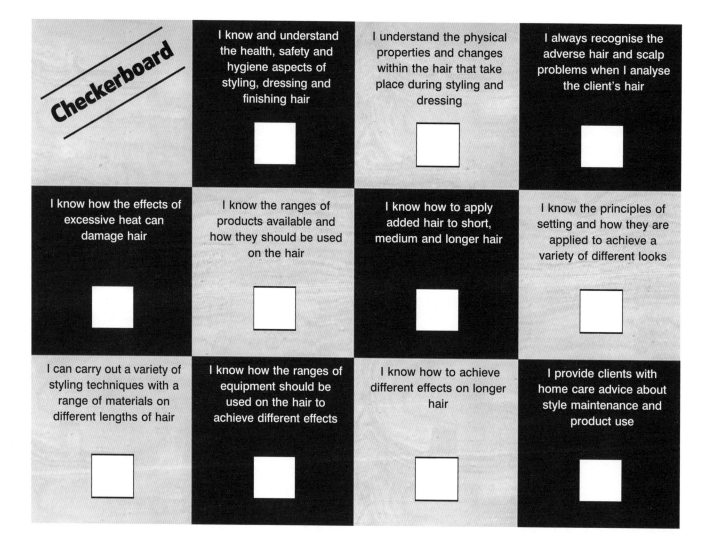

Checkerboard

I know and understand the health, safety and hygiene aspects of styling, dressing and finishing hair

I understand the physical properties and changes within the hair that take place during styling and dressing

I always recognise the adverse hair and scalp problems when I analyse the client's hair

I know how the effects of excessive heat can damage hair

I know the ranges of products available and how they should be used on the hair

I know how to apply added hair to short, medium and longer hair

I know the principles of setting and how they are applied to achieve a variety of different looks

I can carry out a variety of styling techniques with a range of materials on different lengths of hair

I know how the ranges of equipment should be used on the hair to achieve different effects

I know how to achieve different effects on longer hair

I provide clients with home care advice about style maintenance and product use

Revision questions:

Quick quiz: A selection of different types of questions to check your knowledge.

Q1 A _____ pleat is a type of vertical roll.   Fill in the blank

Q2 Humidity in the atmosphere will make a set drop.   True or false

Q3 Which of the following dressings are traditionally, long 'hair up' styles ?   Multi selection

Plaits	☐	1
Knots	☐	2
Twists	☐	3
Rolls	☐	4
Braids	☐	5
Pleats	☐	6

Q4 Unstretched hair is said to be in the alpha state.   True or false

Q5 What condition is created by excessive tension being made on the root   Multi choice
area of the hair?

Alopecia areata	○	a
Male pattern baldness	○	b
Traction alopecia	○	c
Alopecia totalis	○	d

Q6 Heated rollers are a quick way of setting dry hair in to style?   True or false

Q7 Hair styled with tongs, produces which of the following results and   Multi selection
effects?

Increased body at the roots	☐	1
No body at the roots	☐	2
Movement at the ends	☐	3
Straighter effects	☐	4
Wavy effects	☐	5
Same as blow dried effects	☐	6

Q8 On long hair, a chignon is a form of _____.   Fill in the blank

Q9 Which item of equipment would provide spiraled curls on long hair?   Multi choice

Curling tongs	○	a
Ceramic straighteners	○	b
Crimping irons	○	c
Blow-dryer	○	d

Q10 'Hair ups' are easier to perform on hair that has just been washed,   True or false
conditioned and dried off.

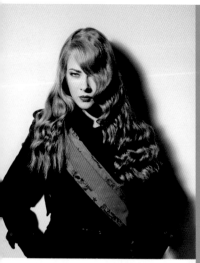

Chapter**ten**
Hair extensions

GH23

GH23.1

GH23.2

GH23.3

GH23.4

GH23.5

GH23.6

CREDIT VALUE FOR UNIT GH23
8 Credits

▶ **More information** See Unit G22 Monitor procedures to safely control work operations

- Personal hygiene GH19 (eku15)
- Contact dermatitis GH23 (eku7)
- General salon hygiene

See also Appendices for following relevant legislation:

- COSHH GH23 (eku5)
- Electricity at Work Regulations GH23 (eku4)

Hair extensions: quick overview

Unit title

GH23 Provide creative hair extensions services

This is a **optional** unit for students taking hairdressing level 3, it is made up of six main outcomes

Main outcomes

GH23.1 Maintain effective and safe methods of working when adding hair extensions

GH23.2 Plan and prepare to add hair extensions

GH23.3 Attach hair extensions

GH23.4 Cut and finish hair with extensions

GH23.5 Maintain and remove hair extensions

GH23.6 Provide aftercare advice

What do I need to do for GH23.1?

- Take adequate precautions in preparing yourself and the client before any hair extension procedure
- Work tidily, safely and effectively at all times
- Maintain standards of personal health and hygiene
- Use a range of tools and equipment suitable for preparing and attaching extensions
- Work to time and maintain client records

What do I need to do for GH23.2?

- Consult the client and examine their hair
- Look for contra-indications to hair extension services

- Carryout tests to determine service suitability
- Record details arising from the consultation
- Apply added hair to achieve the desired effect
- Confirm the length and look required
- Order materials suitable for achieving the effect
- Prepare the materials prior to application

What do I need to do for GH23.3?

- Confirm the look before starting the service
- Section and divide the hair accurately
- Use appropriate attachment system to achieve the desired effect
- Maintain an even tension and systematic approach to the work
- Identify and resolve problems as they arise

What do I need to do for GH23.4?

- Adapt your cutting techniques to creatively style the completed extensions
- Use products when and where necessary to achieve the desired effect
- Confirm the finished effect with the client

What do I need to do for GH23.5?

- Remove extensions according to the manufacturer's instructions
- Use the correct tools and products to remove the extensions
- Clean and prepare the hair ready for the next service

What do I need to do for GH23.6?

- Give the client recommendations and advice for maintaining their hair extensions at home

What aspects do I need to cover for GH23.1, GH23.2, GH23.3, GH23.4, GH23.5 and GH23.6?

- Both hot and cold attachment systems
- A variety of cutting tools and techniques suitable for finishing the effect
- A variety of factors and tests that influence the hair extension service
- The contra-indications associated with hair extensions
- The advice that you need to give to clients who have had extensions

Keywords

Contra-indication
Any factor or state (of the hair or skin) that will affect the planned service for a client

Blending
A technique for mixing different colours of hair extension fibres to create more naturally occurring effects, multi-toned effects, highlighted effects

Synthetic fibre extensions
A range of alternative, fibrous materials (nylon, acrylic, kerakalon etc.) used for extending hair

Real hair extensions
Naturally occurring hair types derived from organic proteins found in humans and animals used for extending hair

Traction alopecia
A condition that is caused by the excessive pulling of hair at the root, it is often associated with longer hair worn in plaits, twists and hair extensions

Information covered in this chapter

- The range of materials used in hair extension services
- How to mix/blend extensions prior to attachment
- The attachment systems that you can use
- The consultation aspects that you must cover before starting

- The ways of working safely and effectively during the application of hair extensions
- The advice you should give to clients in order to maintain their own hair extensions
- How to remove hair extensions safely and professionally

EKU statement

GH23 (eku1) Your salon's requirements for client preparation

GH23 (eku6) Your salon's image and expected standards of service

GH23 (eku8) The range of protective clothing that should be available for clients

GH23 (eku9) The type of personal protective equipment that should be available and used by yourself

GH23 (eku10) Why it is important to use personal protective equipment

GH23 (eku12) How the position of your client and yourself can affect the desired outcome and reduce fatigue and the risk of injury

GH23 (eku14) Why it is important to avoid cross-infection and infestation

GH23 (eku17) Methods of working safely and hygienically and which minimise the risk of cross-infection and cross-infestation

GH23 (eku19) The importance of personal hygiene

What do I need to know for GH23.1, GH23.2, GH23.3, GH23.4, GH23.5 and GH23.6?

- Your salon's requirements in relation to salon policies and current legislation
- How to work safely and hygienically when extending the client's hair
- How to use a range of tools and materials for hair extension services
- How and when to conduct tests prior to the service
- The ways in which hair extensions can be damaging to the client's hair and skin
- How to prepare and work with the materials for different hair extension systems
- The advantages and disadvantages of different hair extension services
- How to style the hair after the extensions have been applied
- How to recommend or provide advice to the client on hair maintenance at home

Introduction

Hair extensions are now accepted as a routine hairdressing service. What was once a specialism for just a few has grown so much in popularity that it is now a core service for the comprehensive salon that prefers to provide a wide variety of service options for its clientele.

This chapter provides the essential knowledge for the application, styling and maintenance of both real hair and synthetic fibre hair extensions.

GH23.1 Maintain effective and safe methods of working when adding hair extensions

Preparation for extension services is somewhat different to that of other salon services, although the aspects that affect your safety and that of the client are very similar to any salon procedure.

The factors that affect your client in relation to comfort are particularly important as most hair extension services involve a lot of sitting in one position for long periods of time. Because of the length of time spent standing, you are also at risk from injury from poor posture.

Take care with personal health and safety and make sure that you don't cross-infect your client from poor hygiene.

In addition to this you must take every care in the way that you handle and use the following equipment as:

- it is easy to spill bonding chemicals on to the client
- you may be using hot equipment that could easily burn you or your client
- you will need to keep an even tension upon the client's hair whilst you work, without putting too much pressure upon their hair or scalp.

Potential risks with different hair extension methods

Hot bonded extension systems

The tools used with this system reach very high temperatures, and can cause serious burns when used incorrectly or accidentally touched. The heated tools have a high operating temperature ranging from 120°C–250°C.

When applying the system ensure that the client's gown is securely fastened, this will protect clients from accidental spillage of the hot polymer resins dispensed from the extension tools. Do not bring the hot applicators that dispense heated resins directly to the client's head, use scalp protectors or scalp shields when working closely to the client's head.

And whilst you work, ensure that the heated extension tools such as dispensers, applicators and heat clamps are placed safely on a flat work surface, capable of withstanding the high operating temperatures.

Cold fusion extension system

These systems can cause allergic reactions. Always conduct a skin sensitivity test before applying this system on a client.

Braided/plaited extensions

The braiding extension system can cause injury by putting too much tension on to small areas of the scalp. These tension spots are at the very least painful and at worst can cause traction alopecia. Tension spots are created when the hair is pulled excessively at the scalp, putting a strain on the hair root. Tension spots easily become infected, as the hair follicles are opened by the excessive tension, and bacteria can enter and multiply. It can cause the client severe discomfort and medical treatment may be required.

Sewn-in hair extensions

When working with a sewn in system, take particular care as the needles are very sharp and could inadvertently pierce a client's skin. Where possible use a curved needle as this reduces the risk of any injury.

Sewing with thread can put excessive tension on the scalp area causing tension spots, so again, traction alopecia is also a risk with this system.

EKU *statement*

GH23 (eku51) The advantages and disadvantages of the different methods of attachment

EKU *statement*

GH23 (eku33) The potential consequences of excessive tension on the hair

GH23 (eku34) How to identify the signs of traction alopecia

EKU *statement*

GH23 (eku3) Your salon's and legal requirements for disposal of sharps and waste materials

GH23 (eku11) Why it is important to protect clients from hair clippings

GH23 (eku15) Why it is important to keep your work area clean and tidy

GH23 (eku16) Methods of cleaning, disinfection and/or sterilisation used in salons

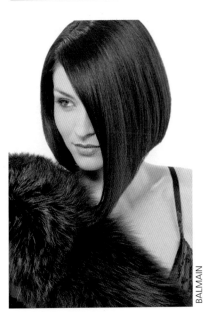

BALMAIN

Remember

Traction alopecia
The tension on the hair is increased with the use of added hair; this can exert exceptional pressure on the hair follicle particularly on scraped back hairstyles or on free hanging effects.

In extreme cases hair loss may be caused by this continued pulling action; areas of hair become thin and even baldness may result!

EKU *statement*

GH23 (eku13) The safety considerations which must be taken into account when adding hair extensions (e.g. possible reaction to adhesives, removal solutions, traction alopecia etc.)

GH23 (eku18) The correct use and maintenance of tools and equipment

GH23 (eku37) The types of hair extension products available and their respective advantages and disadvantages

GH23 (eku44) The manufacturer's preparation instructions for the system(s) in use in your salon

GH23 (eku45) The hair extension systems and attachment methods with which you may need assistance

GH23 (eku52) The range of specialist equipment necessary for each attachment method and how these are used

TUTOR SUPPORT

Discussion 10.1: Health and safety

General health and safety considerations

- Keep your nails trimmed, hands clean and hand jewellery to a minimum; as there is the risk of cross-infecting the client by passing on infections with dirty hands and nails.

- Nails and jewellery can easily get caught in the extension hair, which is uncomfortable and painful. If jewellery gets caught in the extension hair it may result in having to cut it out.

- Wear comfortable clothes that are not too tight as working with hair extensions involves a lot of standing for long periods of time.

- Always wear comfortable shoes that will enable you to stand for long periods of time.

- Consider your posture and work position. Avoid bending over or down to the client – use a hydraulic or gas lift chair to adjust the client to the correct working height. This will lessen your chances of any skeletal injury, fatigue or repetitive strain.

- The work area must be kept scrupulously clean. Workstations, hairdressing trolleys, any work surfaces and the surrounding floor area must be spotless.

- Extension hair can be a hazard if it falls to the floor and is not swept up, you or others could slip on it.

- When applying the hair extension service on a client ensure that gowns or capes are worn so that the client is protected from hair clippings, accidental spillage of hot polymer resins, cold fusion products or removal solutions. All of these products can cause burns or an allergic reaction.

- Any extension hair that has fallen on the floor must *not* be applied into a client's natural hair.

- Always ensure tools are sterilised and cleaned when they have been in used *before* using them on another client.

- If you use a razor for restyling the hair after, make sure that you dispose of used blades in a sharps container.

- Ensure that the working environment is adequately ventilated so that vapours or odours from hair extension materials do not make you, your client and the other staff feel ill.

- Clear up any spillages of chemicals or materials immediately.

- Wear appropriate PPE (apron and disposable vinyl gloves) if you are handling chemicals or hazardous substances.

Activity
There are different ways of bonding extensions to natural hair. You can complete this activity by filling in the missing information in the table below. Keep the information for future use within your portfolio.

Extension system	What precautions should you take?
Hot bonded extensions	
Cold fusion extensions	
Plaited extensions	
Sewn-in extensions	

Products and equipment for hair extensions

The products and equipment required to perform the hair extension service are many and varied and depend upon which application technique you choose to work with.

The following is a list of products and equipment needed when working with several extension systems.

Hair extension connector tools

1 Professional heat clamp   Heat clamps are designed to attach and seal fibre extensions. (They will not attach real hair extensions.) This tool has two heated tips that melt fibre hair at a specific temperature. This tool heats from 140°C to 220°C. When the fibre has melted it creates a hard heat seal bond that holds a fibre extension in place at the root area or seals the end of a fibre extension when the stylist has created a braid or dreadlocks (see below).

2 Professional bonding applicator   This tool allows for pre-shaped polymer resin adhesive sticks to be inserted into the tool. This tool heats to a temperature of 180°C. The resin is then dispensed from a nozzle of the applicator, enabling the stylist to deposit the resin on to real hair or fibre hair and then attach an extension in place by creating a polymer resin bond.

3 Heated pre-bonded extension applicator   This tool has one or two heated tips that reach a temperature of 100°–140°C. This tool melts pre-bonded extensions, which are extension strands with a wax, protein or keratin polymer resin already applied to the end of a piece of extension hair. Pre-bonded applicators melt the resin on to the natural hair, creating a bond that attaches the extension in place. Pre-bonded applicators will attach pre-bonded fibre hair and pre-bonded real hair.

4 Needle and thread   A curved mattress needle can be used to sew weaves or wefts on to hair. The weave is sewn on to a scalp plait or corn braid. The thread used is designed to sew weaves on to hair. It is a silk thread that can be purchased in a variety of colours.

Good practice/Health and safety
- Perform a skin test before using cold fusion liquids as some of these products can cause allergic reactions.
- Read the manufacturer's instructions contained with these tools and products before using them.

Remember

Bonding applicator tools must be placed on a flat stable work surface when in operation as the heated resin that drips from this tool will deliver serious burns if accidentally spilled on skin.

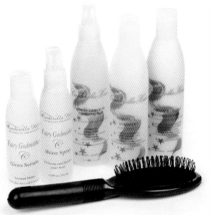

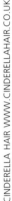

CINDERELLA HAIR WWW.CINDERELLAHAIR.CO.UK

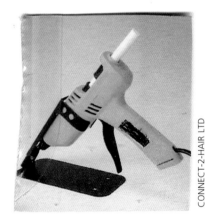

A bonding applicator

CONNECT-2-HAIR LTD

Hair extension connector products

1 Liquid, cold fusion adhesives   These products vary greatly from gum to rubber or latex-based liquids. They are applied from bottles that have brushes attached to the lids, similar to the application of a nail polish. Cold fusion liquids will attach fibre hair and real hair in place by painting the liquids on to the real hair and extension hair, then placing the two hair types together. These products are not heated.

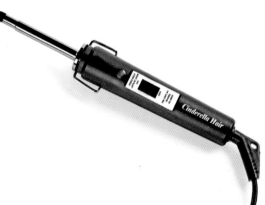

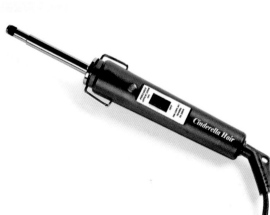

CINDERELLA HAIR WWW.CINDERELLAHAIR.CO.UK

A heated extension applicator

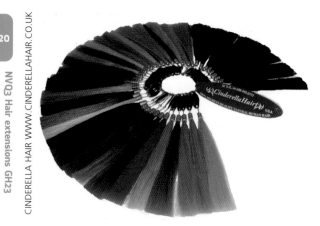

BALMAIN

2 Polymer resin adhesive sticks
This is a resin stick inserted into a bonding applicator that is melted and then dispensed from the applicator. Designed to create extension bonds on individual fibre or real extension hair.

3 Synthetic acrylic fibre hair
This extension hair is made from acrylic and designed to be used for extension hairstyles. The fibre is manufactured in a variety of deniers (thickness or fineness). The deniers are designed to look and feel as similar to natural hair as possible with an acrylic. Fibre hair is manufactured in specific colours that once produced cannot be altered. The fibre comes in a variety of structures – straight, soft wave, deep wave, braids and dreadlocks and crinkled structures that mimic straightened African hair textures. Fibre structure can be changed using heat from a hot hairdryer or heated rollers. Fibre hair will be damaged or melted when excessive heat is applied to it.

Fibre can be purchased in lengths from 35–160 inches, and comes in more than 100 colours ranging from natural colours to neon fantasy colours. Fibre is packaged in 100 gram bales or packets or it is sewn into weaves/wefts. The weaves/wefts are sold in 4 oz packets.

4 Real human extension hair

- *Asian hair* – Asian real hair comes mainly from China or India. This hair is cleansed in a caustic soda solution to remove bacteria or infestation. It is then rinsed and dried, bleached and coloured to match manufacturer's colour shade charts. When wavy or curly structures are required, the Asian hair is permed. After the chemical treatments have been carried out, the cuticle layer of the Asian hair is damaged and must be treated as chemically damaged hair when applied into natural hair. Asian hair is coarse in structure and very strong, which is why it is used for extensions, wigs, toupées and hair pieces. Asian hair comes in a variety of lengths from 10–24 inches. It is normally packaged in 4 oz packets or sewn into weaves/wefts. The weaves/wefts are sold in 4 oz packets.

- *European hair* – This hair comes mainly from former Soviet states such as Russia. It is coloured to match extension colour shade charts. If a wave or curl structure is required it is permed. European hair is finer than Asian hair and should be treated as chemically processed when applied into natural hair. It comes in a variety of natural colours and fantasy colours plus several lengths from 10 to 24 inches. It comes in 1 oz packets and is sometimes sewn into weaves/wefts in 1 oz packets. European virgin hair has had no chemical treatment. It comes in only natural colours and structures. This hair comes in lengths from 10 to 24 inches. It is very rare and very expensive. It comes in 1 oz packets and is sometimes sewn into weaves/wefts in 1 oz packets.

Remember

Real hair prepared for hair extensions is root point correct. It is important that the roots and tips are aligned together or tangling of this loose hair will occur.

Remember

Real hair that is not prepared on weaves or wefts comes loose. This loose hair is tied in 1 oz or 4 oz bundles called *bulk hair*.

Remember

 Do not use heated electrical hairdressing tools on fibre hair, e.g. tongs or straighteners, as this will melt the fibre and cause irreparable damage.

Remember

Neon-coloured fibre hair will glow under ultraviolet lights.

5 Pre-bonded extensions These are strands of fibre or real hair with wax, protein or keratin resin applied at the root end of an extension at the manufacturers. These are applied using a heated pre-bonded tool. These extensions come in a range of structures and a variety of colours and lengths. Pre-bonded extensions come in packets of 5, 10, 20 or 25 strands.

6 Silicone pads These are small pieces of heat-resistant silicone sheet measuring 2 cm by 4 cm. They are used during the application of bonded extensions. The silicone pads protect stylists' fingers from the intense heat of resin bonds and are used to roll resin into bonds at the root area of the natural hair attaching extensions in place.

7 Scalp protectors or scalp shields These are circular plastic discs 4 cm in diameter. They are placed at the root area of an extension. They are secured on to the natural hair before attaching an extension in place. Scalp protectors have a small hole in the centre where natural hair feeds through. This strand of natural hair will have the extension attached. Scalp protectors prevent loose strands of natural hair becoming trapped in an extension bond and keep the natural hair sections clean and neat.

8 Soft bristle brush This is a brush that has a padded face and soft bristles which protrude from the padded base. Soft bristle brushes should be used when blending, mixing and brushing extension hair.

9 Mixing mats Mixing mats are designed to hold real hair root point correctly and they assist in the blending of real hair colours. They are used to hold real hair safely whilst applying extensions. They are two square mats, 6 × 6 inches. Each mat has small wire teeth or pins protruding from one side. These teeth are slightly bent. They are bent backwards (away from you) on the bottom mat and forwards (towards you) on the top mat. The two mats are then placed together so that the teeth can interlock, trapping the real hair in between. The real hair is then drawn out of the mats in small pieces the size of an extension. This hair then has a resin bond dispensed on the root end of the real hair ready to be attached to the natural hair as an extension.

10 Removal tool This tool is similar to a small pair of pliers. It crushes and breaks extension seals and resin bonds during the removal of extension.

11 Removal solutions These are acetone, alcohol, oil- or spirit-based solutions that are recommended by the extension product companies to break down the resins, acrylics, rubber, latex and wax bonds which attach extensions in place.

12 Resin drip tray A metal dish or silicone mat the size of an ashtray is placed underneath the nozzle of a bonding applicator to catch dripping resin.

13 Client aftercare products

- *Clarifying shampoo* – shampoo designed to remove sebum, oil, wax, styling products and pollutants from the extension hair and natural hair. This shampoo must be oil and silicone free.

- *Light conditioner* – a conditioner specifically designed for fibre hair and natural hair. It is manufactured by extension product companies and designed to coat the fibre hair, forming a surface barrier and protecting the fibre from any heat or friction damage caused by brushing and styling. It is a light conditioner for the natural hair.

- *Daily maintenance spray* – a spray mist that is applied to the mid-lengths and ends of the fibre. It untangles the fibre and protects the fibre from heated appliances used for styling. The spray is manufactured by extension product companies. The daily maintenance spray must be used before brushing fibre and before any heated styling tools are used to style the fibre.

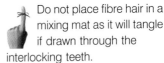

TUTOR SUPPORT

Project 10.2: Fibres and hair that can be used in applying extensions to the hair

Good practice/Health and safety
Stylists should wear protective disposable gloves when using removal solutions to protect their hands. Always use these products in well-ventilated areas. Do not smoke or have naked flames near these products as some of them are highly inflammable.

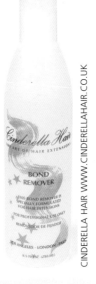

CINDERELLA HAIR WWW.CINDERELLAHAIR.CO.UK

Remember
Do not place fibre hair in a mixing mat as it will tangle if drawn through the interlocking teeth.

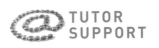

TUTOR SUPPORT

Project 10.3: Equipment and product list and health and safety issues

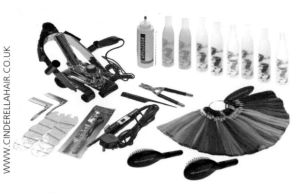

EKU *statement*

GH23 (eku31) The factors that must be taken into consideration prior to adding hair extensions (e.g. hair density, hair and skin disorders, etc.)

GH23 (eku43) How to conduct an examination of the hair and scalp to recognise factors which will affect the hair extension service

GH23 (eku60) The courses of action to take in the advent of the presence of the contraindications in the range (i.e. when to encourage the client to seek medical advice, when to explain the service is not possible, when a modification to the service will be necessary)

Remember

Do not use your best pair of hairdressing scissors as extension hair will blunt scissors.

• *Reconstructive conditioner* – a conditioner that works within the hair shaft designed to strengthen and rebuild hair. Reconstructive conditioners are manufactured by extension product companies specifically for real hair extensions.

• *pH balanced rinse* – an acid balanced rinse that has the same pH as hair and skin (4.5–5.5). This product is diluted in water: 1 part rinse to 10 parts water. It is used after shampooing and conditioning and applied through the mid-lengths and ends of the hair. The acid balanced rinse is designed to close the cuticle layers of the real hair, therefore reducing tangles and matting that can occur when the real hair is wet. A pH balanced rinse is manufactured by extension product companies specifically for real hair.

14 Colour ring or swatch

15 Cutting comb, pin tail or tail comb

16 Hairdryer or air styler

17 Flat sectioning clips

18 Hairdressing scissors, pair of thinning scissors, razor and razor blades

19 Selection of round brushes or blow-drying brushes

20 Flat stable work surface on which to place heated bonded tools and a hairdressing trolley.

Activity

Explain in your portfolio what each of these pieces of equipment does.

Item of equipment	What is it for?	What does it do?
Heat clamp		
Bonding applicator		
Heated pre-bonded extension applicator		

GH23.2   Plan and prepare to add hair extensions

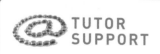

TUTOR SUPPORT

Project 10.4: The length of the client's hair

Consultation

A pre-service, thorough hair extension consultation is essential; it is one of the most important parts of the hair extension service as there are many issues to cover and explain. A consultation appointment should be booked for a minimum of 30 minutes although you may need longer.

During the analysis, you will be checking the client's hair condition to see that the natural hair is strong and healthy enough to hold an attachment of extension hair in place for a three-month period of time.

You will be looking at the first 2–4 inches of the client's natural hair as this area is where an extension will be secured. The analysis should establish whether the client's hair is normal, fine, coarse, dry or greasy. If a client has a greasy hair condition that necessitates shampooing on a daily basis, then a hair extension service is *not* suitable. The sebum will either break down the bonds securing the extension in place or make the natural hair too slippery and the attached extensions will slip down the hair shaft and fall out.

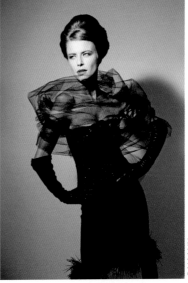

BALMAIN

Remember

You have to be satisfied that a client's fine hair will be strong enough to hold a secured extension in place for up to three months.

Consultation considerations

- The first question that should be asked is what hair extension hairstyle is to be achieved – length, thickness, volume, body, colour, decoration or texture?

- It is vital to establish what style is to be achieved before embarking upon this service as this will determine which hair extension application technique can be used and whether the client's natural hair length, condition and porosity is suitable for the required hairstyle.

- A client's natural hair should be a minimum of 8 cm (3 inches) long to apply a textured extension hairstyle.

- A client's natural hair should be a minimum of 10 cm (4 inches) long to apply hair additions that create decorative looks, e.g. crystal strands, highlights or flashes of colour.

- A client's natural hair should be a minimum of 13 cm (5 inches long) to create volume and thickening extension hairstyles.

- A client's natural hair should be a minimum of 15 cm (6 inches) long to create a natural-looking lengthened extension hairstyle. When applying a weave or weft extension to African hair types, the client's natural hair must be long enough to enable the stylist to create a continuous and firm tight corn braid or scalp plait.

Remember

The porosity of the client's natural hair has to be assessed throughout the hairshaft from root to point, to check whether the client's hair is normal, dry, chemically treated or bleached.

EKU *statement*

GH23 (eku36) How the contra-indications in the range can affect the delivery of hair extension services to clients

You need to establish whether the client's natural hair is strong enough to withstand extension hair attached at the root area and whether the mid-lengths and ends of the client's hair will withstand the friction and wear and tear of added extension hair for up to three months. If the client's natural hair is delicate or broken then it will not be strong enough to wear a hair extension hairstyle. (See hair tests for hair extension services p. 224.)

Contra-indications for hair extensions

The following are the contra-indications (issues that adversely affect a service being performed) to hair extensions these factors must be taken into account during a hair extension consultation.

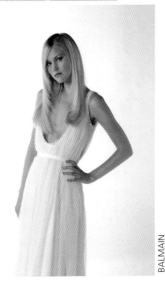

BALMAIN

Remember

The price of the extension hair normally increases as the length of the hair increases.

EKU *statement*

GH23 (eku23) The types and purposes of tests in the range

GH23 (eku24) The importance of following manufacturers' instructions for testing

GH23 (eku25) The methods of and reasons for conducting pull tests

GH23 (eku26) When and how tests should be carried out and the expected results

GH23 (eku27) How the results of tests can influence all aspects of the service

GH23 (eku28) The potential consequences of failing to carry out tests

GH23 (eku29) The courses of action to take in the event of adverse reactions to tests and when the contra-indications in the range are encountered (i.e. when to encourage the client to seek medical advice, when to explain the service is not possible, when a modification to the service will be necessary)

GH23 (eku30) Why it is important to record test results

EKU *statement*

GH23 (eku41) The general differences in preparation requirements between human hair and man-made extensions

Diversion See Unit G21 Provide hairdressing consultation services (see pp. 20–23 for more information on contra-indications and hair tests).

Do not provide hair extensions when your client:

- is suffering hair fall or who are having medication or treatment for hair fall
- shows signs of alopecia
- shows signs of thin or thinning hair
- has any breakage through the first 2–4 inches of their hair at the root area
- has weakened or damaged hair
- is taking medication or having treatment for cancer
- is pregnant or during the first six months after giving birth
- shows signs of psoriasis or eczema on the scalp
- has skin allergies or excessive skin sensitivities
- has excessively oily hair and scalp.

Remember

Hair extension hairstyles can take from 30 minutes to 10 hours to apply. During the consultation clients should be informed about the length of time needed to apply their hairstyle.

As part of the consultation and prior to any extension service you will need to test the hair for:

- strength and any weakened hair/hair damage
- its ability to stretch and return in length.

You will also need to test the client's skin for sensitivity or allergies to the attachment and removal chemicals that you may be using.

Hair tests for extension services

Tests	What does this test do?
Pull test	A pull test will identify whether the hair has sufficient capability of retaining the root within the hair follicle. If you pull a single hair and it comes away from the scalp it could be indicating that the hair is either in a catagenic stage (see hair growth pp. 19 and 29) or unable to sustain any additional weight. Either way, this is a contra-indication to hair extension services.
Elasticity test	By taking a hair between the fingers and stretching it you can assess the amount of spring it has. Hair without spring has no elasticity and lacks sufficient strength or structure to enable extensions services to take place.
Skin test	The skin test is used to assess the reaction of the skin to chemicals or chemical products. To find out whether a client's skin reacts to the chemicals in the removal agent, a skin test should be carried out at least 24 hours prior to the chemical process.

Choosing extension hair

After establishing that the client's hair condition, porosity and length are suitable for the requested hair extension hairstyle, you must then choose what extension hair is suitable for the client.

Real human hair, either Asian or European hair (real hair), or synthetic acrylic fibre hair (fibre) can be applied. The choice of extension hair to be used to create the extension hairstyle depends on the client's budget, suitability of the client's natural hair or the choice of application tools and attachment techniques.

Real hair is sold in different lengths from 10–24 inches. Synthetic fibre is sold in various lengths from 35–60 inches.

Establish the length of extension hair needed for the required style to be achieved. Real hair is supplied in several structures: straight, soft wave, deep wave, curly or spiral curled. Synthetic hair is supplied in several structures: straight, soft wave, deep wave. Pre-made dreadlocks, braids and crimped hair can be purchased. During the consultation establish the correct structure suitable for the client extension hairstyle. After establishing the extension hair that is to be used – either real hair or synthetic hair – the extension hair colour must be selected.

Using a colour ring or colour shade chart, select the base colour, major tone and minor tone required (see colour selecting, mixing and blending section pp. 227–229).

During the consultation, the stylist should educate the client about the home aftercare products and procedures that need to be followed throughout the duration of the extension hairstyle (see advice and home-care maintenance pp. 245–246). There are two different product ranges and procedures to follow, depending on whether the client is wearing real extension hair or fibre extension hair.

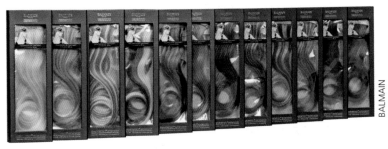

BALMAIN

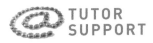

TUTOR SUPPORT

Discussion 10.2: Contra-indications that may prevent hair extensions

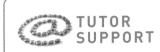

TUTOR SUPPORT

Discussion 10.3: Type of hair extension and colour

Activity

Explain in your portfolio what each of these extension products is for.

Product	What is it for?
Liquid adhesive	
Polymer resin sticks	
Silicone pads	
Scalp shields	
Mixing mats	
Removal tool	
Resin drip tray	

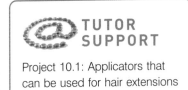

TUTOR SUPPORT

Project 10.1: Applicators that can be used for hair extensions

TUTOR SUPPORT

Discussion 10.4: Safety issues when cutting and styling hair with added extensions

EKU *statement*

GH23 (eku32) The average rate of hair growth

GH23 (eku35) The potential effects on the client's hair of wearing extensions over a long period of time

EKU *statement*

GH23 (eku46) How to estimate the length of time the hair attachment processes in the range are likely to take

EKU *statement*

GH23 (eku2) Your salon's expected service times for adding hair extensions

Remember

All hair extension hairstyles should be removed from the client's natural hair after three months' wear. All removal should be conducted in the salon by a professional trained person as the removal of extensions, if poorly performed, will break and damage the hair.

EKU *statement*

GH23 (eku20) The importance of questioning clients to establish any contra-indications to hairdressing services

GH23 (eku21) Why it is important to record client responses to questioning

GH23 (eku22) The legal significance of client questioning and of recording the client's responses

Maintenance appointments

Each hair extension hairstyle needs regular maintenance appointments at the salon. These appointments are every two, four or six weeks depending on the hairstyle, application technique and extension hair used to create the style. During the consultation the client should be informed about the maintenance appointments required for their hairstyle.

Remember

Natural loss of hair

Each person loses 80–100 hairs per day in natural hairfall. Whilst wearing extensions this hair cannot fall out and becomes trapped at the root area above the extension attachment. If the extension strand is left in the hair for more than three months, the trapped hair will begin to mat. When the matting occurs it becomes impossible to remove an extension hairstyle without damaging the natural hair.

Remember

Hair growth

The rate of hair growth is an important factor in assessing how long extensions will last; as they grow away from the root area at the same rate as the natural hair; that being an average of 1.25 cm per month.

If the hair is allowed to grow too far away from the scalp the extensions will become very difficult to manage and should be professionally removed.

How long will it take?

To get a rough idea of how long a hair extension service will take, you could time how long it takes to apply one extension then multiply that by the total amount that you will use to create the whole effect.

On average a trained extension stylist should take one minute to apply one extension. A lengthened hairstyle needs approximately 150–250 single extensions. The time of each appointment will be dictated by the amount of extensions to be applied and the hairstyle required.

Consultation: Points to remember

- Analyse the client's natural hair condition, porosity, strength, length and required style.
- Select the type of extension hair, the style, length, colour and structure.
- Advise the client about the correct aftercare products, maintenance appointments and removal procedures.
- Work out the length of time need to provide the service.
- Provide a quote of the total price, including application, maintenance appointments and removal service and aftercare products.

- Book the correct time for each appointment and ensure that you have the trained support staff available to complete the service.
- Order the correct extension hair materials, length and colour for the client.

Finalising the consultation and completing the records

Make sure that you quote the price of the extension service:

- recommend the products that will be required to maintain the look
- explain that a deposit needs to be taken in order to book the service
- remember the time that needs to be allowed for the service
- tell the client how long the extensions will last before they need to be removed.

Finally, book an appointment date and time and make sure that the record is completed, covering all the following aspects.

The client record will:

- assist the salon reception when booking the appointment time, maintenance appointments and the removal appointment
- help in the ordering of materials; i.e. the extension hair required and the correct aftercare products
- provide evidence of the responses given to you by the client at the time that the consultation was carried out.

EKU *statement*

GH23 (eku38) The principles for blending added hair

GH23 (eku40) How to prepare hair extensions ready for use following manufacturers' instructions

GH23 (eku42) How the client's hair should be prepared for each of the hair attachment techniques in the range

Activity
Aftercare advice and maintenance is a very important part of the total extension service.
In your portfolio, explain the benefits for each of the products listed in the table below.

Aftercare product	What benefits does it provide
Clarifying shampoo	
Light conditioner	
Daily maintenance spray	
Reconstructive conditioner	
pH balanced rinse	

Diversion Records are an essential back-up if something goes wrong; see GH17 Recording the events p. 268 for more information.

Selecting and blending extensions and colours together

Creating extension hairstyles requires learning new skills over and above the stylist's existing hairdressing knowledge. Selecting, mixing and blending fibre hair and real hair is an additional skill that requires a new understanding of selecting colours. When applying

Remember

Fibre extension hair is packaged in 100 g bales. Real extension hair is packed in 4 oz bulk or weaves/wefts.

Remember

It is very rare to find extension hair that matches natural hair exactly. Often a second or third colour will have to be selected and mixed into the base colour to get an exact match of natural colour. A natural head of hair is not one colour but made up of several colours. Extension hair must mimic this natural phenomenon.

EKU *statement*

GH23 (eku39) How to mix a number of added hair colours (e.g. to give block colour and highlighting effects)

Remember

Special note

Do not place the root of the human hair at the tip end of the human hair. It is vital that real hair is always placed root point correct – this means roots together and tips together. If the real hair is mixed with root and tips lying in opposite directions then the hair will severely mat, locking together as tightly as velcro. When real hair is in this state it is virtually impossible to separate or untangle.

a natural-looking extension hairstyle it is important to create extension hair which is the same colour as the natural hair. If there is seen to be even a fractional difference in colour the extension hairstyle will look false. Therefore selecting, mixing and blending colours are a vital new skill for you to learn with this service.

Selecting extension hair colours to match to the natural hair colour

Take a hair extension colour ring or shade chart. Place the colour ring swatches of hair colour against the client's natural hair. Select the extension hair colour that is the nearest colour to the client's own hair colour. This is the *base colour* or *first colour*. Use the colour ring to identify the second colour that is the nearest colour to the client's own hair colour. This is the major tone or *second colour*. Use the colour ring and look closely for the *third colour* that matches the hue (glint) of the client's natural hair colour. This is the minor tone or third colour.

You have now selected the base colour, major tone and minor tone of the natural hair. Blending the extension colours in their correct proportions to match natural hair is a very visual technique. However, find below a formula to follow that will assist you in calculating the correct proportions of colour to mix in order to make an exact colour match.

Colour formula for mixing extensions

Adding 25 per cent (25 g or 1 oz) of a second colour to the base colour will lighten or darken the base colour.

Adding 12.5 per cent (12.5 g) of a second colour to the base colour will give a strong tone.

Adding 6 per cent (6 g) of a second colour to the base colour will give a hue or glint of colour.

Adding equal amounts (25 g + 25 g) of two different extension hair colours together will change the base colour.

Blending extensions together

Remove the selected base colour of extension hair from its packaging, then divide 25 per cent, 12.5 per cent or 6.25 per cent of the second colour and third colour from the packing (using the formula above). After selecting the quantities of extension hair, place the colours together. Ensure the ends of the extension hair are together. When blending fibre hair colours together, hold the fibre hair in the centre. Lightly spray fibre with a daily conditioning spray. Use a soft bristle brush to blend the fibre hair colours together. Start brushing from the ends of the fibre, working towards the centre.

When blending real hair colours together, always place real hair in a mixing mat with the root ends together.

Place the first colour or base colour onto the mixing mat. Then place the second colour and third colour on top of the base colour. Place the lid of the mixing mat on top of the selected colours. As you draw the real hair out of the mixing mat during application the colours will mix together.

Multi-mixing

Megamixing is the process of mixing a number of colours together until the fibres are totally blended.

1 Decide on the colour or colours to be achieved.

2 Select the appropriate fibres to be mixed. Carefully remove the required amounts of fibre from the packs.

3 Take the base colour – the greatest amount – and place the fibres in the palm of your hand, holding them near one end. Place any secondary colours – the lesser amounts – on top. Close your fingers and hold the fibres tightly in your hand.

4 With your thumb, fan out the fibre along your first finger.

5 Now, using a bristle brush, brush the fibre downwards. This will tend to mix the fibres.

6 Hold the opposite end of the fibres in your palm and repeat this process. This will mix the fibres further.

7 Continue brushing and changing ends until the colours have been totally blended and the final colour is uniform.

Block colour

Block colouring gives a more defined colour or highlighting effect.

1 Take the base colour – the greater amount – and hold it centrally in the palm.

2 Lay the secondary colour – the lesser amount – on top, keeping the ends together.

3 Starting with your hands about 20 cm apart, bring your hands together. Divide the fibre into two equal amounts and separate your hands. Slight mixing will have occurred.

4 Again, place the fibre in one hand on top of the fibre in the other. The fibre is now all in one hand, partially mixed.

5 Bring your hands together and again divide the fibres into two. Further mixing will have occurred, but the fibres will still be in blocks of colour.

6 Repeat until the colour is sufficiently mixed.

7 Gently brush the fibre to remove any tangles, but not so as to mix the fibres further.

Remember

Do not attempt to brush real hair colours together in order to blend the colours as most of the real hair will stay in your brush or fall on the floor.

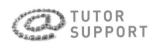

TUTOR SUPPORT

Project 10.5: Methods of mixing extension hair colour to achieve different effects

EKU *statement*

GH23 (eku50) How the attachment systems in the range secure hair extensions into the client's hair

GH23 (eku53) The generally accepted sequences of working for the hair attachment systems in the range

GH23 (eku54) The manufacturer's instructions for the attachment of extensions for the system(s) in use in your salon

GH23 (eku55) Why it is important to maintain a correct and even tension when adding hair extensions

GH23.3   Attach hair extensions

Adding hair extensions

There are a number of different methods of attaching extensions to natural hair. The method chosen by a stylist and client will vary depending on whether the stylist is attaching fibre or real-hair extensions.

In the following section of this book you will find a number of step-by-step guides to the process of adding hair extensions. They include a step-by-step guide to attaching synthetic hair, a step-by-step guide to attaching real hair and pre-bonded method, which can be used to attach either synthetic or real hair.

You will also find in this section, descriptions of two extension hairstyles and diagrams that will demonstrate how to undertake the planning and placement of extensions to create hairstyles from synthetic fibre or real hair.

Step-by-steps

Attaching synthetic fibre extensions

1 Prepare the fibre to be used.

2 Prepare the heat-sealing device – clean it, select the temperature setting, and plug into the power point.

3 Prepare other tools and materials: combs, clips, brushes, scissors, styling sprays and bonding solution (if required).

4 For hair extensions over the whole head, section the head into five areas.

5 Leave a 7 mm section of natural hair out around the hairline.

6 Start at the nape area. Take a band of hair above the hairline; secure the remainder out of the way with clips.

7 Starting in the centre of this band, take a section of hair 5 mm by 5 mm and again clip the remainder out of the way.

8 Divide the section of natural hair into two.

9 Your assistant now takes a similar amount of fibre and lays it centrally in between, forming a cross.

10 Cross the two pieces of natural hair over, right over left and hold the hair apart while your assistant crosses left over right.

11 Cross again, right over left.

12 Your assistant leaves the top weft of fibre out and subdivides the bottom weft into two, pulling these apart so that you can cross over between them.

13 You both continue crossing until you have 12 mm of braided 'hair'.

14 With your assistant holding the top of the plait between thumb and index finger, wrap the weft of fibre left out (step 12) around the braid.

15 With the heat sealer, close the tips over the bound braid approximately 20 mm down the braid. To close the tips, gently press them on to the fibre for 2 seconds. Lift the top tip and give a half turn, then close your tips again. Remove the heat after 2 seconds.

16 Pinch and roll the heated area between your fingers. Ensure that you have a smooth, round seal.

17 Repeat steps 1–16.

18 When the nape row is complete, continue up the head row by row.

19 After all the extensions have been applied, cut and dress the hair into the desired style.

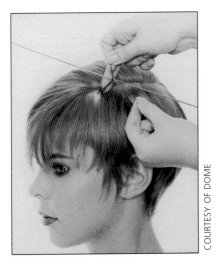

COURTESY OF DOME

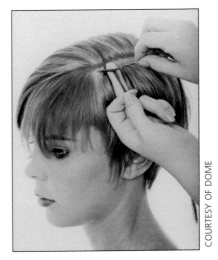

COURTESY OF DOME

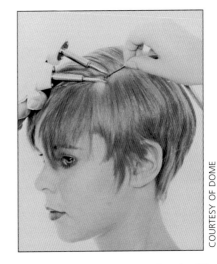

COURTESY OF DOME

Step 1 A section of hair is taken and divided into two, Monofibre is then taken, to the same amount of the section and placed centrally on the head in the opposite direction. The four stem braid is then made by the stylist crossing right over left and the assistant crossing left over right. After the first crossing the stylist divides the weft into two and leaves the top weft out. They continue crossing for approximately 2 cms

Step 2 The stylist clasps the four wefts together, hands it to the assistant and divides the top weft left out at the beginning of the crossing into two. The stylist then wraps one piece of the divided weft around the braid

Step 3 The Stylist then applies the C2, with its controlled heat to the braid, which then reconstitutes itself into the heat seal

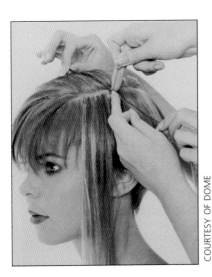

COURTESY OF DOME

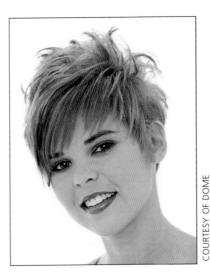

COURTESY OF DOME

Step 4 The stylist then squeezes the heat seal and takes the other weft left out to cover the heat seal

Step 5 The Stylist then cuts and styles the Extensions into the desired style

Steps for attaching Monofibre™: Hair Extension from Dome Cosmetics

Attaching real hair

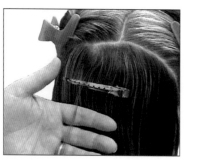

Step 1 Take a ½ cm square section of natural hair, approximately the size of a highlight. Place a section clip underneath this section to keep the area clean from travelling hairs

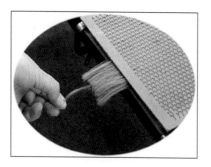

Step 2 Draw a small amount of real extension hair from the mixing mat. Select the same quantity of real extension hair to natural hair, approximately the size of a highlight

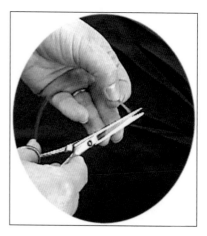

Step 3 Blunt cut and level off the root end of the real hair

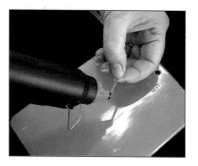

Step 4 Take the real hair to the nozzle end of the applicator and dispatch a small drop of resin onto root area. Wipe excess resin off onto the nozzle of applicator

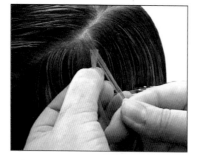

Step 5 Take the real extension hair to the root area of the client's natural hair. Place the resin underneath the natural hair section. Place it 1 cm away from the scalp. In one hand hold both pieces of hair together, leaving your other hand free to pick up a silicon pad and place this underneath the resin

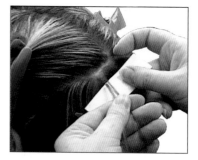

Step 6 Gently press and push the resin through the natural hair. This ensures even coverage of resin through real and extension hair

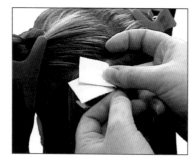

Step 7 Use the silicon pad gently to mould and roll the resin into a bond that is the size of a small bead. The bond must be closed at the bottom

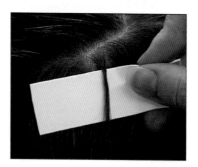

Step 8 The bond takes 30 seconds to cool down, creating a secure attachment holding real extension hair onto the client's hair for up to three months

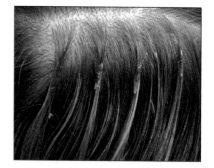

Step 9 Extensions are applied into the natural hair in rows that are 1–2 cm apart. A row of natural hair is left out in between a row of extension hair. Each extension attachment should lie flat to the head

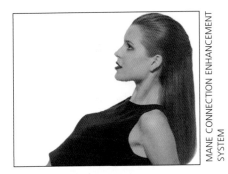

MANE CONNECTION ENHANCEMENT SYSTEM

Hair by Theresa Bullock, photography by Ozzie Rizzo from *eXtensions: The Official Guide to Hair Extensions*

Step 10 Finished look

Attaching pre-bonded hair extensions

Natural hair extensions bought from the supplier arrive prepared by the manufacturer. They are available in a variety of strand colours, sizes and types – finer strands are for use around hairlines and partings, thicker strands are for use in other areas. You can also choose between straight, wavy and curly hair types. The wefts of hair are 'gummed' together with a polymer resin, so no colour blending is required. They are ready to attach to the hair.

Although the procedures for natural hair extensions may seem similar to those for synthetic hair extensions, in reality the processes are quite different. The polymer resin is activated by a device which emits ultra-high-frequency sound waves: once activated it moulds around the section of hair and creates a strong permanent bond.

Natural hair extensions can be styled by blow-drying, tonging or using heated rollers. It is possible to use semi-permanent or temporary colours, but perming and colouring are not recommended.

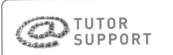

TUTOR SUPPORT

Project 10.6: Applying different extensions

Attaching processed hair extensions

1 Prepare the high-frequency equipment according to the manufacturer's instructions.

2 Prepare the other tools – the plastic strand shield, brushes, combs, clips and whatever else you will need.

3 For hair extensions over the whole head, section the head into five working areas.

4 Leave a 7 mm section of hair out around the hairline.

5 Start at the nape area. Take a band of hair above the hairline. Secure the remainder out of the way with clips.

6 Starting in the centre of this band, take a section of hair 5 mm by 5 mm and again clip the remainder out of the way.

7 Slide on the plastic protection shield and push it near to the scalp area.

8 Place the polymer-bonded end of the extension into the centre of the hair section, approximately 12 mm from the scalp and forming a V-shaped wedge of hair around the bond. An even distribution of natural hair should surround the bonded end of the hair extension, to prevent uneven tension or breakage.

9 Place the grooved tip of the high-frequency device below the hair section.

EKU *statement*

GH23 (eku47) How to judge the quantity of hair to be added to achieve a balanced and well proportioned look

10 Wait for the polymer to bubble before rolling it smoothly between your index finger and thumb. (Bubbling will occur in just a few seconds.)

11 Check that the bottom end of the bond is adequately sealed.

12 Continue the process, repeating steps 1–11 until the complete row is finished.

13 Continue working up the back of the head until the section is complete.

14 After all the extensions have been applied, cut and dress the hair into the desired style.

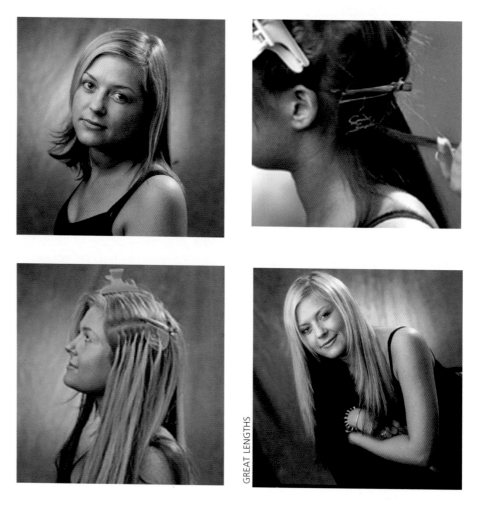

GREAT LENGTHS

Planning and placement

So many extension hairstyles can be created with this service using fibre hair and real hair. Once the principles of the planning and placement of the extensions are understood, virtually any style can be created.

Sectioning of client's natural hair

This diagram shows the sectioning of the client's natural hair and the areas where extensions can be placed. Hair extensions are applied in the interior of the natural hairstyle. They are placed 1–2 cm behind the hairline, parting and crown area. The natural hair is sectioned into six areas.

Area 1 is the nape section. Take a section using a tail comb from the top of the ear to the top of the ear across the occipital bone.

Area 2 is at the back section of the head above the occipital bone up to the crown. Take a section using a tail comb from the top of the ear to the top of the ear over the top of the head and through the crown area.

Area 3 is at the right-hand side or temple area section of the head from the ear to the top of the recession area. Take a section from the top of the recession at the front hairline straight back to the crown area.

Area 4 is from the top of the right-hand recession to the client's parting and reaching back to the crown area.

Area 5 is the left-hand side or temple area section of the head from the ear to the top of the recession area. Take a section from the top of the recession at the front hairline straight back to the crown area.

Area 6 is from the top of the left-hand recession to the client's parting and reaching back to the crown area.

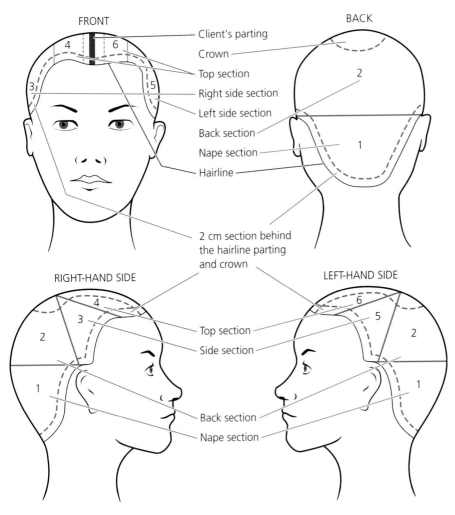

Sectioning of client's natural hair

Extensions are placed in the interior of a hairstyle always placed 1–2 cm away from the hairline and placed 1–2 cm away from the parting and crown.

Planning and placement of extensions

This diagram shows a natural-looking lengthened hairstyle using fibre. The extensions are placed 2 cm behind the hairline. The natural hair is divided into six sections. A heat clamp was used creating individual extensions held in place with fibre heat seals.

Area 1   has two rows of extensions applied. They are placed 2 cm away from the hairline. A 2 cm section of natural hair was left extension free across the occipital bone. This section is left extension free. If extensions are applied on this bone they will protrude and create a distorted shape.

Area 2   has three rows of extensions applied right up to the crown, placing the extensions 2 cm away from the crown area.

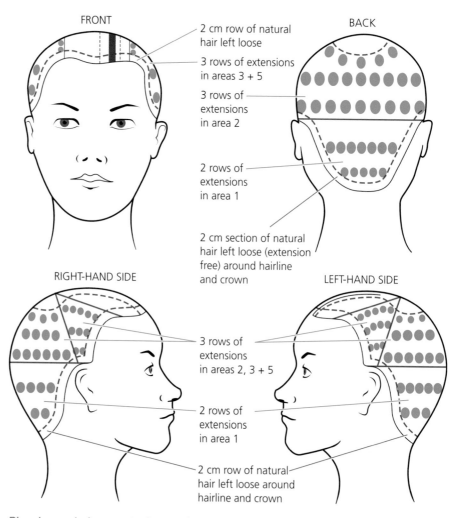

Planning and placement of extensions

Areas 3 and 5   have three rows of hair extensions applied. A 1 cm section of hair is left extension free in Areas 3 and 5 above the second row. This area is the widest point of the head and is often left loose as extensions applied here will protrude and distort the hairstyle shape.

There are 100 extensions in this hairstyle. It takes three hours to apply these extensions, using 150g of fibre hair, which is one-and-a-half packets. The colours used are 50g or pale blonde, 50g of cool blonde/ash blonde, 25g of light brown, 25g of gold.

The fibre is blow dried using a warm hairdryer. The style was cut using scissors, point cutting the perimeter lines and slide cutting to create some layers at the front of the hairstyle. This hairstyle has to be completely removed after three months' wear.

Textured extension hairstyle

The diagram shows the planning and placement of extensions to create a large curly, textured extension hairstyle. This is a lengthened spiral curled look. The extensions are placed 1 cm behind the hairline. A heat clamp was used creating individual extensions held in place with fibre hot seals. Two stylists were required to work on this hairstyle (see attaching synthetic fibre extensions, pp. 230–231). The natural hair is sectioned into six sections.

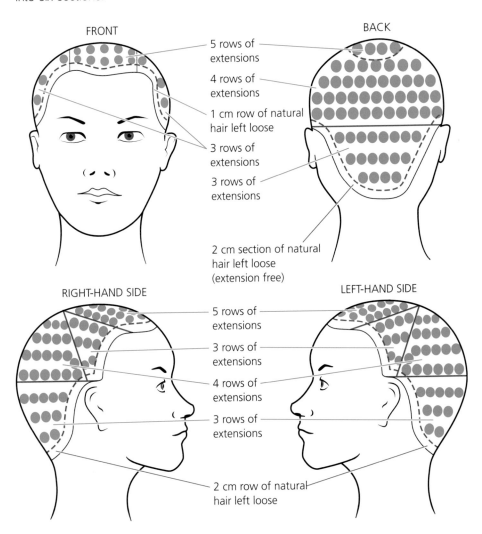

FRONT

BACK

5 rows of extensions

4 rows of extensions

1 cm row of natural hair left loose

3 rows of extensions

3 rows of extensions

2 cm section of natural hair left loose (extension free)

RIGHT-HAND SIDE

LEFT-HAND SIDE

5 rows of extensions

3 rows of extensions

4 rows of extensions

3 rows of extensions

2 cm row of natural hair left loose

Application of hair extensions

Area 1 has three rows of extensions applied. They are placed 1 cm away from the hairline. A 2 cm section of natural hair was left extension free across the occipital bone. This section is often left extension free. If extensions are applied on this bone they will protrude and create a distorted shape.

Area 2 has four rows of extensions applied right up to the top of the head.

Areas 3 and 5 have three rows of hair extensions applied. A 1 cm section of hair is left extension free in Areas 3 and 5 above the second row. This area is the widest point of

EKU *statement*

GH23 (eku48) How the intended final styling can affect the hair extension process

GH23 (eku49) How the attachment systems in the range can affect the way extensions are added and cut

GH23 (eku61) The reasons for establishing and following guidelines

GH23 (eku62) Why and how hair sectioning needs to be adapted when hair extensions are present

GH23 (eku63) How to creatively carry out cutting techniques in the range to blend the client's own hair and the hair extensions to suit the style requirements

GH23 (eku64) Why and how cutting techniques in the range should be adapted when hair extensions are present

GH23 (eku65) Why and how checking methods for cutting should be adapted when hair extensions are present

the head and often left loose as extensions applied here will protrude and distort the hairstyle shape.

Areas 4 and 6 have five rows of extensions applied covering the whole top area right back and over the crown.

There are 250 extensions in this hairstyle. It takes four hours to apply these extensions, using 300g of fibre hair, which is in three packets. The colours used are 50g of white, 50g of light blonds, 100g of cool/ash blonde, 50g of light brown, 25g of ginger and 25g of gold.

The fibre is curled on heated bendy rollers. The style was cut using scissors. The curled fibre was blunt cut and shaped visually. Gel is used to reduce fizzy ends and hold the curls in shape. The fibre has to be re-curled every 4–6 weeks as the curl will drop. This hairstyle has to be completely removed after three months' wear.

Activity

Knowing when or if an extension service can be carried out is critical to the success of the service and the ongoing repeated business.

In your portfolio answer the following questions:

1 What is traction alopecia?

2 What things should you do when conducting a consultation for an extensions service?

3 What things would be contra-indications to an extension service?

4 What preparations should you make?

5 How would you go about selecting the colour(s) of fibre for a client?

6 How do you mix the fibres together?

7 What aftercare advice should you give to clients?

GH23.4 Cut and finish hair with extensions

Cutting extension hairstyles

Remember

If the extension hair is wet or damp whilst cutting, when it dries it will shrink into a distorted finished result. Fibre hair has no elasticity and therefore needs no tension whilst cutting. Real hair is chemically damaged and will therefore stretch when wet. If cut whilst wet it will dry in uneven lines.

The cutting tools that can be used on extension hair are hairdressing scissors, a razor, clippers and thinning scissors. All extension hairstyle cutting is performed on dry extension hair as creating the styles are visual haircuts using soft blending techniques and not technical blunt haircuts. The principles of hairstyle balance and proportion must be retained in creating a finished result.

Use a razor or clipper on very straight extension hair as these tools will create soft lines in the hairstyle. If scissors are used on straight fibre it will exaggerate blunt or straight lines that are cut into them which can make the finished hairstyle look very false.

Use hairdressing scissors or clippers on wavy or curly extension hair as these tools will give a soft line in the wavy or curly hair without thinning the ends of the extension hair to such a degree that the ends will frizz, mat or tangle.

Most of the cutting techniques recommended for cutting extension hair can be used on natural hairstyles. These cutting techniques are designed to create soft, thinned, tapered or graduated blending results that are most suitable for extension hair, ensuring that the finished hairstyle looks natural.

TUTOR SUPPORT

Project 10.7: Cutting techniques for extension hairstyles

Cutting techniques for extension hairstyles

1 **Blunt or club cutting**. This is a technique that cuts a heavy straight line and is created using scissors.
2 **Soft tapering**. This technique cuts a soft, thin layer into the mid-lengths and ends of the extension hair and is created using a razor or thinning scissors.
3 **Spiral tapering**. This is a technique that cuts uneven lengths through the mid-lengths and ends of extension hair and is created using a razor or scissors.
4 **Layering**. This is a technique used to connect short hair into long hair by sliding a razor or scissors down the hair length creating a soft lightly layered profile line.
5 **Surface graduated layering**. This is a technique used to layer extension hair without removing weight and bulk from the extension hair and is created using scissors or clippers.
6 **Skim or surface clippering**. This is a technique used to break up surface layers of extension hair or reduce length and bulk at speed and is created using electric clippers.
7 **Point cutting**. This is a technique used to cut an even perimeter line into extension hair without cutting a false looking straight line, created using scissors or thinning scissors.

Diversion For more information relating to controlling the accuracy of the cut see Chapter 4, Unit GH16 Creatively cut hair using a combination of techniques pp. 87–94.

Remember

If wavy or curly extension hair is thinned or tapered too much it will tangle and frizz at the ends.

Styling hair extensions

The tools that can be used to style fibre extension hair are hairdryers or airstylers set at a medium temperature or heated rollers.

The tools that can be used on real extension hair are hairdryers or airstylers, heated rollers, curling tongs, crimpers, hot brushes and straightening irons. Always avoid using heated hairdressing tools onto the bonds that attach extensions in place as the heat will soften the bonds and the extensions will fall out. Whilst styling extensions incorporate the natural hair in with the styling, do not separate the extensions away from the natural hair as this will make blow-drying and setting very difficult. It will also give variable structure to the finished hairstyle, making the result look unnatural.

Wavy or curly fibre extension hair will drop after a couple of weeks. The curl or wave will fall out as the fibre is softened from the heat of the client's body temperature. The fibre will need re-curling regularly throughout the hairstyle's life span of three months.

Remember

- Hot hairdressing tools will melt and irreparably damage fibre hair. Do not use hot hairdryers, heated curling tongs, hot brushes or straightening irons on fibre hair.
- Real extension hair is delicate as it has been chemically damaged. Therefore the stylist must recommend the most appropriate styling tool for the client to ensure that the extension hair is maintained in optimum condition.

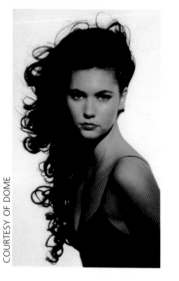

COURTESY OF DOME

Remember

For the best styling results on extension hair, always style the extension hair in a dry or virtually dry state. This will ensure you achieve a stronger set or shape that will hold in place for a long period of time. Setting or drying extension hair from wet will take a very long time to dry and will result in a weak result lasting only a couple of hours.

Remember

Before re-curling fibre hair, smooth the fibre out using a soft bristle brush and warm hairdryer and then re-curl fibre from a virtually straight structure. This will ensure that you do not double-curl the fibre. Double-curling will give a frizzy, unattractive result. Double-curling is achieved when you attempt to curl fibre on top of an existing curl or wavy structure.

EKU *statement*

GH23 (eku57) How to remove hot and cold hair attachment systems

GH23 (eku68) The types of products to use when removing hot and cold hair extensions

Styling products for use on extension hair

- Mousse
- Gel
- Setting lotions
- Hairspray
- Pomade – use sparingly

Apply styling products to the mid-lengths and ends of the extension hair. Avoid the root area as some styling products contain oil, wax, silicone and alcohol ingredients which can break the extension bonds down, making the extension fall out, or making the natural hair very slippery so the extensions slip out down the hair shaft.

GH23.5 Maintain and remove hair extensions

Remember

Do not apply excess tension on the root area by tying tight ponytails.

Remember

Hair extension hairstyles must be dried immediately at the root and bonded area. Do not brush or comb extensions when they are still wet as the bonds can break down and fall out.

Good practice/Health and safety

Some removal solutions can irritate the skin or dissolve nail polish and nail extensions – ensure you wear rubber gloves.

Different hair extension types have differing techniques of removal. You need to check with the manufacturer for more details for their particular hair extension services.

The following information provides general guidelines for the removal of extensions for:

- cold fusion systems
- hot bonded systems
- cold fusion (using adhesive tape)

Cold fusion systems

1 Section the hair so that you can work on the extension weft without getting removal product on the rest of the hair

2 Place a cotton wool pad beneath the weft to protect the scalp

3 Apply the removal chemicals directly from the applicator onto the weft

4 Wipe the weft with the pad to evenly apply the chemical

5 Leave to penetrate through the extension and weaken the bond

6 Heat the weft near to the root area to activate the removal product

7 When the bond has disintegrated, carefully remove the weft by carefully peeling downwards and away from the hair.

Remember

 Put on your disposable vinyl gloves on before handling any removal chemicals.

Hot bonded systems

All hot bonded systems have similar removal techniques, the only differences being in products and removal tools.

1 Section the hair so that you can work on the extension without altering the rest of the hair extensions

2 Using the removal tool, crush the bond throughout the length of the seal

3 Place a cotton wool pad beneath the bond and apply the removal liquid evenly across the seal

4 Leave for a minute or so, so that the chemicals can break down the adhesion to the hair.

5 Re-crush the bond throughout the seal

6 Then remove the extension by pulling it gently along the hair.

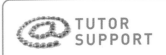 **TUTOR SUPPORT**

Discussion 10.5: Safety precautions that should be observed when removing extensions

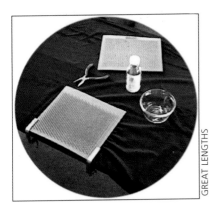
GREAT LENGTHS

Step 1 You need a removal tool, removal solution (if applicable), pad of cottonwool and rubber gloves. If you are removing real hair extensions have a mixing mat available

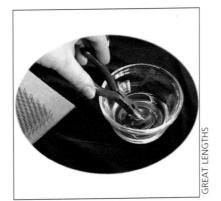
GREAT LENGTHS

Step 2 Dip your removal tool in the removal solution, placing a pad of cottonwool underneath the resin bond. Then apply a drop of removal solution onto the resin bond that attaches the extension in place

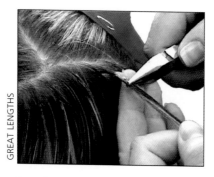

GREAT LENGTHS

Step 3 Crush the resin bond with the removal tool and the bond will begin to crumble

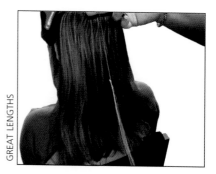

GREAT LENGTHS

Step 4 Holding the end of the extension slide the extension out of the natural hair

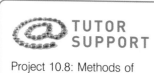

TUTOR SUPPORT

Project 10.8: Methods of removal of hair extensions

There may be some residue of resin left in the client's natural hair. Brushing the natural hair, and shampooing and conditioning it, will easily remove this.

Other systems

Cold fusion (attached by adhesive tape)

Self-adhesive extensions use special chemical sprays or solutions to dissolve the bond attaching them to the hair. When this is applied/sprayed on to the self-cling tape it quickly reduces the adhesion and therefore releases the weft from the hair. The removed weft can then be inspected to see if it is worth keeping or whether it should be thrown away.

The self-cling strips can be removed from the weft in the same way that the extension is removed from the hair and, depending on the quality of the weft, it can be washed, re-conditioned and retained for future use or, otherwise, discarded. If the weft is to be re-used, new, double-sided self-adhesive tapes will need to be applied after the wefts have been dried.

EKU *statement*

GH23 (eku56) How to maintain hot and cold hair attachment systems and why maintenance is important to how long the hair style will last

GH23 (eku58) Why it is important to remove product build up and debris as part of the extension removal process

GH23 (eku66) The types of finishing products suitable for use with hair extensions

GH23 (eku67) The types and purpose of specialist products available for the aftercare of hair extensions

GH23 (eku80) The types of anxieties commonly experienced by clients undergoing the hair extension process

GH23 (eku81) How to help relieve client anxieties in a reassuring way

GH23 (eku82) How to give effective advice and recommendations to clients.

1 Section the hair so that you can work on the extension getting removal product on the rest of the hair

2 Pour a small amount of removal solution onto a cotton wool pad and evenly apply along the length of the adhesive tape

3 Allow the chemicals to penetrate for around 30 seconds

4 Hold the end of the extension weft and pull it down and away from the natural hair.

Sewn-in extensions

On straight hair These can be easily removed by the careful cutting of the stitches that hold the weft in place.

On plaited hair That appears as free hanging braids, simply cut above the hard bond at the ends of the extension and unravel the plaits using the end of a tail comb. After removing the extensions comb the hair through to detangle the lengths and shampoo and condition to prepare the hair for the next service.

GH23.6 Provide aftercare advice

There are two types of extension hair that can be used to create hair extension hairstyles:

- synthetic, acrylic fibre extension hair
- real human extension hair that is either Asian or European hair.

The two hair types need different home-care products. The following client advice and home-care procedures should be given to clients who wear extension hairstyles.

Synthetic, acrylic fibre extension hair

The home care products required for fibres are:

1 *A clarifying shampoo*. This is a shampoo designed to remove sebum, oil, wax, product build-up and pollutants from the extension hair and natural hair. This shampoo must be oil and silicone free.

2 *A light conditioner*. This is a conditioner specifically designed for fibre hair and natural hair. It is normally manufactured by extension product companies and designed to coat the fibre hair, forming a surface barrier and protecting the fibre from any heat or friction damage caused by brushing and styling the fibre. It is a light conditioner which sits on the surface of the natural hair.

3 *A daily maintenance spray*. This is a spray mist that is applied to the mid-lengths and ends of the fibre. It untangles the fibre and protects it from heated appliances used for styling. The spray is only manufactured by extension product companies. The daily maintenance spray must be used before brushing fibre and before any heated styling tools are used to style the fibre.

4 *A soft bristle brush*. This is a brush that has a padded face and soft bristles that protrude from the padded base. Soft bristle brushes should be used when blending, mixing and brushing hair.

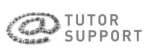

TUTOR SUPPORT

Project 10.9: Information that should be given to client having hair extensions between visits to the salon

Remember

Oil- and silicone-based shampoos can break down the bonds attaching extensions in place. They can also build up on the hair shaft, causing the extension to slip out of the hair.

Remember

Conditioner must not be applied to the root area of the client's hair or directly onto the bonds that attach the extensions in place. If applied to the roots or bonds it will leave a deposit on the natural hair causing the extension to fall out and it can break the bonds down.

Remember

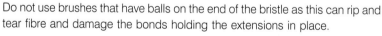

Hair extensions are a big step for the client. If it's their first experience of the service, they will be venturing into the unknown. Explain what takes place and the things that they can expect to happen when they work with their hair themselves.

Above all, look out for signs of uncertainty or doubt; be reassuring and dispel worries or concerns that they might have. That way everyone will be happy with the results!

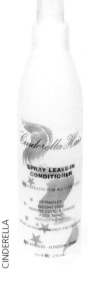

Soft bristle brush

Real extension hair

The home-care products required for real hairs are:

1. *A clarifying shampoo*. This is a shampoo that is designed to remove sebum, oil, wax, styling products and pollutants from the extension hair and natural hair. This shampoo must be oil- and silicone-free.

2. *A reconstructive conditioner*. This is a conditioner that works within the hair shaft, designed to strengthen and rebuild hair. Reconstructive conditioners are manufactured by extension product companies specifically for real hair. Real hair has gone through several chemical processes before application, making it porous and chemically damaged. Reconstructive conditioners should be used to assist in maintaining the strength, shine and manageability. Light conditioners are not recommended for real hair as these products would build up on the real hair, making it dull, lifeless and heavy.

3. *A pH-balanced rinse*. This is an acid-balanced rinse that has the same pH as hair and skin (4.5–5.5). This product is diluted in water 1 part pH rinse to 10 parts water. This product is used after shampooing and conditioning and is applied through the mid-lengths and ends of the hair. The acid-balanced rinse is designed to close the cuticle layers of the real hair, therefore reducing tangles and matting that can occur when the real hair is wet. This rinse can be used as a daily product contained in a water spray and applied to damp down real hair before restyling. A pH-balanced rinse is manufactured by extension product companies specifically for real hair.

4. *A soft bristle brush*. Soft bristle brushes should be used when brushing real hair extension hairstyles.

Remember

Do not use brushes that have balls on the end of the bristle as this can rip and tear fibre and damage the bonds holding the extensions in place.

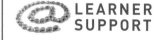 **LEARNER SUPPORT**

Creative hair extensions wordsearch

Remember

All home-care products and tools must be recommended to the client by the stylist who has created the extension hairstyle. Products used on extensions that are not recommended by a stylist could damage or make extensions fall out.

Home-care advice for extensions

This is a step-by-step procedure to be followed consecutively by clients when cleansing conditioning and styling extension hairstyles.

1 Shampoo extension hairstyles at least twice a week, reducing natural oil build-up at the root area.

2 Before shampooing brush gently with a soft bristle brush. Begin brushing at the ends of the hair in downward strokes until you reach the root area. Then brush from the root through to the tips.

3 Using your fingers ensure all the extensions are separated at the root area.

4 Whilst shampooing real hair the head should be in an upright position. Standing in the shower is an ideal position. The hair and water should flow in a vertical downward direction. The water temperature should be warm.

5 Use a clarifying shampoo recommended by your stylist specifically for your hair extension hair. Using your fingertips, stroke the shampoo gently into the hair from the roots to the tips. Do not massage or rub the extensions when wet.

6 Apply a recommended conditioner to the mid-lengths and ends of the extension hair. Then rinse thoroughly.

7 After shampooing and conditioning, wrap a towel around the hair and pat gently to remove excess water. Wrap hair in a towel and leave for 20 minutes for the towel to absorb all the moisture from the extensions and natural hair.

8 Separate the extensions at the root area with your fingers before drying.

9 Dry the extensions with a warm hairdryer using a diffuser if required.

10 After drying the root area, brush gently from the ends towards the root area in a downward direction. Always hold the hair extensions at the roots whilst brushing to avoid placing unnecessary tension on the bonds and root area.

11 Long or lengthened hair extensions must be plaited and secured with a covered band on the ends before going to bed at night. Do not go to bed with damp or wet extensions as matting and tangling will occur.

Remember

Do not allow natural oils to build up at the scalp area as this can break down the bonds and then the extensions slip out.

Styling extension hairstyles do's and don'ts

✔	Always explain the benefits of using professional brushes and styling products.
✔	Always explain to the client the ways that they should be handling their own hair extensions at home.
✔	Always tell the client what sorts of products to use and those that should be avoided and why.
✔	Explain to the client the things that they should look out for in respect to hair damage, weakened hair and traction alopecia.

EKU *statement*

GH23 (eku70) How to correctly detangle hair from point to root using specialised combs and brushes

GH23 (eku71) The importance of following manufacturers' instructions when shampooing and conditioning the hair

GH23 (eku72) Products for home use that will benefit the client and those to avoid and why

GH23 (eku73) How to protect the hair when sleeping and why

GH23 (eku74) How lifestyle can affect the client's choice of style (e.g. active sports, career requirements)

GH23 (eku75) How the use of artificial hair can affect their styling possibilities

GH23 (eku76) How to maintain their agreed style

GH23 (eku77) How long the hair extensions can be expected to last

GH23 (eku78) Removal requirements for attached hair

GH23 (eku79) How to deal with signs of traction alopecia

EKU *statement*

GH23 (eku69) The types of styling and finishing techniques that can and cannot be used with hair extensions and why

EKU *statement*

GH23 (eku59) The types of problems that can occur when adding hair extensions and how to remedy them

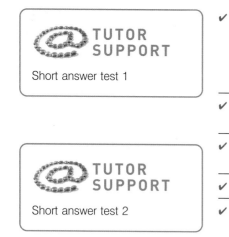

✓	Use hairdryers and heated rollers on the fibre hair. Heat will straighten or curl fibre extensions. Once heated and cooled down the fibre will retain this texture until more heat is applied to re-curl or straighten. Water will not alter the movement of fibre extensions. Do not use curling tongs, curling brushes, straighteners or crimpers directly on the fibre.
✓	Use hairdryers and heated rollers on real hair. Electric curling tongs, straighteners and hot brushes may be used on Asian or European hair extensions.
✓	Always avoid the bonded areas with these heated tools as direct heat will soften the bonds.
✓	Do not backcomb the hair extensions as this will cause irreparable tangling.
✓	Do not use styling products that contain oils, wax, silicone or excessive alcohol as these will break down the extension bonds.

Typical problems with artificial/synthetic hair extensions

Problem	Advice to give
Hair extensions tend to tangle or get knotted easily	Suggest suitable products and tools that will help to make grooming and brushing easier. Explain that the longer lengths should always be combed from points to roots. Long hair and particularly synthetic hair needs to be disentangled by working and freeing up from the ends back through the lengths towards the bonded area of the weft with a wide tooth comb rather than a brush.
Hair lengths tend to get matted when they are shampooed	Suggest conditioning products that are designed to work on synthetic/artificial hair. Sometimes the conditioners for acrylic hair are best applied before the hair is wetted; this reduces the locking and matting result caused by the action of rubbing during shampooing. Suggest that the hair is shampooed in a different way along the lengths by a smoothing action, rather than rubbing at the scalp.
Longer lengths get matted or knotted during sleep/ overnight	People who are more restless during sleep may find that the rubbing action of the hair on the pillow makes the extensions lock together overnight. Suggest tying the hair in ponytail with a soft fabric ribbon. This reduces the movement and the effects caused by chafing on the pillow. Alternatively, if the hair is very long, you can advise wrapping the hair in a silken scarf. This holds the lengths together and stops any chance of knotting.
Hair gets in the way at work or in sport	Clients who are used to shorter hair will not be familiar with the problems associated with long hair. Explain the benefits of wearing hair up as opposed to down during work/sport as this may have a more professional or beneficial effect.
Limited styling options after extensions have been applied	When artificial extensions have been applied to the hair, the options available to the client for future styling/finishing in other ways are limited. Synthetic hair does not respond well to hot styling: the hair can't be moulded or shaped in the same ways that you would style natural hair. You must make the client aware of this from the outset. Any excess heat applied to the hair will cause it to distort, mat together or melt. When this occurs, the only course of action is to cut the damaged lengths off or to remove them altogether! This can be avoided as long as you point out the problems before they leave the salon.

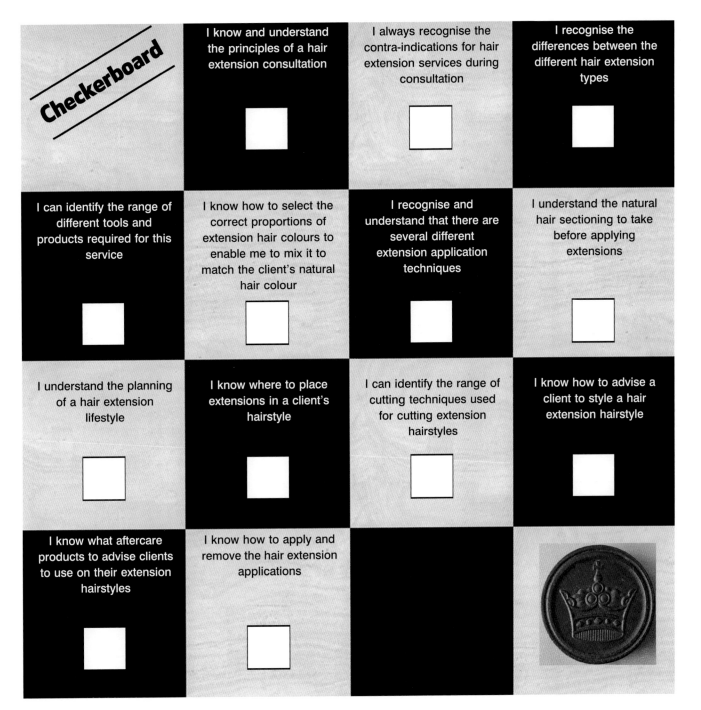

Checkerboard

Checkerboard	I know and understand the principles of a hair extension consultation	I always recognise the contra-indications for hair extension services during consultation	I recognise the differences between the different hair extension types
I can identify the range of different tools and products required for this service	I know how to select the correct proportions of extension hair colours to enable me to mix it to match the client's natural hair colour	I recognise and understand that there are several different extension application techniques	I understand the natural hair sectioning to take before applying extensions
I understand the planning of a hair extension lifestyle	I know where to place extensions in a client's hairstyle	I can identify the range of cutting techniques used for cutting extension hairstyles	I know how to advise a client to style a hair extension hairstyle
I know what aftercare products to advise clients to use on their extension hairstyles	I know how to apply and remove the hair extension applications		

Assessment of knowledge and understanding

Revision questions

Quick quiz: a selection of different types of questions to check your knowledge.

Q1 The condition of the client's hair near the _____ is particularly important when considering a hair extension service.   Fill in the blank

Q2 Clients who have to wash their hair on a daily basis are suited to hair extension services.   True or false

Q3 Which of the following are contra-indications for hair extensions?   Multi selection

Psoriasis	☐	1
Dandruff	☐	2
Alopecia	☐	3
Excessive oily scalp	☐	4
Infection	☐	5
Gel, mousse or hair wax	☐	6

Q4 Artificial fibre and synthetic fibre are the same thing.   True or false

Q5 A full head of extensions would on average amount to: Multi choice

75–125 single extensions	○	a
150–250 single extensions	○	b
300–500 single extensions	○	c
500–1000 single extensions	○	d

Q6 The cost of real hair extensions is proportional to their length.   True or false

Q7 Which of the following are not connector products for hair extensions?   Multi selection

Heated pre-bonded extension applicator	☐	1
Cold fusion adhesive	☐	2
Polymer resin adhesive sticks	☐	3
Mixing mats	☐	4
Acetone	☐	5
Spirit based solutions	☐	6

Q8 In making colour choices the main or first colour is known as _____ colour.   Fill in the blank

Q9 Which of the following is not recommended as home-care maintenance for real hair extensions?   Multi choice

Washing the hair with a clarifying shampoo	○	a
Refreshing the hair with a daily maintenance spray	○	b
Applying conditioners to the root area	○	c
Drying the hair with a warm drier	○	d

Q10 You should always hold the hair extensions at the roots whilst brushing.   True or false

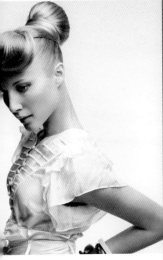

Chaptereleven
Colouring hair

GH17

GH17.1

GH17.2

GH17.3

GH17.4

GH17.5

**CREDIT VALUE
FOR UNIT GH17
12 Credits**

> **More information** About contra-indications, tests, consultation and customer care see Unit G21 Provide hairdressing consultation services

> **Diversion** Your responsibilities under COSHH regulations GH17 (eku6) and Electricity at Work
> GH17 (eku7) See Unit G22 Monitor procedures to safely control work operations
> Your responsibilities for customer records under Data Protection Act GH17 (eku5) See Appendix 4

Creative colouring: quick overview

Unit titles

GH17 Colour hair using a variety of techniques

This is a **optional** unit for both hairdressing and barbering at level 3, it is made up of six main outcomes

Main outcomes

GH17.1 Maintain effective and safe methods of working when colouring and lightening

GH17.2 Prepare for colouring and lightening services

GH17.3 Creatively colour and lighten hair

GH17.4 Lighten hair

GH17.5 Resolve basic colouring problems

GH17.6 Provide aftercare advice

What do I need to do for GH17.1?

- Make sure that the client is adequately covered, protected and prepared for the service
- Make sure that the working position is comfortable and safe for both you and the client
- Keep the work area clean and tidy and that waste materials are disposed of properly
- Work without causing risks to you or your client's health and safety
- Work efficiently and effectively at all times
- Accurately maintain the client's treatment records

Keywords

Artificial colour

The term refers to any form of colour that is not a naturally occurring pigment. These could be semi, quasi or permanent (para-dyes)

Synthetic colour

Another professional term that can be used instead of artificial colour

Para-dyes

A term that refers to permanent colours containing paraphenylenediamine or PPD. This is chemical compound that people can have a sensitivity to, or allergic reaction to on contact with the skin

Skin test

A test done 24–48 hrs prior to colouring to establish whether a client has a sensitivity or reaction to PPD or colouring products

Pre-pigmentation

Part of a larger process, colouring back, where missing pheomelanin (yellow/red pigments) are replaced first, so that the final target shade can be achieved without unwanted ashen 'green' tones being present

Pre-softening

A process of softening resistant white hair with hydrogen peroxide so that the colour coverage is improved

What do I need to do for GH17.2?

- Ask questions to identify any contra-indications to colouring and/or lightening
- Accurately record the responses to your questions
- Carry out suitable tests and record the outcomes
- Select and prepare your products and tools appropriate to your consultations' findings

What do I need to do for GH17.3?

- Explore suitable colour options using visual aids
- Apply products safely, accurately, and innovative ways in line with manufacturers' instructions
- Use appropriate techniques to achieve the expected result
- Monitor the product development by strand testing
- Identify and resolve any problems as they occur

What do I need to do for GH17.4?

- Confirm the desired result before the lightener is applied
- Apply lightening products quickly, safely and accurately in line with manufacturers' instructions
- Continually monitor the lightener development, hair condition, the client's scalp and the condition of the product whilst processing
- Remove the lightener to minimise discomfort, leaving the scalp free of product
- Apply toners if necessary to achieve the desired effects

What do I need to do for GH17.5?

- Resolve basic colouring problems
- Identify correct courses of action for colour correction procedures
- Ensure that the finished result meets the client's expectations

What do I need to do for GH17.6?

- Give accurate constructive advice on how the client can maintain their hair colour

What aspects do I need to cover for GH17.1, GH17.2, GH17.3, GH17.4, GH17.5 and GH17.6?

- Quasi- and permanent hair colouring products, lighteners and toners
- A variety of contra-indications to colouring and lightening services

- The necessary tests as and when they are needed

- A range of factors that influence or limit the way in which colouring and lightening is carried out

- A variety of innovative colouring techniques i.e. slicing, block colour and weaving

- A variety of lightening techniques i.e. root application, full and partial head

- Colour correction techniques that restore natural depth and tone, neutralise unwanted tones and cover resistant hair

- The advice and recommendations that you should give for the client to maintain their hair at home

What aspects do I need to know for GH17.1, GH17.2, GH17.3, GH17.4, GH17.5 and GH17.6?

- Your salon's requirements for preparation, timings and standards of service

- How to work safely, effectively and hygienically when colouring and lightening hair

- The different factors that can affect or influence successful colouring and lightening services

- The questions that you must ask and the tests that need to be done prior to and during the colouring services and the records that you must make

- The courses of action that you should take in the event of adverse reactions to tests or unexpected results during development

- The principles of colouring and lightening and the effects of these products upon the hair

- How natural and synthetic pigments differ and how light changes their appearance

- How different strengths of hydrogen peroxide affect hair and how they can be diluted

- How pH is affected by colouring products and how hair is balanced after processing

- How and when to pre-soften and pre-pigment hair

- The range of tools, equipment and materials and how these used

- A variety of techniques that can be used to achieve creative colouring results

- The types of problems that can be encountered during processing and how these can be resolved

- The aftercare advice and recommendations that you should give to clients

Information covered in this chapter

- The preparations that you must make before carrying out any colouring service

- Basic colour correcting methods and problem solving

- The tools and equipment used during colouring and lightening services, their maintenance and the preparations that you should make before colouring hair

- The factors that influence successful results in colouring and lightening services

- A range of innovative colouring and lightening techniques on differing hair lengths and types

- How to correct simple, routine colouring problems and faults

- The aftercare advice that you should give

Introduction

Colouring is arguably the most exciting and often the most difficult aspect of modern fashionable hairdressing. The increasing demands and expectations of clients have made colouring and in particular the application of special colour effects the 'must-have' of hairdressing.

Our clients are getting more informed about hair styling, hair condition and the benefits of product usage. But colouring for them has a compulsory 'magnetic' but still elusive draw, techniques and products are developing all the time and the possibilities are boundless, so dare to create a little magic!

Foreword

If you have continued into level 3 after completing NVQ level 2 then quite a lot of the basic principles covered there will still be fresh in your mind and much of the first part of this chapter will be familiar to you.

However, if there has been a gap in your training then you will be able to refresh your memory by reviewing this information again. This is not intended to be a repetition of what you have already learned; but is a necessary aspect of the essential knowledge elements for colouring and lightening hair at level 3.

Note

If you have recently completed your NVQ level 2 you will already be familiar with the underpinning principles and knowledge for colouring and lightening hair.

If you want to refresh your memory for this topic continue from this point onwards; alternatively, jump forwards to:

EKU *statement*

GH17 (eku1) Maintain effective and safe methods of working when colouring and lightening
GH17 (eku2) Prepare for colouring and lightening services
GH17 (eku3) Creatively colour and lighten hair
GH17 (eku4) Lighten hair
GH17 (eku5) Resolve basic colouring problems
GH17 (eku6) Provide aftercare advice

The principles of colour and colouring

Seeing colour

When you look at an object, what you are actually seeing is light reflected from it. White light is really a mixture of many colours – that is why sunlight refracted through falling rain can produce a rainbow. This splitting of white light creates what we see as seven different colours: red, orange, yellow, green, blue, indigo and violet. (**R**ichard **O**f **Y**ork **G**ave **B**attle **I**n **V**ain.)

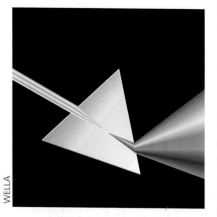

WELLA

The colour spectrum from visible light

A white object reflects most of the white light that falls upon it; a black object absorbs most of the light falling on it. A red object reflects the red light and absorbs everything else.

Hair colour depends chiefly on the pigments in the hair, which absorb some of the light and reflect the rest. The colour that we see is also affected by the light in which it is seen, and (to a lesser extent) by the colours of clothes worn with it.

- White light from halogen bulbs and full daylight will show the hair's natural colour.
- Yellowish light emitted from standard electric light bulbs adds warmth to hair colour, but neutralises blue ash or ashen effects.
- Bluish/green light from fluorescent tubes reduces the warmth of red/gold tones in hair.

Mixing colours

The colours of the pigments in paints arise from three primary colours – red, blue and yellow. Pairs of these give the secondary colours – i.e. red and blue mixed together creates violet, yellow and blue creates green and yellow and red create orange. White and black can be added to vary the tone of the colour.

The primary colours in light are different – red, green and blue. (These are the three colours used in video cameras, computer screens and television.) The secondary colours are yellow, cyan and magenta.

The ways in which colour pigments are mixed together in paint to produce other new colours is similar to that used in hairdressing. Like paint, permanent hair colours can be mixed together to create different shades.

Natural hair colour

The natural colour of hair is determined by the colour of pigments within the hair's cortex. These are formed when the hair is in its germinating stage of growth.

Hair colour pigments – **melanin** – are deposited into the hair shaft at the region of the papilla and germinal matrix. The pigments responsible for black and brown hair are called **eumelanin**; those responsible for red and yellow hair are called **pheomelanin**. (There are in fact others, but these are the main pigments.) The hair colour you actually see is affected by the amount and proportion of the pigments present, by the light in which the hair is seen and – to a certain extent – by the colours of the clothes and make-up worn.

With age, or after periods of stress, the production of natural pigments may be reduced. The hairs already on the head will not be affected, but the new ones will. As hairs fall out and are replaced, the proportion that have the original pigmentation diminishes and the hair's overall colour changes. It may become lighter. If no pigment is produced at all, then the new hairs will be white.

The proportion of white hairs among the naturally coloured ones causes the hair to appear grey. Grey hair or greyness (**canites**) is often referred to as a percentage; for example, '50 per cent grey' means that half of the hairs on the head are white and the rest are pigmented.

It is not uncommon for young people to exhibit some grey hairs – this does not necessarily mean that they will go grey, or completely white, at an early age.

EKU *statement*

GH17 (eku36) and GH18 (eku33) How the type and distribution of melanin creates natural hair colour

GH17 (eku38) How the natural pigmentation of hair affects the colouring and lightening process

Remember

In vibrant red or bright auburn hair, nearly all the melanin is present in the form of pheomelanin; however, another alpha-amino pigment is present in a complex iron compound called trichosiderin. (In 100 g of red hair, there are 40 mg of trichosiderin.) The trichosiderin changes the colour make-up of hair, giving it the rich, attractive colour of a genetically Celtic origin.

Colouring this particular type of red hair is difficult because of this different pigmentation. Lightening red hair is especially hard as this compound is very difficult to remove.

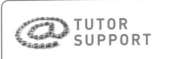

TUTOR SUPPORT

Project 11.1: Assessing the client's natural colour

EKU *statement*

GH9 (eku34) and GB2 (eku35) The principles of colour selection, including the International Colour Chart (ICC)

Depth and tone

Hair science/Depth and tone

When we talk about colour we often use the words *depth* and *tone*. Depth is used to describe how light or dark the colour is and tone is used to describe the colour or hue that we see such as brown golden red etc.' Depth = how light or dark it is. Tone = the colour or hue – ashen, golden, mahogany, etc.

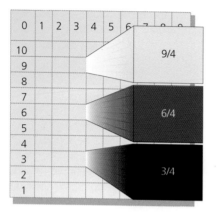

Depths and tones

These terms are easier to understand if we tabulate them in the following way.

Depth	Very light			
	Light			
	Medium			
	Dark			
	Very Dark			
		Gold	Red	Violet
	Tone ⟶			

Taking this principle further, the International Colour Chart (ICC) offers a way of defining hair colours systematically (although charts may vary between manufacturers). Shades of colour are divided and numbered, with black (1) at one end of the scale and lightest blonde (10) at the other. Tones of other colours (/1 /9 or also stated as .1 .9) are combined with these, producing a huge variety of colours. Charts are usually arranged with shades in rows down the side and tones in columns across the top. To use them, first identify the shade of your client's hair: that row of the chart then shows the colours you could produce with that hair.

For example, if your client has medium blonde hair (depth 7) and you colour with a copper tone (.4), the result should be a rich copper blonde (7.4). The possibilities are almost endless, as these examples indicate:

● to produce ash shades, add blue

● to produce matt shades, add green

● to produce gold shades, add yellow

● to produce warm shades, add red

● to produce purple or violet shades, add mixtures of red and blue.

Activity
Depth and tone – warm and cool shades
The natural 'depth' of hair refers to how light or dark it is, whereas 'tone' refers to colouration e.g. red, blue or green.

Task 1. (Working with depth)
With your colleagues and using the salon shade chart, take it in turns to select the nearest natural shade for each of them. (Tip: don't make the mistake of looking at the rest of the chart; just keep to the natural bases.)

Task 2. (Working with tone)
Again in a group work through your salon's shade chart and for each shade note down its shade name, number or code, then decide as a group whether it is a warm tone or a cool tone.

Keep the information from both of these tasks in your portfolio for future reference.

1 How many warm shades were there?

2 How many cool shades were there?

3 How many were neither warm nor cool?

4 Did you find any surprising results?

L'Oréal Majirel shade chart

10	Lightest blonde							
9	Very light blonde	Very Light Natural Ash Blonde 9,1		Very Light Deep Golden Blonde 9,33	Very Light Natural Copper Blonde 9,04			Very Light Natural Cool Blonde 9,07
8	Light blonde		Light Iridescent Blonde 8,2	Light Golden Blonde 8,3				
7	Blonde	Ash Blonde 7,1			**Deep Copper Blonde 7,44**		Extra Iridescent Red Blonde 7,62	
6	Dark blonde		Dark Deep Iridescent Blonde 6,22	Dark Natural Golden Blonde 6,03	**Dark Copper Red Blonde 6,46**	Dark Mahogany Golden Blonde 6,53	Dark Extra Red Blonde 6,66	Dark Natural Cool Blonde 6,07
5	Light brown	Light Deep Ash Brown 5,11			Light Extra Copper Red Blonde 5,46	Light Mahogany Iridescent Brown 5,52	Light Red Brown 5,6	Light Cool Ash Brown 5,71
4	Brown		Extra Burgendy Brown 4,20	Golden Brown 4,3		Mahogany Ash Brown 4,51		
3	Dark brown							
1	Black							
	Natural/Basic ,0	Ash ,1	Mauve ,2	Gold ,3	Copper ,4	Mahogany ,5	Red ,6	Metallic ,7

Remember

Compound henna

Compound henna is not pure vegetable henna; it is mixed with other element oxides and is therefore incompatible with modern colouring and perming materials!

EKU *statement*

GH17 (eku34) and GH18 (eku31) The principles of colour selection, including the International Colour Chart (ICC)

Remember

Incompatibles

Always check with your client what they have been using on their hair previously. Often men will use a simple lotion to stain over greying hair. Many of these types of dye are metallic-salt-based and are therefore incompatible with modern colouring and perming products.

EKU *statement*

GH17 (eku40) and GH18 (eku35) The effects on the hair of different colouring products and lighteners

GH17 (eku48) What makes hair resistant to artificial colour

GH17 (eku51) and GH18 (eku48) The different types of colouring products and lighteners available and how and when to use them

In the table above we see how the L'Oréal shades are positioned within the colour table. Row 1 containing 'Black' denotes the *darkest* shades. These gradually go up in numbers to Row 10 which contains 'Lightest Blonde' (10.0) and 'Lightest Ash Blonde' (10.1) and 'Lightest Beige Blonde' (10.13). These denote the *lightest* shades.

Within the table, two shades 'Dark Copper Red Blonde' (6.46), 'Deep Copper Blonde' (7.44) are defined in blue. These two examples identify additional colour properties. These shades are denoted, as are many others in the table, with having a second number after the comma.

Shade	Depth	Primary tone	Secondary tone
Dark Copper Red Blonde	6 •	4	6

1 The primary tone denotes the range that the shade is in.
2 Secondary tone indicates the additional pigmentation within the shade. This provides lots of extra colouring permutations.

Sometimes colour manufacturers want to increase a shade's intensity and vibrancy. This is achieved by adding double the tone to the particular shade, doubling the tonal effect.

Shade	Depth	Primary tone	Secondary tone
Deep Copper Blonde	7 •	4	4

Colour types

Semi-permanent colour

Semi-permanent colours are ready to use straight from the bottle. Always check the manufacturer's instructions to ensure that you know which type of colour you are going to use.

Semi-permanent colours contain pigments which are deposited in the hair cuticle and outer cortex. The colour gradually fades each time the hair is shampooed. Some colour will last through six washes, others longer.

Generally, these colours are not intended to cover large percentages of white hair – for instance, black used on white hair would not produce a pleasing result. Choose colours carefully.

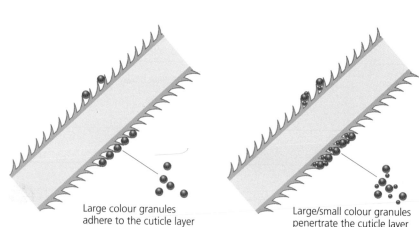

Large colour granules adhere to the cuticle layer

Large/small colour granules penetrate the cuticle layer

Note. Some salons (incorrectly) dilute permanent colour for use as semi-permanents. These products may contain skin sensitisers, however, so skin tests must be performed before hair colour is used in this way. Check manufacturer instructions for more information.

Features and benefits Semi-permanent colours are ideal for those people who want to try colour but are not ready yet to take a big step forward into the maintenance of permanent colour effects. They last up to six or eight shampoos and do not produce any regrowth; the hair loses the colour on each subsequent shampoo so the effect fades over time. As part of the colouring package they always contain conditioning agents that add shine and improve style manageability while the colour is deposited on to the hair. They also provide an ideal solution for livening up faded mid-lengths and ends for clients who have permanent colours; this is particularly useful if the hair is not really ready yet for another treatment of peroxide-based colours.

Semi-permanents will colour white/grey hair to some extent, although the penetration doesn't extend beyond the cuticle layer, so colour density is relatively poor. (White hair tends to have a very smooth cuticle so there is less spaces for the pigments to bond on to.) The colour range is varied, ranging from fashion effects to many of the shades you would expect to see in a standard shade chart. They are simple to use and require no developer and hence no mixing.

TUTOR SUPPORT

Project 11.8: Match base shades on the shade chart

Features and benefits

Feature	Benefits
Have large molecules that sit on the surface of the hair whilst other smaller ones penetrate deeper into the hair	A great way to introduce clients to colour without long-term commitment. Fairly easy to remove as they are washed away in six or eight shampoos
Come in a variety of types as mousses, liquids, gels, creams	Easy to apply, normally require no mixing, take a short time and leave no regrowth
Come in a variety of colours as fashion effects or as standard shade chart references	Can be used as a fashion statement or alternatively as a trial for a permanent colour effect.
Can be used in colour correction work	A simple and quick pre-filler and pre-pigmentation shade
Add tone to white/grey hair	Provides some masking/coverage for unwanted greys
Provides a different alternative to permanent colour	Can provide a colour choice for those people who because of sensitivity or allergy may not be able to have permanent colours

Points to remember

- Only lasts for up to six or eight washes
- Often difficult to remove totally from hair that is extremely porous or lightened
- You can not lighten hair with semi-permanent colour
- Will not colour white/grey hair with 100 per cent coverage
- Covers with far better results than temporary colours

Longer-lasting colour

Now that 'frequent use' shampoos have become popular, semi-permanent colours fade quickly. Therefore a new generation of longer lasting, quasi-permanent colour has been introduced which are more practical and economical. These colours allow for a greater coverage of white hair and last for up to 12 washes.

Quasi-permanent colour

Quasi-permanent colours are nearly permanent – they last for a longer period of time than semi-permanent colour but not as long as the true permanent colour. When using them, follow the manufacturer's instructions carefully.

Features and benefits

Quasi colours are used a lot in the home retail sector. They are not true permanent colours but do require the mixing of colour with a low strength developer. They last for at least 12 washes and anything up to 24 and, regardless of advertisers' claims, *they can leave a regrowth*. These types of colours do have a better ability to cover white/grey hair and this is the main reason why they are so popular as home colours.

Quasi colours should be treated like permanent colours or lighteners; they do require a skin test 24–48 hours beforehand.

Feature	Benefits
Are processed with a developer and have similar molecules that penetrate deeper into the hair	Easy solution for all-over colouring; lasts a long time, generally up to 12–24 shampoos
Come as gels or creams	Require mixing with developer and made easy to apply for home use. Leaves a regrowth
Come in a variety of colours as fashion effects or as standard shade chart references	Can be used as a fashion statement or as an alternative to more permanent-based colour
Can be used in colour correction work	As an alternative longer-lasting pre- pigmentation shade
Add depth and tone to white/grey hair	Provides up to 50 per cent coverage for unwanted greys
Provide a different alternative to permanent para-dyes	Tend to be used regularly and more often than salon-provided treatments
Good conditioning properties, add shine and improve manageability	Leaves hair in good condition, manageable and adds shine

Points to remember

- Always requires a skin test
- Lasts for 12 washes, leaves a regrowth
- Can only be removed by colour reduction (not removable by colour or lightener)
- Often provides the basis for colour correction work if wrongly used at home
- Good coverage, colours white/grey with better saturation than semis
- Similar effects to permanent colours

EKU *statement*

GH17 (eku35) What is meant by the term 'oxidation'

Permanent colour

Permanent colours are made in a wide variety of shades and tones. They can cover white and natural-coloured hair to produce a range of natural, fashion and fantasy shades.

Hydrogen peroxide is mixed with permanent colour. This oxidises the hair's natural pigments and joins the small molecules of synthetic pigment together, a process called 'polymerisation'. The hair will then retain the colour permanently in the cortex. Hair in poor condition, however, will not hold the colour and colouring could result in patchy areas and colour fading. (This is because any damaged or missing areas of cuticle will allow pigments to be released during shampooing.)

The use of modern permanent colour can lighten or darken the natural hair colour, or both together in one process. This is achieved by varying the percentage strength of hydrogen peroxide.

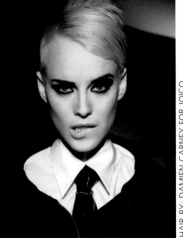

HAIR BY: DAMIEN CARNEY FOR JOICO,
PHOTOGRPAHY: HAMA SANDERS

NVQ3 Colouring hair GH17

Main points to remember True permanent para-dyes are the only colours that cover white/grey hair with 100 per cent saturation/coverage. The colours tend to come in easy-to-dispense tubes as creams or gels which are then mixed with hydrogen peroxide, as the developer, to create lasting effects that have to grow out. Even if the colour used is darker than the natural depth and deposits only, the colour effect will remain until it is either cut or grows.

Tiny colour granules are mixed with hydrogen peroxide – they pass through the cuticle layer into the cortex

Artificial depth and tone are added. Lightening of the natural pigments can occur with some shades

The granules swell and join together becoming permently trapped

The para-dyes contain PPD (paraphenylenediamine). This is a known irritant and it is this compound that necessitates the need for conducting skin or sensitivity tests before any colouring service is carried out. There are other chemicals within para-dyes and they all do different things:

- Ammonia/resorcinol is alkaline and when it comes into contact with the hair it swells the hair shaft in preparation for the pigmentation. It also acts as an **activator** or booster for the hydrogen peroxide by releasing oxygen and starting the **oxidation** process.
- Conditioning agents improve the hair during the colouring process, enabling it to be smoother and shinier as a result.

EKU statement

GH17 (eku41) and GH18 (eku38) How the different strengths of hydrogen peroxide affect the colouring and lightening of the hair

EKU *statement*

GH17 (eku43) and
GH18 (eku41) How to
dilute hydrogen peroxide to
form different strengths of
solutions

EKU *statement*

GH17 (eku1) and
GH18 (eku1) Your salon's
requirements for client
preparation

GH17 (eku4) and
GH18 (eku2) Your salon's
and legal requirements for
disposal of waste materials

GH17 (eku9) and
GH18 (eku7) The range of
protective clothing that
should be available for clients

GH17 (eku10) and
GH18 (eku8) The type of
personal protective
equipment that should be
available and used by yourself

GH17 (eku11) and
GH18 (eku9) Why it is
important to use personal
protective equipment

GH17 (eku12) and
GH18 (eku10) How the
position of your client and
yourself can affect the desired
outcome and reduce fatigue
and the risk of injury

GH17 (eku13) and
GH18 (eku11) Why it is
important to position your
tools and equipment for
ease of use

GH17 (eku18) and
GH18 (eku16) Why it is
important to keep your work
area clean and tidy

GH17 (eku19) and
GH18 (eku17) Methods of
working safely and
hygienically and which
minimise the risk of cross-
infection and cross-infestation

GH17 (eku20) and
GH18 (eku18) The importance of personal hygiene

GH17 (eku22)
and **GH18** (eku20)
Methods of cleaning,
disinfecting and/or
sterilisation used in salons

- During the process hydrogen peroxide oxidises the natural pigments of the hair and this enables the synthetic pigments to bond with them, creating a permanent change within the hair's cortex.

Vegetable-based colour As well as being a popular source for conditioning agents, plant extracts have been used as dyeing compounds for thousands of years. These were the only sources of colour until chemists developed synthetic alternatives. Natural henna (Lawsonia) is still used widely today in many countries and it is used for dyeing skin as well as the hair. Natural plant-based dyes do not present any problems for hairdressing treatments; however, these ingredients are sometimes added to other elements to form compounds. These are mixtures of vegetable extracts and mineral substances. One that is still available is compound henna – vegetable henna mixed with metallic salts. This penetrating dye is incompatible with professional products used in hairdressing salons and will react with professional salon colours and perming products.

Metallic dyes Metallic dyes are surface-coating colour. They are variously known as reduction, metallic, sulphide and progressive dyes. These types of dye are also incompatible with chemical hairdressing services and are still found in men's colour restorers; such as 'Just for Men' and 'Grecian 2000'.

Using hydrogen peroxide

The effects of hydrogen peroxide on hair

Hydrogen peroxide strength	Effect upon the hair (Note. Variations will occur between fine and coarse hair)
20 vol or (6%)	• Assists the deposit of colour into the hair; adding depth, making it darker • Enables coverage of white/grey hair • Will lighten two levels above base 6 (on fine hair) • Will lighten one level below base 4
30 vol or (9%)	• Will lighten hair three levels above base 6 (on fine hair) • Will lighten hair two levels below base 4
40 vol or (12%)	• Will lighten hair four levels above base 6 (with high lift colour)

Remember

Hydrogen peroxide
When hydrogen peroxide lightens hair to any level it will remove the smaller pigments first. The larger warmer pigments (pheomelanin) within the hair are more difficult to remove so unwanted golden or even orange tones are often left within the hair.

Diluting liquid hydrogen peroxide

This illustration shows you how the strengths that you have in stock can be diluted to make lesser strength hydrogen peroxide.

The first column refers to the strength peroxide that you have, the second refers to the peroxide you want to create. The last three columns show you how many parts of the peroxide you need and how many parts of distilled water you need to add to it.

Diluting liquid hydrogen peroxide

Strength you have	Strength you want to create	Peroxide	Add	Water
40 vol (i.e. 12%)	30 vol (i.e. 9%)	3	+	1
40 vol	20 vol (i.e. 6%)	1	+	1
40 vol	10 vol (i.e. 3%)	1	+	3
30 vol (i.e. 9%)	20 vol (i.e. 6%)	2	+	1
30 vol	10 vol (i.e. 3%)	1	+	2
20 vol (i.e. 6%)	10 vol (i.e. 3%)	1	+	1

Remember

Mixing colour Don't mix permanent colours together until you are ready to use them. Mix the colours carefully, making sure that you measure the amounts accurately. If the proportions are wrong the final effect will be wrong!

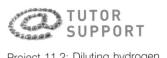

TUTOR SUPPORT

Project 11.2: Diluting hydrogen peroxide

GH17.1 Maintain effective and safe methods of working when colouring and lightening

Safety and preparation

Although Chapter 15 covers many of the general aspects that you need to know, each technical procedure has specific things that relate to that area of hairdressing alone. Hair colouring is particularly problematic as it involves the application of a variety of potentially harmful chemicals. Therefore the care that you take in handling products and preparing yourself and the client is absolutely critical to safe and successful colouring.

Records Should be found and put ready at the beginning of the day. The appointment book identifies all the expected clients, so all their treatment history – dates of visits, who provided the services, previous chemical services, records of any tests and any addition comments – can all be collated long before the clients arrive.

Similarly, when clients have been in, any results of tests or notes following treatments must always be updated. The records are essential for keeping things going smoothly;

Diversion For more information on sterilising tools and equipment see Unit G22, Health and safety pp. 388–389 and 392–393.

Diversion For more information on tests see pp. 266–268.

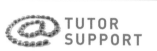

TUTOR SUPPORT

Project 11.4: Risk assessment for colouring service

EKU *statement*

GH17 (eku4) Your salon's and legal requirements for disposal of waste materials

Remember

Salon cleanliness is of paramount importance the work area should be clean and free from clutter or waste items. Any used materials should be disposed of and not left out on the side; it

(a) is unprofessional and

(b) presents a health hazard to others.

by maintaining services even if key staff are away. Let alone if things go wrong and they are needed in any legal action taken against the salon.

Tests   Collect together the results of any tests carried out prior to the appointment. If there have been any adverse reactions or contra-indications no permanent colour service can be carried out. Have you made this clear to the client and made plans for alternative services such as temporary or semi-permanent colouring?

Materials   After the records have been found it is advisable to get all tubes, cans or bottles of colour put aside and ready along with the client's record information. Doing this earlier has several benefits. It can save valuable time later when you need to mix them, particularly if you are running on a tight schedule. But it has useful benefits for the salon's stock control systems too: when products are removed from stock you can see when certain colours are running low. These can be noted and the relevant person made aware.

Gowning   Always make sure that the client and the client's clothes are adequately protected before any process is started. Most salons have special 'colour-proof' gowns for colouring and lightening processes. These gowns are resistant to staining and are made from finely woven synthetic fabrics that will stop colour spillages from getting through onto the client's skin or clothes. When you gown the client, make sure that the free edges are closed and fastened together. On top of this and around the shoulders you can place a colouring towel.

Using barrier cream   Barrier cream can be used as physical barrier to prevent staining around the client's face/hairline. It is also particularly useful if the client has any general sensitivity to chemical-based products. Remember. It is not an excuse for poor slapdash application; allowing you to extend the colour application beyond the hairline area to the skin. But it will help in areas where colour seeps off the hair – onto the skin.

Apply barrier cream to the skin with a finger or cotton wool close to the hairline, taking care not to get it onto the hair; as this could stop the colour from taking evenly.

It can be removed later after you have shampooed the colour from the hair and before any other services are conducted.

Seating position   The chair back should be protected with a plastic cover. If this is not available a colouring towel can be folded lengthwise and secured with sectioning clips at either end. The client should be seated comfortably, in an upright position, with their back flat against the cushioned chair pad.

Trolley   You should have your colouring trolley prepared and at hand with the materials you will need. Foils for highlighting should have been previously prepared to the right lengths and combs, brushes, sectioning clips etc. should be all cleaned and sterilised and ready for use.

You   Your personal safety is also important. The care you take in preparing for work should be carried through in everything you do and this is made even more important when you are about to handle hazardous chemicals. Put on a clean colouring apron and fasten the ties in a bow. Then take a pair of disposable vinyl gloves and put them on ready for the application. (See below for preventing dermatitis.)

Use your time effectively; each salon allocates different times for different services. For example, a re-touch may only take 20 minutes to apply on shorter hair whereas a long hair set of full head woven highlights could be booked for an hour.

Preventing dermatitis

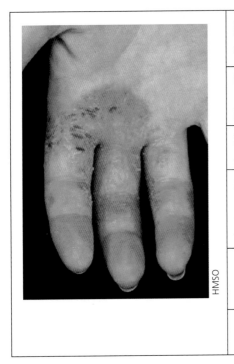

HMSO

Five steps to preventing dermatitis

Step 1. Wear disposable vinyl gloves when rinsing, shampooing, colouring, bleaching, etc.

Step 2. Dry your hands thoroughly with a soft cotton or paper towel.

Step 3. Moisturise after washing your hands, as well as at the start and end of each day. It's easy to miss fingertips, finger webs and wrists.

Step 4. Change gloves between clients. Make sure you don't contaminate your hands when you take them off.

Step 5. Check skin regularly for early signs of dermatitis.

EKU *statement*

GH17 (eku8) and GH18 (eku6) What is contact dermatitis and how to avoid developing it whilst carrying out colouring and lightening services

What do you do if you think you have dermatitis?

Dermatitis is an occupational health hazard for hairdressers it is avoided by wearing non-latex disposable gloves for all processes or services that involve contact with chemicals. If you think you are suffering from dermatitis, then you should visit your doctor for advice and treatment. If you believe it has been caused or made worse by your work as a hairdresser, then you should mention this to your doctor and you must also tell your employer as they are required by law to report a case of work-related dermatitis amongst their staff.

Activity

For this activity complete the missing information in the table below to create the correct liquid hydrogen peroxide strengths.

Strength you have	Strength you want to create	Peroxide	Add	Water
40 vol (i.e. 12%)	30 vol (i.e. 9%)	?	+	1
40 vol	20 vol (i.e. 6%)	?	+	?
40 vol	10 vol (i.e. 3%)	1	+	?
30 vol (i.e. 9%)	20 vol (i.e. 6%)	?	+	1
30 vol	10 vol (i.e. 3%)	?	+	?
20 vol (i.e. 6%)	10 vol (i.e. 3%)	?	+	1

EKU *statement*

GH18 (eku14) The safety considerations which must be taken into account when colouring and lightening hair

EKU *statement*

GH17 (eku49) and
GH18 (eku46) How and
why the contra-indications
in the range can affect the
delivery of the colouring
service to clients
GH17 (eku52) and
GH18 (eku49) How and
why the factors in the range
can influence your choice of
product and/or application
techniques
GH17 (eku58) Sources of
creative information and
inspiration (eg historical,
cultural and fashion)

Colouring preparation checklist

✔	Find the client's treatment record/or prepare a new one.
✔	Make sure that the styling section and chair is clean, safe and ready to receive clients.
✔	Make sure that the seat is lowered, providing easier access for the clients whether they be young, old or with physical conditions.
✔	Make sure that the client is well protected with a clean fresh gown a colouring towel and cape.
✔	Make sure you comb or brush the hair thoroughly before you start to remove tangles, see if all product can be removed and check for cuts or abrasions on the scalp
✔	Carry out your consultation using visual aids.
✔	Look for contra-indications and conduct your tests.
✔	Record the responses to your questions (and update the treatment history).
✔	Note If you need to do a skin test then no further action can be taken until the results of the tests are available.
✔	Make sure that you have your tools and products prepared and close at hand.
✔	Make sure that you have checked the equipment that you need to use and it is ready and safe.

GH17.2 Prepare for colouring and lightening services

Consultation

Your choice of colour is crucial: take time to make it carefully. A hurried choice may give disastrous results!

A number of questions need to be answered before the final choice of colour is made.

Activity

Building a portfolio of creative looks

Visual aids are essential for showing clients themes, ideas and impressions as they go a long way in showing what can be achieved.

The diversity of colouring effects available for your client is only limited by your imagination. When you are trying to convey an idea from your mind, what would be a better solution than a visual one?

Build a creative portfolio of effects so that you can use it with your clients.

You can find sources for your ideas from the internet, style magazines, colour swatches or almost anywhere.

What does the client require?

Clients look to colour as a solution for many things.

Many clients requesting a permanent colour are seeking to disguise their greying hair. A client who wants something to tone a few grey hairs may be successfully assisted with temporary, semi-permanent or longer-lasting colourants. However, if the client is really longing simply to be young again it is difficult to help much with any type of colour, though it may well be possible to help them to look a little more youthful.

Most colour work undertaken within the salon has been stimulated by fashion. The majority of this work now falls into the partial colouring techniques. The multi-toning permutations present a 'boundless' choice of options, carried out by an ever-growing range of techniques and applications. With the decline in full-head colouring (probably much to do with the variety and choice of home colouring products) these partial, varietal colouring options remain a 'professionals only' option for the client.

What other factors are relevant?

During your consultation with your client, you will need to consider the following points:

1 their age and lifestyle
2 their job, if they have one
3 their fashion and dress sense, and the colours they prefer to wear
4 their natural hair colour and their skin colour
5 the hair's texture, condition and porosity
6 the colourant you could use
7 the techniques you would employ
8 the time and cost involved.

When you have taken these points into consideration, you should be able to determine which hair colour shade, colourant and process to recommend to your client.

Natural light vs indoor lighting

Lighting should always be considered when selecting colours with the client. Strong white halogen light may give a true likeness to actual depth and tone. But people seldom stand for long periods of time within these spotlights. Make sure that you point this out during consultation as most clients (and many hairdressers!) don't look closely enough at hair images in style and fashion magazines. Good photography (and later digital editing) will always deceive the non professional eye; always look closely at the effects within images to see if colours are:

- *realistic* – do the tones that you see within an image result from clever colouring or a lighting effect?
- *achievable* – does the positioning of the colours that you see reflect something that can be adapted into a technique?
- *an enhancement* – would the overall colour of the hair still look as good against the client's skin tones?

Take your visual aids or magazines into natural daylight so that a more realistic colour comparison can be made. This will help dispel any misunderstanding later, particularly if you are matching up a shade from an image created in a studio under specialist lighting for a fashion magazine.

Remember

Health and safety
Before using permanent or any long-lasting colourants, you must always perform a skin (sensitivity) test. If there is any reaction, you cannot carry out the colouring. To do so could result in an allergic reaction and a possible personal injury claim

EKU *statement*

GH17 (eku37) and GH18 (eku34) The effects of light and artificial lighting on the appearance of hair colour

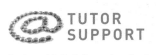

TUTOR SUPPORT

Project 11.3: Influencing factors affecting colours and techniques

Remember

Effects of different types of lighting

- White light from halogen bulbs and full daylight will show the hair's natural colour.

- Yellowish light emitted from standard electric light bulbs adds warmth to hair colour, but neutralises blue ash or ashen effects.

- Bluish/green light from fluorescent tubes reduces the warmth of red/gold tones in hair.

EKU statement

GH17 (eku26) The types and purposes of tests for colouring and lightening services

GH17 (eku31) and GH18 (eku28) The potential consequen-ces of failing to carry out tests

GH17 (eku32) and GH18 (eku29) The courses of action to take in the event of adverse reactions to tests and the contra-indications in the range (i.e. when to encourage the client to seek medical advice, when to explain the service is not possible, when a modification to the service will be necessary)

GH17 (eku33) and GH18 (eku30) Why it is important to accurately record test results

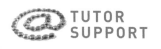

TUTOR SUPPORT

Discussion 11.1: Questions for consultation

Remember

Use the client's records
Make sure that you refer to the client's record if they have been to the salon before, or make out a new card to note down what you decide and the results of any tests.

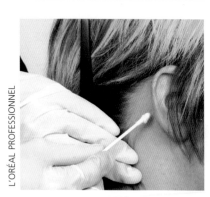

A skin allergy test

L'ORÉAL PROFESSIONNEL

Good practice/Health and safety: Preparing yourself and the client

- Always refer to the results of tests first
- Always gown and prepare your client properly so that she is protected from spillages of chemicals
- Prepare your work area so that you have everything at hand
- Always wear the PPE (i.e. the vinyl gloves and aprons) provided by the salon every time you apply colour
- Apply barrier creams as or where necessary
- Always follow the manufacturer's instructions; never deviate from the tried and tested formulae
- Make sure that your work position is clear and that your posture is correct
- Make sure that the client is comfortable throughout as she will be sitting for some considerable time

Activity
Colour coordination

Colour coordination is an important part of creating a total colour effect. Most clients given the choice would prefer to have colours that suited them and your ability to find colour solutions for them is therefore an integral part of your job.

Create a colour portfolio of themes that cover both harmonising and contrasting effects. You can do this by collecting pictures from magazines and from the internet that show different hair colours worn in different ways.

In your portfolio now answer these questions:

1 Which ones work well and why?

2 Which ones didn't work well together and why?

3 What aspects of colour create harmonising effects?

4 What aspects of colour create contrasting effects?

Colour tests

Don't forget that the following tests are designed to help you identify contra-indications and to protect your client:

- *skin test* – to assess the client's sensitivity to the colour
- *porosity test* – to assess the smoothness or roughness of the cuticle
- *elasticity test* – to determine the hair's state or condition
- *incompatibility test* – if metallic chemicals are present
- *colour test/strand test* – to check the process of colouring.

Tests – why, when and how?

TEST	WHY IS IT DONE?	WHEN IS IT DONE?	HOW IS IT DONE?
Skin test (Patch test)	The sensitivity test is used to assess the reaction of the skin to chemicals or chemical products. In the salon it is mainly used before colouring (although it can be used in other chemical services e.g. extensions, relaxing etc.). Some people are allergic to external contact of chemicals such as PPD (found in permanent colour). This can cause dermatitis (see GH17.1 preventing dermatitis p. 339) or, in even more severe cases, permanent scarring of skin tissue and hair loss. Some people are allergic to irritants reacting internally, and have conditions such as asthma and hay fever. Others may be allergic to both internal and external irritants.	To find out whether a client's skin reacts to chemicals in permanent colours, carry out a skin test 24 to 48 hours prior to the chemical process.	Remove the client's earrings. Behind the ear and, using a cotton-bud, apply a little of the unmixed colourant product sufficient to cover 1 cm^2. Re-apply two or three times allowing it to dry between each application. Leave for 48 hours without washing, covering or touching. If during the 48 hours after the test you or your client notices any abnormal reaction such as intense redness, itching or swelling in or around the test area DO NOT APPLY THE COLOUR. Recommend that your client seeks medical advice before any colour applications area made.
Porosity test	This test also indicates the hair's current condition by assessing the hair's ability to absorb or resist moisture from liquids. (Hair in good condition has a tightly packed cuticle layer, which will resist the penetration of products.) Hair that is very porous holds on to moisture; this is particularly evident when you try to blow dry it. The hair takes a long time to dry.	Before chemical services. If the cuticle is torn or damaged, the absorption of moisture and therefore hydrogen peroxide is quicker therefore the processing time will be shorter. Over-porous hair will quickly take in colour but will not necessarily be able to hold colour as the cuticle is damaged and allows the newly introduced pigments to wash away.	Rub strands of hair between your fingertips to feel how rough or smooth it is. If it feels roughened, as opposed to coarse, it is likely that the hair is porous.
Elasticity test	This determines the condition of the hair by seeing how much the hair will stretch and return to its original length. Overstretched hair will not return to the same length and remains permanently damaged.	Prior to chemical treatments and services. (Ideal for hair that has impaired elasticity such as bleached and coloured.)	Take a couple of strands of hair between your fingers, holding them at the roots and the ends. Gently pull the hair between the two points to see if the hair will stretch and return to its original length. (If the hair breaks easily it may indicate that the cortex is damaged and will be unable to sustain any further chemical treatment.)
Incompatibility test	This will show if there are any chemicals present, such as metallic salts or other mineral compounds, within the hair, which will react against any new proposed services.	Carried out prior to colouring, highlighting and perming treatments.	Place a small sample of hair in a mixture of 20 parts liquid hydrogen peroxide (6 per cent) and one part ammonium-based compound from perm solution. If the mixture bubbles, heats up or discolours do not carry out the service.

TEST	WHY IS IT DONE?	WHEN IS IT DONE?	HOW IS IT DONE?
Strand test	A strand test or hair strand colour test is used during processing to assess the development of the colour on a strand or section of hair. A strand test is also useful when lightening natural pigments from hair or prior to removing synthetic pigments (i.e. decolour or colour reducer) to see how the hair will respond.	Most colouring products just require the full development time recommended by the manufacturer – check their instructions. (However, some hair conditions take on the colour faster than others and a strand test will check the colour development and see if the product needs to come off earlier.)	1. Rub a strand of hair lightly with the back of a comb to remove the surplus colour. 2. Check whether the colour remaining is evenly distributed throughout the hair's length. If it is even, remove the rest of the colour. If it is uneven, allow processing to continue, if necessary applying more colour. If any of the hair on the head is not being treated, you can compare the evenness of colour in the coloured hair with that in the uncoloured hair.

Note. Always follow the manufacturer's instructions when conducting/carrying out tests.

Recording the events

The maintenance of the client's records is an essential part of the service; because the service – in its true sense doesn't end there.

Good customer service is built upon over time, on a repeated basis. *How would you maintain the same level of service in the future without having accurate information of the processes that have already been undertaken?*

Records are not just about filling in a card with what products you have used and how long they were left on for. In more complex, critical areas of work you also need to record what has been *said*.

In a normal client–stylist consultation, you the stylist ask a variety of questions that, depending on the response you receive, make decisions upon a suitable course of action. Fine: what if you ask a client about what they have coloured their hair with and they said a L'Oréal colour from Boots, but in actual fact they have used a metallic-salt-based colour restorer instead?

Unless you have spotted the slight metallic or flat colour that these products produce, you might carry out your planned treatment, oblivious to the disaster that was about to occur!

Accurate records in this situation may prevent a legally provable case of professional negligence being brought against the salon; the records would show that you acted upon the information provided and if you have documented the client's responses, you can demonstrate that neither you nor the salon are at fault.

Consultation checklist

✔	Look at the client's treatment history
✔	Identify any contra-indications by asking questions and looking through the hair for visible signs
✔	Find out what the client wants – use visual aids to establish requirements
✔	Assess suitability and achievability of the desired look

✔	Look for colouring problems or pre-service requirements
✔	Conduct any tests – check the results of hair tests against planned services
✔	Avoid confusing technical jargon; always clarify in simple terms what you mean
✔	Agree on a suitable course of action and give an idea of service timings and costs
✔	Summarise the main points of the consultation and get ready to start
✔	Whilst the service is being done; give them some advice on how to maintain their hair at home and recommend those products that are suitable to use and those that are not
✔	Give them an idea of how long the effect will last (and prompt them to re-book their next appointment before they leave)

EKU statement

GH17 (eku2) Your salon's expected service times for colouring work

GH17 (eku29) How the results of tests can influence the colouring and lightening service

GH17.3 Creatively colour and lighten hair

Colour selection principles: 1. Choice, previous processes and current condition

EKU statement

GH17 (eku50) and GH18 (eku47) The types of tools, materials and equipment used for colouring and lightening hair and how and when to use them

GH17 (eku59) The importance of sectioning hair accurately when colouring

GH17 (eku60) Methods of applying and removing colouring products and lighteners

GH17 (eku65) How and why to adapt the sequence of application to take account of the relevant factors in the range

GH17 (eku69) How and why to neutralise colour tone

Colour selection – the process you go through in choosing the right target shade for your client's hair and the correct mixture of products to achieve that target shade – is based upon:

- the customer's initial choice
- the previous processes on your client's hair (e.g. whether it is already permed, highlighted etc.)
- the current condition of your client's hair.

If the hair has been regularly coloured before and there is a clear regrowth, with ends that have faded, you may only need to do a straightforward regrowth application with the same colour. Then later in the development process the residual colour can be diluted and taken through to the rest to refresh the total effect. So, in this instance, a regrowth that takes 20 minutes to apply can be left for 30 minutes' development, and then in the last 15 minutes it can be taken through to the ends, until it's all ready to be removed. However, if your client's hair has been coloured before, you also need to remember that it will not be possible to make the hair lighter by colouring. Permanent colour does not reduce permanent (synthetic) pigments from the hair. (If this is required you will have to use a colour remover first.)

If you need or want to counteract and neutralise unwanted tones in the hair, you will need to apply the principles of the colour wheel. If the client wants to *calm down* unwanted red tones then you will be choosing a colour slightly darker in *depth* but which has the matt *tones* capable of neutralising the effect of the red. Conversely, if your aim is to eliminate ashen matt tones (the colour often seen on fairer hair colours that are regularly subjected to chlorinated swimming pools) then you will be introducing warmer tones to the hair. So in this situation, a 'greeny'-looking base 6 blonde will be improved by a shade depth 6 but with a tone warmth .03 (for more information see the depth and tone table earlier in this chapter). If you had to reduce a tonal effect that was too yellow, say on a head that had been lightened, then although the principle of toning bleached hair is slightly different, you would still be applying the principles of the colour wheel and therefore using a violet-based ash colour to neutralise the unwanted tones.

The colour circle

Remember

1 Only mix enough
   product to complete
the job as any excess will
be wasted as it cannot be
used again.

2 Always follow the
   manufacturer's instructions
when mixing your colouring
products.

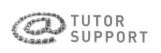

**TUTOR
SUPPORT**

Project 11.5: Selection of the
colour different to target shade

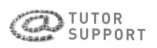

**TUTOR
SUPPORT**

Discussion 11.3: Contra-
indications and how the hair
may react to the colour

If your client has never had any colour on their hair before (virgin hair) then colour targeting is easy. Your client will be able to choose practically any shade on the permanent shade chart, providing it is at the same depth or darker than their natural colour. (It is possible to lighten hair with colour in certain situations. See the bleaching and lightening section later in this chapter.)

If your client has grey or greying (i.e. white) hair then you will have to decide and agree on what reduction of grey is necessary. If the client wants to cover all the grey, then this is only achievable by using or adding base shades to the target colour, i.e. a natural shade or a natural + target shade. The amount of base added to target shade is directly proportional to the amount of grey. Grey hair is referred to as a percentage of the whole head; therefore a client who has about a quarter of their hair that is grey is referred to as 25 per cent grey. Similarly, a client with one tenth of grey hair is 10 per cent grey.

Remember

Formula for mixing base shades to cover grey

- If a client has 25 per cent grey/white then you need $\frac{1}{4}$ of the base shade added to $\frac{3}{4}$ of the target shade.
- If a client has 50 per cent grey/white then you need $\frac{1}{2}$ of the base shade added to $\frac{1}{2}$ of the target shade.
- If a client has 75 per cent grey/white then you need $\frac{3}{4}$ of the base shade added to $\frac{1}{4}$ of the target shade.

Accuracy using measuring flasks and mixing bowls

Amounts of hydrogen peroxide at any strength must be accurately measured; the amount used in relation to colour is a critical factor to a successful and safe outcome. Different types of colour are formulated to be used with particular developers; for example, a Wella *Colour Perfect* should be mixed with *Welloxon* developer. If you use a different developer the consistency will be wrong and this will make the application difficult. All gel and cream colours, when mixed, will be stiff enough not to run on either the brush or the hair. Using unmatched, alternative developers will do the opposite and could be a potential hazard for the client.

When you measure developer into a measuring flask you must make sure that your eyeline is at the same level as the liquid in the flask. If you do put a little too much into the flask the pouring edge will allow you to put back what you don't need.

When you mix developer with colour from tubes, you will notice that all tubes have markings on the side showing the $\frac{1}{4}$, $\frac{1}{2}$ and $\frac{3}{4}$ points. These enable you to squeeze from the bottom of the tube up to these points, knowing that your measurement will be accurate.

If you are mixing two or more shades of colour together, always mix these well in the bowl first before adding any developer. This allows the different pigments to be evenly distributed throughout the colour and also throughout the hair when it's applied!

Pre-softening white hair

Pre-softening is done as a preparation for colouring difficult white/greying hair. In situations where there is a significant amount of white hair to be coloured, it is advisable that the hair is prepared by prior pre-softening. Resistant white hair often has a shiny or glassy look and this is due to the cuticle layer being packed down tightly in a closed, flat position. If you were to apply a permanent colour to this you will find that the colour will have a shadowed or faded look where you will still see the ashen grey underneath. To stop this from happening you need to pre-soften the hair beforehand.

How to pre-soften white hair:

- Pour 30 cc of neat 20 volume (6 per cent) liquid hydrogen peroxide into a colouring bowl.
- Apply the hydrogen peroxide to the resistant, white hair with a colouring brush.
- Place the client under a pre-heated hood dryer or colour **accelerator** for 15 to 20 minutes.
- Then, after the drying has finished, the cuticle layer will have lifted sufficiently for you to be able to apply a permanent colour and it will now deposit properly into the cortex as opposed to lying at or around the cuticle's surface.

Current condition

The hair's existing condition is a major contributing factor in the way in which it will respond when it is coloured. Hair that is too porous will absorb the colour differently. The porosity of hair is never even along the hair length, let alone across the hairs throughout the head. This is because the porosity of the hair is directly related to areas of damaged cuticle. Areas of high porosity occur at sites along the hair shaft where cuticle is torn or missing. At these points, moisture or chemicals can easily enter the inner hair without cuticle layer resistance.

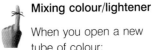
EKU *statement*

GH17 (eku47) and
GH18 (eku39) The reasons
for pre-softening and pre-
pigmenting hair

This changes the rate of absorption, which ultimately affects the final evenness of the colour and the hair's ability to retain colour in subsequent washing etc. pH-balancing conditioners help to even out the hair's porosity and return chemically treated hair back to a natural pH 5.5 which is essential if:

(a) the colour is going to last

(b) the hair is going to stay in good condition.

During processing the only other factors that affect the achievement of an even and expected final colour result (providing your selection is correct) are:

- timing   - temperature.

Pre- and post-colour treatments

The unevenness of porosity is also a major factor in the achievement of good colouring results. If the hair has different porosity levels throughout its length then the resulting colour will also be uneven because the hair will absorb the colour at different rates. In areas along the hair where the porosity is higher, then the colour will take more quickly. Conversely, in areas where the cuticle is intact, then the colour will develop at the normal rate.

This unevenness is counteracted by preparing the hair with a pre-colour treatment. The treatment is applied to dry hair before colouring, throughout the lengths to even out the colour absorption rate and enable the hair to achieve an even colour result.

A post-colour treatment can also be used in order to seal areas of damaged or missing cuticle; helping the colour to reduce fading by locking in the synthetic para-dye pigments. These treatments will also neutralise the action of hydrogen peroxide upon the hair by:

- removing excess oxygen as an anti-oxidant (anti-oxidising agent) another factor in reducing colour fade
- closing the cuticle layer
- balancing the pH of the hair by returning it to pH 5.5.

Timing

The level of colour saturation is proportional to the length of time that that the hair is exposed to colour. Under-processed hair will not achieve the same saturation as hair that has had full development. In other words, the longer that colour is left on, the more density the colour will have.

This can be explained in another way: imagine that you wanted to redecorate a plain, smooth, white wall. First of all, you choose the colour and shade of paint that you want it to be. Then after some preparation, you take a brush and start by applying the first coat. When this is dry you look at the colour, only to find that the effect is uneven and patchy. You can see that the tone you wanted is there but it is often thin and almost transparent in places. So you repaint the wall. When the extra layer of paint dries, the saturation of colour is better and more even but still a little patchy in places. Finally you apply a third coat to the areas that are still patchy and when it dries the colour has an even density throughout. This effect is called *saturation*; it is achieved by the evenness of the density of the colour application throughout the hair.

Temperature

Temperature is also a major contributing factor to colour development. The warmer the colour environment the quicker the hair will take and the term *colour environment* is important here. The colour environment can be localised to the client or relate to the whole salon: the salon temperature may be cool but putting the client under a Climazone or Rollerball accelerates the colour.

We know that when colour is introduced to heat it takes more quickly. However, you do need to remember that the human body produces heat too. In fact, up to 30 per cent of body heat is emitted through the top of your head! (This is why wearing a hat in winter keeps you warm.) This heating effect has a dramatic impact on the development of colour and is even more critical when lightening or bleaching!

So, with this extra heat around the scalp area, you can see there are potential problems of controlling the colour and aspects to the client's safety. To help control this process you must make sure that when the colour is applied to the root area, the hair is lifted away from the scalp and the air is able to circulate and ventilate the scalp evenly. This ensures that there are no 'hot spots' anywhere that would take more quickly or become a safety hazard to the client.

TUTOR SUPPORT

Project 11.6: Pre-softening and pre-pigmenting

EKU *statement*

GH17 (eku63) How to place colour in a way to complement a hair style

Colour selection principles: 2. Harmonising and contrasting effects

Understanding how colours harmonise or contrast in a hairstyle is fundamental to colour selection. In the illustrations below the same colours have been used in a variety of different ways. Note how the effects convey very different images. In each of the illustrations, the same two colour combinations have been used. But the way in which they have been used differs in each case. (Each of the possible colour variables is denoted in *italic* type.)

TUTOR SUPPORT

Project 11.7: Contrasting result and harmonising result

1 (Far left) Illustration depicts the balanced *light* and *dark* effect that is created when *vertical*, yet *uniform* sections of *contrasting* colour are *evenly* applied to a plain gold background.

2 (Centre left) This is the predominately *darkened* result when *more vertical* and *varying* sections of *contrasting* colour are *randomly* applied to a plain gold background.

3 (Centre right) This predominantly *lighter* effect is produced when *fewer vertical* and *varying* sections of *contrasting* colour are *randomly* applied to a plain gold background.

4 (Far right) This *darkened* effect results from *more vertical* yet *uniform* sections of *contrasting* colour being *evenly* applied to a plain gold background.

Before looking at the next illustration we should remember the technique variables having an impact in this scenario. (See table below.)

	Effect	Sections	Direction	Amount	Positioning	Intensity
Technique variables	Light	Uniform	Vertical	Less	Even	?
	Dark	Varying	?	More	Random	Contrasting

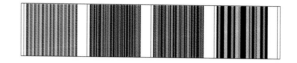

In this series of illustrations, new variables have been introduced; they have a major impact on the total effect too. Here a *third*, yet *harmonising* colour is added. This new addition harmonises with its companion colours in two ways:

It provides a mid-tone, somewhere halfway between the light gold and the dark brown.

It has a natural, tonal 'fit' i.e. it harmonises with the two other colours.

The purpose of the illustration is to show that the same background is totally changed with just the addition of one other shade. Stark contrasts of colour are softened by the addition of a harmonising tone. The reverse happens when the added tone does not harmonise with its background. There are two other aspects to now consider:

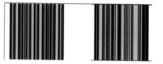

1 The dimension of other directions.
2 Uneven background colour.

The next illustration introduces these criteria.

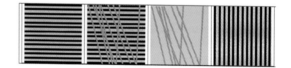

- We can now see that in the first illustration (far left) the image has changed direction. The colours are exactly the same but the resultant effect is very different.
- This is compounded in the next image where the third colour is reintroduced again, but now appears multi-directional.
- The next depicts the removal of contrast colour, just leaving random directional movement.
- Finally, there is the added dimension of uneven colour background.

This is aesthetics – there are no rules here; well, certainly not written ones. However, there are a number of points that have a bearing on taste, good design, artistic appreciation and therefore your colour planning.

Taste is subjective; whatever you find appealing may not be acceptable to others. In colour consultation you must get a feel of what the client finds attractive.

Good design is again subjective; the images displayed within the text bear no relationship to hair colouring. Or do they? The planning of styles, particularly new fashions, must originate from something. Fashion in clothes starts on the designer's drawing board and the collections you see created for top competitions like the British Hairdressing Awards are also based on a theme. The theme is the inspiration behind the design; therefore, in principle, simple geometry becomes the underlying components of style construction.

Hairdressing is not self-indulgent *fine art* – well not for the majority of us. It happens to be a form of commercial art. Commercial artists produce work – commission – for paying clients. Hairdressers do a very similar thing. The commercial artist finds out what the client wants, produces some visual examples, and then, on agreement, undertakes to complete the task in hand. Therefore, bearing this analogy in mind, we do exactly the same. Our clients use our artistic knowledge and skills to get what they want.

Wherever your inspiration comes from, remember, it has to be applied in a commercial context, unless it is purely for promotional purposes and in that case the sky's the limit.

Bearing this information in mind here are the variables that you need to consider before colouring hair.

Effect	monochrome	duo-toned	multi-toned	light/dark	subtle	strong
Sections	uniform	varied	narrow	wide	blocked	
Direction	vertical	horizontal	angled			
Amount	singles	less than 20%	20–40%	40–60%	over 60%	
Positioning	evenly placed	randomly placed	over other colours	with other colours	below other colours	
Intensity	harmonised	contrasting	vibrant	muted		

Step-by-steps

Full head colour

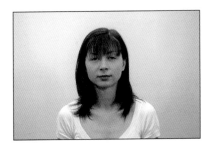

Step 1 Before

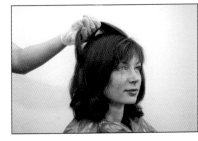

Step 2 Starting at the back apply the colour to the mid length and ends first

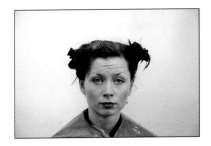

Step 3 Keep the client clean by securing the hair out of the way

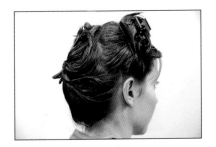

Step 4 Leave to develop for 20 minutes

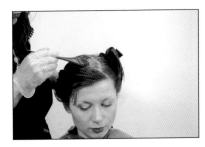

Step 5 Start applying the colour at the roots

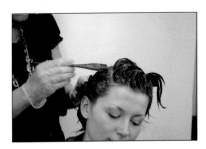

Step 6 Make sure that all the hair is covered

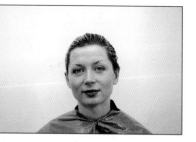

Step 7 Comb the colour through to spread the colour evenly

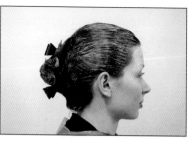

Step 8 Secure and leave to develop for another 20 minutes

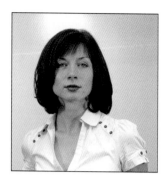

Step 9 Finished effect

Replacing missing natural tones

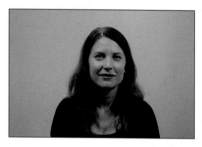

Step 1 Before

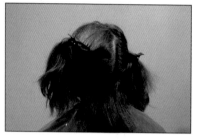

Step 2 Start the highlight foils at the bottom

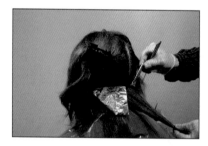

Step 3 Work up the back with the low-lights

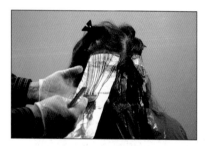

Step 4 With the back done, re-colour the interleaves back to the client's natural depth

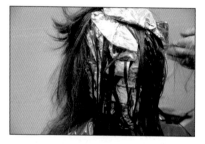

Step 5 Continue placing the foils into the sides and top

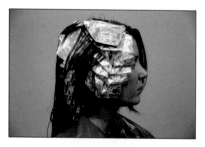

Step 6 Foils in place

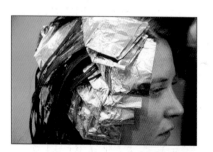

Step 7 Interleave colour applied

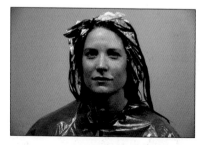

Step 8 Monitor the development

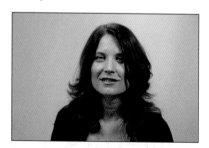

Step 9 Finished effect

Slices

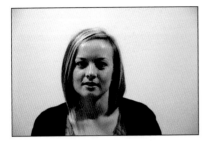

Step 1 Before

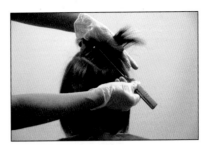

Step 2 Section off the lower back

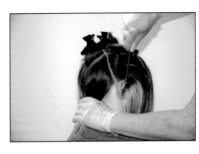

Step 3 Divide and section the sides and secure into place

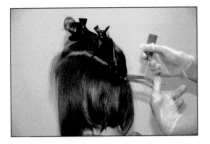

Step 4 Start your darkest meshes at the lower back

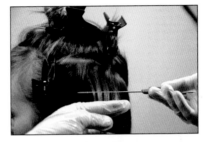

Step 5 Apply contrasting lighter colours as you work up the sides

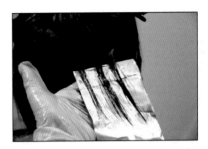

Step 6 Dark tones

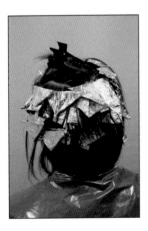

Step 7 80% complete

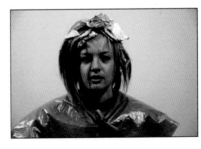

Step 8 Leave until all have developed (some colours may need removing before others)

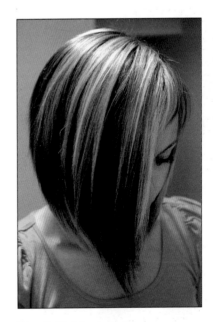

Step 9 Finished effect

Colour slice 2

A similar slice colour technique with strong contrast colour

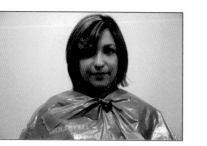

Step 1

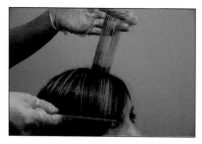

Step 2

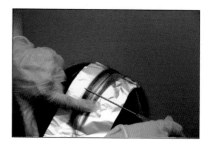

Step 3

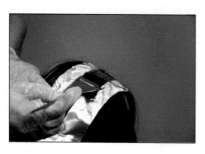

Step 4

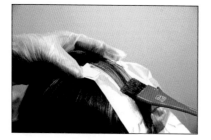

Step 5

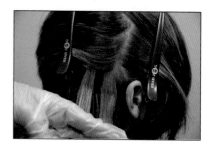

Step 6

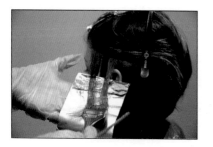

Step 7

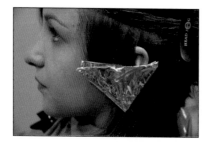

Step 8

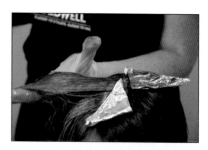

Step 9

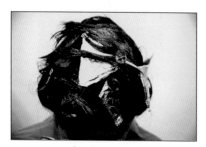

Step 10

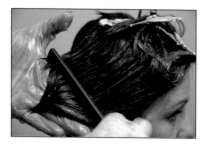

Step 11

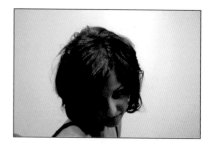

Step 12

Lightening hair

Lighteners and bleaches have chemicals within them that achieve lightened effects by dissolving the natural tones (pigments) within hair. Similar to para-dyes, lightening products are mixed with hydrogen peroxide to activate the oxidising process, and they are used in three main forms:

- *high lift colour* – which is a process that adds tone, whilst lightening natural hair all in one process for partial or whole head applications
- *powder bleach* – which is used for highlighting and partial lightening techniques
- *gel/oil bleach* – which is suitable for whole head applications including the scalp.

EKU *statement*

GH17 (eku16) and
GH18 (eku14) How to use lighteners safely

GH17 (eku39) The reasons for pre-lightening

GH17 (eku44) and
GH18 (eku42) The pH values of different colouring products and lighteners

GH17 (eku70) The potential problems of using colouring products and lighteners on previously chemically treated hair

Activity

Lightening effects upon hair

To check how bleach or high-lift colour acts upon the hair, collect hair cuttings from the salon sweepings and bond samples together. Then apply a lightener to it, be careful to time and observe the process throughout the development.

You should be able to find out exactly how much lightening the hair can take and what the resultant effects are.

Keep a record of the experiment and your responses to the following questions in you portfolio:

1 Try lightening it with different strengths of peroxide: what results did you achieve?

2 Try lightening the hair with different products: what differences did you notice?

3 Try leaving the lightener on the hair beyond the manufacturer's specified timings: what happened then?

(Remember that if the hair contains a lot of red/yellow pigment, it must not be lightened too much – the hair's breaking point will quickly be reached.)

The alkaline compound acts upon the hair by swelling and opening up the cuticle, this enables the peroxide at 6 per cent or 9 per cent to release oxygen and oxidise the natural pigments of melanin from within the cortex. This creates oxymelanin and is seen as it reduces the natural colour through the different degrees of lift. (See the bleach toning table.)

The colour control during lightening is not the same as with colouring though. Often when full head lightening is done the result is quite yellow. (Although the control of warm pigments during lightening is better with high lift colour.)

EKU *statement*

GH17 (eku35) and
GH18 (eku36) What is meant by the term 'oxidation'

The chemistry of bleaching/lightening

Powder bleach contains ammonium/potassium persulphate and sodium/magnesium silicate. These chemicals bleach the hair by oxidation: i.e. oxygen is added to the chemical pigments. Various types of bleach will do this and the most common is hydrogen peroxide (H_2O_2).

EKU *statement*

GH17 (eku69) How and why to neutralise colour tone

EKU *statement*

GH17 (eku21) and GH18 (eku19) Why it is important to check electrical equipment used to aid the colouring and lightening process

GH17 (eku30) The importance of constantly monitoring the development of lightener

GH17 (eku61) How the application and removal of lightener should be adapted to minimise scalp sensitivity and hair damage

GH17 (eku66) Why it is important to avoid disturbing areas still processing when removing products from developed areas

Hydrogen peroxide is available in cream, foam and liquid forms. It acts in stages. First the bleaching agent causes the hair to swell: the cuticle begins to lift. The bleach can then penetrate to the hair cortex, where the liberated oxygen acts on the pigment, lightening the hair.

Longer times or stronger bleaches may be required for hair of different colours. Just how long is required, and what strength of bleach must be used, can be determined using a test cutting.

Toning table

Level of depth	Tone required	Tonal quality	Pre-lighten to
10	Silver, platinum, mauve/violet	Cool	Very pale yellow
9	Ashen blondes, light beige blonde	Cool	Pale yellow
8	Beige blonde	Cool	Yellow
8	Sandy blonde	Warm	
7	Golden blonde	Warm	
7	Chestnut, copper gold	Warm	Orange
6	Red copper	Warm	
5	Mahogany	Cool	Red/orange
4	Burgundy, plum	Cool	

Toning is the process of adding colour to previously bleached or lightened hair. A variety of pastel shades, such as silver, beige and rose, are used to produce subtle effects. Different types of toners are available; read the instructions provided by their manufacturers to find out what is possible.

Types of lightener

High lift colour

All manufacturers produce a special range of colours that are used to lighten hair. As these are mixed with 6 per cent or 9 per cent volume peroxide their ability to achieve very high lift results are limited by the natural depth that you are starting with. The colour control and condition of the hair is generally better than that of using bleach since the colour can deposit ashen, beige or warm tones as the colour works and the hair lightens. And because you are using a hair colour and not bleach, less moisture is removed from the hair during the process, so a better condition is guaranteed at the end.

High lift colours use an alkaline component (e.g. resorcinol) which swells the hair shaft enabling a better penetration of the chemicals into the cortex and hence able to lighten as well.

Removing high lift colour You can remove high lift colour by emulsifying the colour by adding a little warm water to the colour and gently massaging all over, this mixes the colour with the water and helps to release the products from the hair enabling you to use a lighter action within the shampooing process. The hair can be conditioned as normal at the end or an anti-oxidant can be applied to help close the cuticle and lock in the colour results.

Emulsion bleach

Emulsion bleach is slow acting. It is made up of two compounds that are added together and then mixed with hydrogen peroxide:

- oil or gel bleach
- activators, boosters or controllers.

This type of bleach is specially formulated for use directly onto the roots of the hair, and is suitable for contact with the scalp. It is kinder and gentler during the lightening process and is mixed with 20 vol. hydrogen peroxide for root, mid-length and ends application. The lift through the undertone shades is aided and controlled by the addition of activators. These boost the power of the bleach whilst maintaining relatively low hydrogen peroxide strength.

Emulsion bleaches also contain additives which control the resultant colour as the bleach lightens the hair. As mentioned earlier, these tend to make hair yellow, so they have matt emulsifiers which neutralise unwanted yellow tones whilst the lifting process takes place. Heat may be used during the development of the process, but the client must be monitored closely (particularly if a colour accelerator or steamer is used to aid development) as these types of bleach can often be more viscous and mobile and might drip!

Removing emulsion bleach Make sure that when the bleach is removed you rinse without massaging with only tepid or warm water. The client's scalp has been subjected to chemicals and could be sensitive; the cooling action of the rinsing will stop the lightening process and make the client more comfortable. After the emulsion has been rinsed away the hair can be shampooed with a mild colour shampoo and conditioned with an anti-oxidising treatment.

Powder bleach

Powder bleach can be mixed with 6, 9 or 12 per cent hydrogen peroxide, depending upon the level of lift required. Powder bleaches are fast acting and are used for a variety of highlighting techniques. When they are mixed in the bowl the consistency is that of a thick, 'porridge-type' paste. The stiffness of the consistency prevents spillages and enables the bleach to work like a poultice. As the process continues the bleach/peroxide mix will expand. This action is speeded up more if accelerated by heat, so a careful eye should be kept on the development timings.

Removing powder bleach Again, as with emulsion bleach, make sure that when the bleach is removed from the hair you rinse it without massaging, using only tepid or warm water. The removal of powder bleach can be far more problematic than that of emulsion bleach and this has more to do with the colouring technique that has been used. If different coloured highlights have been done with Easy Meche, foil, wraps, etc. these need to be removed carefully and individually as one colour may affect another.

Although the client's scalp has not been subjected to chemicals, it still might be sensitive from the colouring technique; again, the cooling action of the rinsing will stop the lightening process and make the client more comfortable. Afterwards the hair can be shampooed with a mild colour shampoo and conditioned with an anti-oxidising treatment.

EKU *statement*

GH17 (eku46) and GH18 (eku45) Why it is important to leave the hair and scalp free of colouring products and lighteners

EKU *statement*

GH17 (eku17) and GH18 (eku15) The precautions that must be taken when handling powder lighteners

Remember

The principles for removing bleach lightener are exactly the same for any colour removal in that the task must be completed thoroughly so that all colouring products are removed from the hair and scalp. This will stop further processing and eliminate any possibility of discomfort or irritation.

Remember

The degree of lift required in emulsion bleach is controlled by the number of activators added into the mixing bowl with the oil. It is not boosted by stronger hydrogen peroxide levels. Always follow the manufacturer's instructions when using lightening products.

EKU *statement*

GH17 (eku64) How to carry out a full head and regrowth application using lighteners

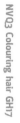
Step-by-steps

Full head lightening and toning

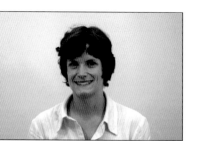

Step 1 Before

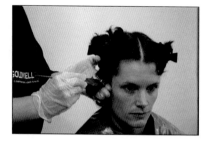

Step 2 Apply lightener to mid lengths and ends first

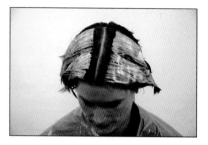

Step 3 Colour showing development

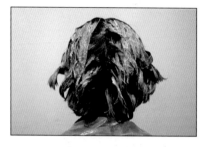

Step 4 Leave until colour has passed the 'orange' stage

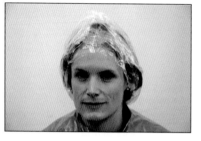

Step 5 Envelope the hair in a plastic cap to help keep the heat in and to aid faster processing

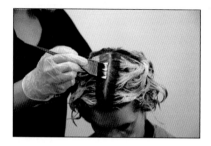

Step 6 With ends now at dark yellow, apply lightener to the root area

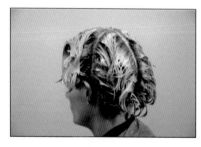

Step 7 Take care not to agitate the scalp

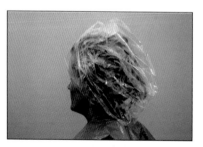

Step 8 Re-apply the plastic cap to aid development

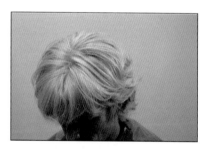

Step 9 Wash off and dry

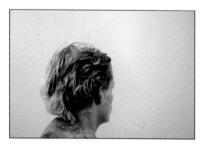

Step 10 Mix and apply the ash toner to all of the hair

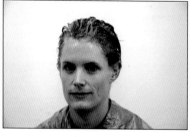

Step 11 Leave until full development is complete

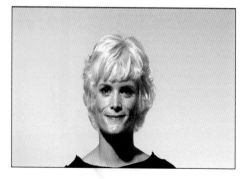

Step 12 Finished ash blonde effect

Contemporary men's colouring

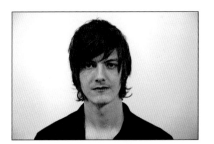

Step 1 Before

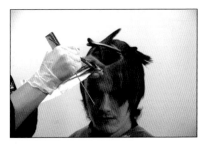

Step 2 Section off hair that is not being lightened and apply lightener to the hair

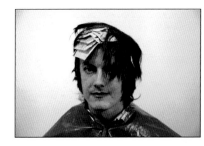

Step 3 Leave to develop

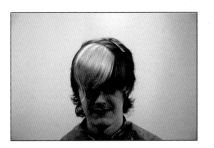

Step 4 Wash and dry hair prior to colouring

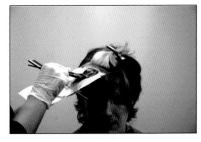

Step 5 Apply contrast colour roots to ends

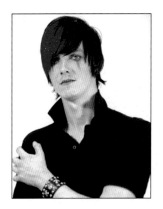

Step 6 Final effect

Remember

Avoid inhalation of powder bleach
Be very careful when you dispense powder bleach into a bowl. The particles are very small and tend to 'dust' into the air very easily; this is a hazardous chemical compound which can cause respiratory conditions. You must avoid contact through inhalation; wherever possible only use 'dust-free' powder bleach.

EKU *statement*

GH17 (eku15) and **GH18** (eku13) The dangers associated with the inhalation of powder lighteners

---

Lightening service required	What you need to check for	Technique/application	Lightener/bleach type
Full head (on virgin hair)	**Test results:** • (Skin tests etc.) **Natural hair depth** • Bleaches will lift five levels quite happily on hair with brown/ash pigments. However, strong red content will be difficult to remove. • Hair beyond base 5 will not lift safely beyond base 9. Suggest other colouring options. **Hair length** • Lengths up to 10 cm lighten evenly, provided the manufacturer's instructions are followed. • Lengths over 15 cm are not recommended, as evenness of colour will be difficult to guarantee.	Bleach mixture must be applied to mid lengths and ends first. A plastic cap should envelope the contents and can be developed with gentle heat until ready. When the bleached hair has lightened, two to three levels of lift the root application can be applied: • Always follow the manufacturer's instructions.	Only emulsion bleach is suggested for application to the scalp. These are used with 6 per cent hydrogen peroxide and sachet controllers to handle levels of lift.

Lightening service required	What you need to check for	Technique/application	Lightener/bleach type
(Full head on virgin hair *continued*)	**Hair texture** • Finer hair needs extra care and lower hydrogen peroxide strengths i.e. 6 per cent • Medium and coarser hair present fewer technical problems **Hair condition** • Only consider hair in good condition for bleaching. Bleaching removes moisture content during the process, and hair that is porous or containing low moisture levels has insufficient durability for bleaching	RUSH LONDON	
Full head (on previously coloured)	Not recommended		
Root application (pre-lightened ends)	**Existing client?** • **Yes,** check previous records and current hair condition and carry out service. • **No,** new client, go through all the checks in the full-head application table and find out the previous treatment history.	Roots only without overlapping previous lightened ends. • Always follow manufacturer's instructions.	Only emulsion bleach is suggested for application to the scalp.
Highlights (fine even meshes on virgin hair) **Note:** The success of highlights on coloured hair is very poor in comparison. This work is often undertaken in salons, but ends seldom lighten effectively, while the roots lighten very quickly. (Colour should be removed with a synthetic colour remover; see section on colouring problems later in this chapter.)	**Test results** • (Skin tests etc.) RUSH LONDON **Natural hair depth** • Bleaches will lift five levels quite happily on hair with brown/ash pigments. However, strong red content will be difficult to remove and require stronger developer and/or additional heat. • Hair beyond base 5 will not lift safely beyond base 9. Suggest other bleaching technique. **Hair length** • Hair length will have an impact on evenness of colour. However, a small tolerance is acceptable and visually indistinguishable on longer hair lengths. **Hair texture** • Finer hair needs extra care and lower hydrogen peroxide strengths i.e. 6 per cent. • Medium and coarser hair present fewer technical problems but generally take longer.	• Plastic self-grip meshes (e.g. Easy Meche L'Oréal). • Foil meshes. • Colour wraps. RUSH LONDON	High lift powder bleach with suitable hydrogen peroxide developer at 6 per cent, 9 per cent or for highest lift 12 per cent (providing no product is allowed to contact the skin/scalp)

Lightening service required	What you need to check for	Technique/application	Lightener/bleach type
(Highlights *continued*)	**Hair condition** • Only consider hair in good condition for bleaching. Bleaching removes moisture content during the process hair that is porous or containing low moisture levels has insufficient durability for bleaching.		
Slices, blocks and slab, bleaching (on virgin hair)	**Test results** (skin tests etc.) **Natural hair depth** • Bleaches will lift five levels quite happily on hair with brown/ash pigments. However, strong red content will be difficult to remove. • Hair beyond base 5 will not lift safely beyond base 9. Suggest other colouring options. **Hair length** • Lengths up to 10 cm will lighten evenly, provided manufacturer's instructions are followed. • Lengths over 15 cm are not recommended, as evenness of colour will be difficult to guarantee. However, if the technique used will allow for bleaching of mid lengths and ends first, then the problem may be overcome. **Hair texture** • Finer hair needs extra care and lower hydrogen peroxide i.e. 6 per cent. • Medium and coarser hair present fewer technical problems **Hair condition** • Only consider hair in good condition for bleaching. Bleaching removes moisture content during the process; hair that is porous or containing low moisture levels has insufficient durability for bleaching.	• Plastic self-grip meshes (e.g. Easy Meche L'Oréal). • Foil meshes. • Colour wraps.	High lift powder bleach with suitable hydrogen peroxide developer at 6 per cent, 9 per cent or, for highest lift, 12 per cent (providing no product is allowed to contact the skin/scalp).

GH17.5 Resolve basic colouring problems

Colouring problems

Colouring and lightening are complex chemical processes and even senior, experienced stylists can make mistakes. The following list provides the main reasons for faults that can occur during processing.

A. Poor consultation

- not finding out what is really needed in the first place
- lack of experience in dealing with the technical issues

EKU *statement*

GH17 (eku67) The types and causes of colouring and lightening problems and how to rectify them (e.g. over and underprocessing, overlapping, skin staining, deterioration of hair condition, uneven results and product seepage)

GH17 (eku72) The types of problems which require specialist colour correction

Diversion For more information see Unit GH18 Provide colour correction services pp. 291–319.

TUTOR SUPPORT

Short answer test 1

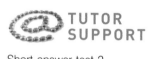

TUTOR SUPPORT

Short answer test 2

EKU *statement*

GH17 (eku75) How to maintain hair colour and condition

GH17 (eku76) Products for home use that will benefit the client and those to avoid and why

GH17 (eku77) How lifestyle can affect the client's choice of colour (e.g. active sports, career and job requirements)

GH17 (eku78) How the continual use of heated equipment can damage the hair

GH17 (eku79) The recommended time intervals between colouring and other services

GH17 (eku74) How to give effective advice and recommendations to clients

- not understanding what you see
- not understanding what the client sees or wants

B. Poor execution of the service

- incorrect choice(s) of colour(s)
- incorrect choice of hydrogen peroxide strengths
- incorrect or careless application
- unrealistic timescale allowed for the service (rushed service)
- unnecessary handling or disturbance during processing
- poor removal of colour products (colours mix or merge causing discolouration)

C. Processing/development

- insufficient time allowed for product development (taking off too soon)
- poor heat/air ventilation around all areas that need processing (hot spots)
- too much heat (causing over-development hair damage or breakage)
- too much time (causing over-processing, hair damage or breakage)

Colouring problems

Problem	Possible causes	Action
Uneven colour	Poor application Section too large Incorrect mixing	Spot-bleach Recolour Strip colour and recolour if necessary
Dark ends	Ends under-bleached Toners too dark Toner over-processed Dark colour remains	Re-bleach Remove using lighteners After removal, time accurately Remove and tone
Too yellow	Under-bleached Base too dark Wrong toner used Wrong bleach	Re-bleach Try stronger bleach Use violet toner Use other than oil bleach
Too red	Under-bleached Too much alkali Wrong toner used	Re-bleach Use different bleach Use green matt or olive
Dark roots or patches	Poor application Toner too dark	Re-bleach evenly remove using lightener
Roots not coloured	Under-bleached Under-timed Toner too dilute Unclean or coated	Re-bleach Re-bleach Reapply Clean and reapply
Colour fade	Over-porous Harsh treatment Overexposure	Condition Advise on hair care

Problem	Possible causes	Action
Hair breakage	Over-processed Incompatibles present Harsh treatment Sleeping in rollers Tied back long hair	Recondition remaining hair Re-test to make sure Provide hair care advice Provide hair care advice Provide hair care advice
Discolouration	Under-processed Excessive exposure Home treatment	Colour match or develop further Recondition and keep covered Provide hair care advice
Green tones	Incompatibles Blue used on yellow Too-blue ash used	Test hair Use warm or red shades Use violet
Too orange	Under-processed Pigment lacking	Apply blue ash Add blue
Too yellow	Under-processed	Add violet and/or bleach further
Hair tangled	Over-bleached Raised cuticle/over-porous	Use anti-oxidants/treatment reconditioners
Colour not taking	Over-porous Chemicals masking the hair Colour bounce/red pigment grabbing at roots	Recondition and pre-fill hair Use deep cleanser to remove build-up Recolour with brown ash pigments (not deposited into hair correctly)
Colour build up	Over-porous Excessive over-application	Recondition and pre-pigment Consider colour removal

Diversion For more information and pictorial explanations of colour correction see Unit GH18 Provide colour correction services pp. 291–319.

TUTOR SUPPORT

Project 11.9: Hair colouring faults

TUTOR SUPPORT

Discussion 11.2: Commitment that will follow colouring for the first time

GH17.6 Provide aftercare advice

Clients need your help to look after there hair at home, you need to give them the right advice so that they can make the most of their new colour and style between visits.

You should tell them what sorts of products that they could use that would make their colour last and reduce the risk of fading. Also make a point of telling them what they should avoid: some products will reduce the effects of your colouring, causing it to fade prematurely or lose its intensity or vibrancy.

Explain the benefits of maintaining their hair in good condition, as hair in good condition is easier to manage, it looks better and is noticeable to everyone else as well.

Home- and aftercare checklist

✔	Talk through the colour effect as you work; tell them how they can maintain their hair by optimising both the look and the condition of their hair
✔	Explain how lifestyle factors can effect their hair colour and ways that they can combat these factors
✔	Show and recommend the products/equipment that you use so that the client gets the right things to enable them to get the same effects

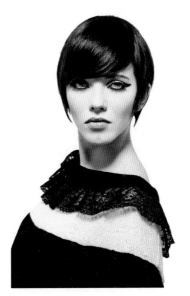

HAIR BY TERRY CALVERT AND THE CLIPSO ARTISTIC TEAM

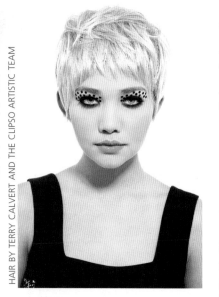

✔ | Tell the client how long the effect can be expected to last and when they need to return for re-colouring

✔ | Warn them about the products that will have a detrimental effect on the colour by telling them what these products would do

✔ | Warn the client about how incorrect handling or styling may reduce the length of time that the new effect will last

Explain how routine styling tools can have detrimental effects

Maintaining the hair in good condition is the single, most important factor for making the most of new colouring effects. You know how difficult it is to make dry, damaged hair look good and your clients can recognise the difference between good and poor condition. Given the choice, they will always choose hair that has; lustre, shine flexibility and strength.

Knowing this, you would be doing an injustice to your clients if you didn't warn them of the pitfalls of incorrect use of hot styling equipment, so make a point in asking them if they use them at home too. If they say that they use heated straighteners or tongs on a daily basis then tell them about the benefits of using heat protection sprays or treatments.

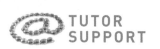

TUTOR SUPPORT

Discussion 11.4: Aftercare colour/lightening service

EKU *statement*

GH17 (eku73) How to give clear instructions to those with less technical knowledge and experience than yourself

GH17 (eku74) How to give effective advice and recommendations to clients

Remember

The condition and look of their hair is directly proportional to the amount of heat applied to it. So if your clients are locked into using heated styling tools their hair is going to need the correct products to maintain it too.

Show and recommend the products/equipment that you use

As you talk about the ways in which you have styled the hair, make a point of talking through the products that you have used as well. You know by experience the products that you would use on their hair to achieve different results and you also know the ones that you would avoid! Well, make a point of telling the client too, because they haven't had the benefit of your training and they don't know.

Be patient though, be sympathetic and avoid technical jargon, nobody likes a 'Clever Dick.' Keep things simple, clear and avoid misunderstandings.

And when you use a particular product, why not hand it to them so they can have a closer look. This way they get to see, smell and feel the product too and subconsciously, this has a very powerful effect on them. By doing this you are involving the client in what you are doing by giving them a greater experience of the service.

This way they will be able to see a direct link between; the effects that you are achieving on their hair, with the added benefits of buying those particular products that will help them to recreate a similar effect.

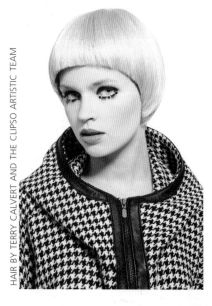

Demonstrate the techniques that you use

Clients want to be able to recreate the effects that you achieve in the salon and this is your chance to show them how to do it. Clients haven't had the benefit of your training; they don't know the little tricks and techniques that make it seem so simple.

Show the client how to do the routine things of; applying conditioner, combing and detangling, blow-drying and styling. We know what happens if these are not done properly, so make a point of giving them a few tips on how the can achieve similar results themselves and how long they can expect it to last.

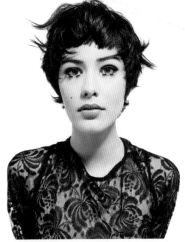

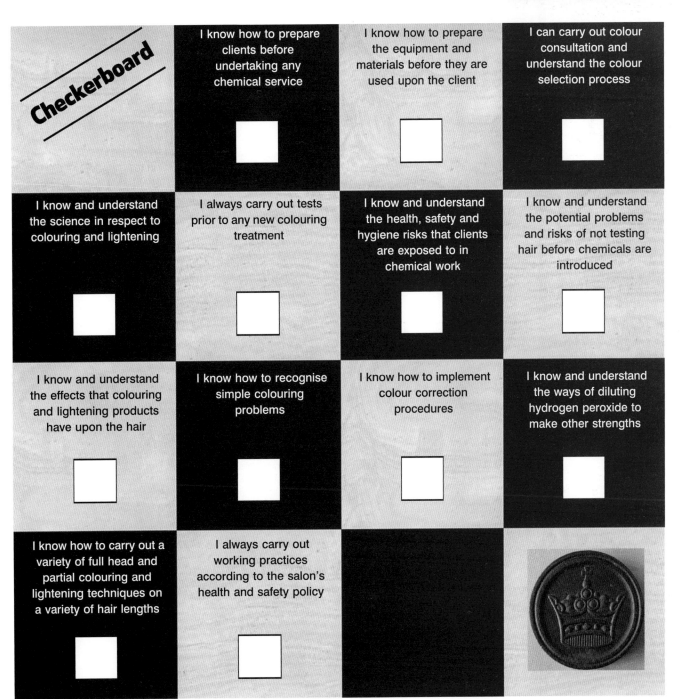

Checkerboard

| I know how to prepare clients before undertaking any chemical service ☐ | I know how to prepare the equipment and materials before they are used upon the client ☐ | I can carry out colour consultation and understand the colour selection process ☐ |

| I know and understand the science in respect to colouring and lightening ☐ | I always carry out tests prior to any new colouring treatment ☐ | I know and understand the health, safety and hygiene risks that clients are exposed to in chemical work ☐ | I know and understand the potential problems and risks of not testing hair before chemicals are introduced ☐ |

| I know and understand the effects that colouring and lightening products have upon the hair ☐ | I know how to recognise simple colouring problems ☐ | I know how to implement colour correction procedures ☐ | I know and understand the ways of diluting hydrogen peroxide to make other strengths ☐ |

| I know how to carry out a variety of full head and partial colouring and lightening techniques on a variety of hair lengths ☐ | I always carry out working practices according to the salon's health and safety policy ☐ | | |

Assessment of knowledge and understanding

Revision questions

Quick quiz: A selection of different types of questions to check your knowledge.

Q1   A _____ test will identify a client's sensitivity to colour products.   Fill in the blank

Q2   A quasi-permanent colour lasts longer than a semi-permanent colour.   True or false

Q3   Which of the following products are likely to be an incompatible?   Multi selection

Permanent colour containing PPD   ☐   1

Retail permanent colour containing PPD   ☐   2

Vegetable henna   ☐   3

Compound henna   ☐   4

Single-step applications for covering grey i.e. 'Just for Men'   ☐   5

Single-step toners for application to bleached hair   ☐   6

Q4   Bleaches and high lift colours are the same.   True or false

Q5   Which of the following tests do not apply to colouring services?   Multi choice

Skin test   ○   a

Incompatibility test   ○   b

Porosity test   ○   c

Curl test   ○   d

Q6   Permanent colours alter the pigmentation of hair within the cortex.   True or false

Q7   Which of the following colouring products do not require the addition of hydrogen peroxide as a developer?   Multi selection

Powder bleach   ☐   1

Semi-permanent colour   ☐   2

Quasi-permanent colour   ☐   3

Temporary colour   ☐   4

Vegetable henna   ☐   5

High lift colour   ☐   6

Q8   Green tones within hair are neutralised by adding _____ tones.   Fill in the blank

Q9   Hair lightened from natural base 7 should be capable of maximum lift to: Multi choice

White   ○   a

Pale yellow   ○   b

Yellow   ○   c

Yellow/orange   ○   d

Q10   Lightened hair that appears too yellow can be neutralised by adding mauve.   True or false

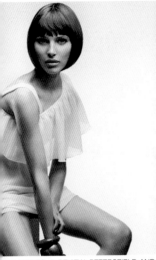

Chapter**twelve**
Colour correction

GH18

GH18.1
GH18.2
GH18.3
GH18.4
GH18.5

CREDIT VALUE
FOR UNIT GH18
13 Credits

 More information
About contra-indications, tests, consultation and customer care

See Unit G21 Provide hairdressing consultation services

 Diversion Your responsibilities under COSHH regulations GH18 (eku5) and Electricity at Work

GH18 (eku4) See Unit G22 Monitor procedures to safely control work operations

Your responsibilities for customer records under Data Protection Act GH18 (eku3) see Appendix 4

Colour correction: quick overview

Unit titles

GH18 Provide colour correction services

This is a **optional** unit for both hairdressing and barbering at level 3, it is made up of five main outcomes

Main outcomes

GH18.1 Maintain effective and safe methods of working when colour correcting hair

GH18.2 Determine the problem

GH18.3 Plan and agree a course of action to correct colour

GH18.4 Correct colour

GH18.5 Provide aftercare advice

What do I need to do for GH18.1?

- Make sure that the client is adequately covered, protected and prepared for the service

- Make sure that the working position is comfortable and safe for both you and the client

- Keep the work area clean and tidy and that waste materials are disposed of properly

- Work without causing risks to you or your client's health and safety

- Work efficiently and effectively at all times

- Accurately maintain the client's treatment records

What do I need to do for GH18.2?

- Find out by question and examination what the problem is

- Ask questions to identify any contra-indications to colour correction services

- Accurately record the responses to your questions

Keywords

Colour stripper

A name given to colouring product that is specially formulated to remove synthetic/ artificial colour from previously coloured hair

Banding

An unwanted effect that appears as distinct bands of uneven colour generally a problem found on longer hair associated with poor colour application/execution or as a result of poor hair condition

Discolouration

An unwanted effect that appears as shadowing or blotches often associated with incompatibles

Colouring back

A process of re-colouring previously lightened hair (e.g. highlights) back to the hair's natural hair depth and tone

Pre-pigmentation

Part of a larger process, colouring back, where missing pheomelanin (yellow/red pigments) are replaced first, so that the final target shade can be achieved without unwanted ashen 'green' tones being present

De-colouring

see *colour stripper* A process which removes synthetic colour from hair by using a colour reducer (*not* bleach)

- Carry out suitable tests and record the outcomes
- Select and prepare your products and tools appropriate to your consultations' findings

What do I need to do for GH18.3?

- Explore suitable colour options using visual aids
- Provide suitable options and alternatives to the client
- Explain what sort of results can be expected
- Explain the likely costs and timings for the service

What do I need to do for GH18.4?

- Select the appropriate materials to carry out the colour correction service
- Apply products safely and accurately in line with manufacturers' instructions
- Use appropriate techniques to achieve the expected result
- Modify or adapt your plan as and when the process requires it
- Remove products from the hair when ready without disturbing areas that are still processing
- Ensure that the finished result meets the client's expectations

What do I need to do for GH18.5?

- Give accurate constructive advice on how the client can maintain their hair colour

What aspects do I need to cover for GH18.1, GH18.2, GH18.3, GH18.4 and GH18.5?

- Quasi-permanent and permanent hair colouring products, lighteners and toners
- A variety of contra-indications to colouring and lightening services
- The necessary tests as and when they are needed
- A range of factors that influence or limit the way in which colouring and lightening is carried out
- A variety of corrective processes and techniques using a range of materials
- A range of hair colour problems on different hair types, textures and conditions
- Colour correction techniques that require pre-pigmentation and restore natural depth and tone, remove colour banding, remove artificial colour and correct highlight/lowlighting problems
- The advice and recommendations that you should give for the client to maintain their hair at home

What aspects do I need to know for GH18.1, GH18.2, GH18.3, GH18.4 and GH18.5?

- Your salon's requirements for preparation, timings and standards of service

- How to work safely, effectively and hygienically when correcting hair colour

- The different factors that can affect or influence successful colour correction services

- The questions that you must ask and the tests that need to be done prior to and during the corrective services and the records that you must make

- The courses of action that you should take in the event of adverse reactions to tests or unexpected results during development

- The principles of colour correction and the effects of the colour correction products upon the hair

- How natural and synthetic pigments differ and how light changes their appearance

- How different strengths of hydrogen peroxide affect hair and how they can be diluted

- How pH is affected by colouring products and how hair is balanced after processing

- How and when to pre-soften and pre-pigment hair

- The range of tools, equipment and materials and how these used

- A variety of techniques that can be used to achieve satisfactory colour correction results

- The types of problems that can be encountered during processing and how these can be resolved

- The aftercare advice and recommendations that you should give to clients

Information covered in this chapter

- The preparations that you must make before carrying out any colour correction service

- Routine colour correction problems and the ways in which they can be resolved

- The materials used during colour correction services and the preparations that you should make before colouring hair

- The factors that influence colour correction services

- A range of colour correction techniques on differing hair conditions and types

- How to adapt and modify your plans if you encounter unexpected problems

- The aftercare advice that you should give

Introduction

Colour correction is, as previously mentioned in the Chapter 11, (Unit GH17 Colour hair using a variety of techniques) is becoming more frequent within the salon. However, it is still quite some way from becoming a basic, routine service. On the contrary, it is work that is specially tailored to suit the needs of the individual client and therefore it is different every time, in every case.

Your experiences with colour correction will continue to build your confidence; the more that you are involved with the service the better prepared you will be in undertaking this essential work.

The main thing is knowing what you are dealing with and fully understanding the situation in hand.

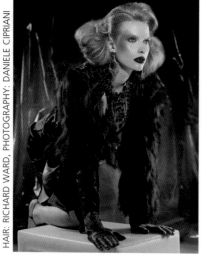

HAIR: RICHARD WARD, PHOTOGRAPHY: DANIELE CIPRIANI

Foreword

You must conduct a thorough consultation to find out exactly what has taken place and over what period of time. Planning a course of corrective action is imperative, unless you understand what you are seeing, you cannot hope to stumble on the correct course of action.

Remember, there will be times when what you see before you doesn't make sense. In other words, there is a discrepancy between what you see and what your client claims has taken place. Clearly, some vital information is missing. This could happen for a number of reasons but it could also be the result of embarrassment on your client's part over things they have done but don't wish to admit.

In order for you to get as much 'honest' information as possible, don't make an issue of the situation. You will get a lot more help if you don't apportion blame or look for someone to be the scapegoat. If this is a new client to you, you have a unique opportunity to forge a professional relationship that is built on respect, which, if you get it right, should last and last.

GH18.1 Maintain effective and safe methods of working when colour correcting hair

Diversion A student who undertakes this optional colour correction unit at level 3 will almost certainly be undertaking the creative colouring unit too.

So, for more colour correction information you will find:

A lot of the essential knowledge underpinning colour correction work is the same as creative colouring and therefore to avoid unnecessary duplication, please note that your attention is diverted to Chapter 11, Unit GH17 Colour hair using a variety of techniques, in a number of places within this chapter.

Diversion If you are unfamiliar with the safety and preparation aspects of colour correction work please see Unit GH17 Colour hair using a variety of techniques, pp. 261–269 for more information.

Preparation and safety

The safety and preparation needed for both you and your client for colour correction work is the same as the procedures for colouring hair.

Records   It is unlikely that you will have a record for your client covering the same colour correction work twice, as each colour correction process is unique and dependent on the problems that are apparent at the time of the visit. However, the maintaining of clients records is particularly important and you should make sure that you provide a full detailed account of any work undertaken.

> **Remember**
>
> The records are essential for:
> - monitoring the effectiveness of any colour correction work undertaken
> - keeping things going smoothly and for maintaining services even if key staff are away
> - a back-up if things go wrong and they are needed as evidence in any legal action taken against the salon.

Tests   Undertake your tests to find the contra-indications that confirm your visual and verbal information. In most cases the hair will be in a poorer condition than that of unprocessed (virgin) hair so testing for elasticity, porosity or signs of damage are vital to the success of the operation. It is very unlikely that a skin test will be required as you will be correcting a previous colour problem and your salon records should show when this test was previously carried out.

Materials Sometimes the products or materials needed for colour correction work will be out of stock. Check your materials to see that you have everything that you need. Where items are missing make sure that you bring this to your managers' attention so that they can be ordered and ready for use.

Gowning Always make sure that the client and the client's clothes are adequately protected before any process is started. Most salons have special 'colour-proof' gowns for colouring and lightening processes. These gowns are resistant to staining and are made from finely woven synthetic fabrics that will stop colour spillages from getting through onto the client's skin or clothes. When you gown the client, make sure that the free edges are closed and fastened together. On top of this and around the shoulders you can place a colouring towel and over this a plastic cape. This needs to be fastened but loose enough for the client to be comfortable throughout the service, Remember that this may be a couple of hours or so.

Using barrier cream Barrier cream can be used as physical barrier to prevent staining around the client's face/hairline. It is also particularly useful if the client has any general sensitivity to chemical based products.

Apply barrier cream to the skin with a finger or cotton wool close to the hairline, taking care not to get it onto the hair as this could stop the colour from taking evenly.

It can be removed later after you have shampooed the colour from the hair and before any other services are conducted.

Seating position The chair back should be protected with a plastic cover. If this is not available a colouring towel can be folded lengthwise and secured with sectioning clips at either end. The client should be sat comfortably, in an upright position, with their back flat against the cushioned chair pad.

Trolley You should have your colouring trolley prepared and at hand with the materials you will need. Foils for highlighting should have been previously prepared to the right lengths and combs, brushes, sectioning clips etc. should be all cleaned and sterilised and ready for use.

Protecting yourself Your personal hygiene and safety is also important. The care you take in preparing for work should be carried through in everything you do and this is made even more important when you are about to handle hazardous chemicals. Put on a clean colouring apron and fasten the ties in a bow. Then take a pair of disposable non-latex gloves and put them on ready for the application.

For more specific information on the following, please note that these essential knowledge and understanding statements below are covered in Chapter 11, Unit GH17 Colour hair using a variety of techniques.

Remember

If the client is new and not from your salon you will need to undertake a skin test and that is regardless that you can see that the hair is coloured. You must protect the salon and yourself legally in the event of something going wrong.

Diversion For more information on tests see pp. 266–268.

Remember

It is not an excuse for poor, slapdash application, allowing you to extend the colour application beyond the hairline area to the skin. But it will help in areas where colour seeps off the hair onto the skin.

Diversion See Unit GH17 Colour hair using a variety of techniques for preventing dermatitis.

Essential knowledge look-up table: The following listed EKU are addressed in Unit GH17 Colour hair using a variety of techniques	See pages
SAFETY AND PREPARATION	
GH18 (eku1) Your salon's requirements for client preparation	260
GH18 (eku2) Your salon's and legal requirements for removal of waste materials	260
GH18 (eku6) What is contact dermatitis and how to avoid developing it whilst carrying out colour correction services	263

Essential knowledge look-up table: The following listed EKU are addressed in Unit GH17 Colour hair using a variety of techniques		See pages
SAFETY AND PREPARATION		
GH18 (eku7)	The range of protective clothing that should be available for clients	260
GH18 (eku8)	The type of personal protective equipment that should be available and used by yourself	260
GH18 (eku9)	Why it is important to use personal protective equipment	260
GH18 (eku10)	How the position of your client and yourself can affect the desired outcome and reduce fatigue and the risk of injury	260
GH18 (eku11)	Why it is important to position your tools and equipment for ease of use	260
GH18 (eku13)	The dangers associated with the inhalation of powder lighteners	283
GH18 (eku14)	How to use lighteners safely	263 and 279
GH18 (eku15)	The precautions that must be taken when handling powder lighteners	281
GH18 (eku16)	Why it is important to keep your work area clean and tidy	260
GH18 (eku17)	Methods of working safely and hygienically and which minimise the risk of cross-infection and cross-infestation	260
GH18 (eku18)	The importance of personal hygiene	260
GH18 (eku19)	Why it is important to check electrical equipment used to aid the colour correction process	280
GH18 (eku20)	Methods of cleaning, disinfecting and/or sterilisation used in salons	260
GH18 (eku21)	The importance of questioning clients to establish any contra-indications to the colour correction service	268
GH18 (eku22)	Why it is important to record client responses to questioning	268
GH18 (eku23)	The legal significance of client questioning and of recording the client's responses	268

EKU *statement*

GH18 (eku6) What is contact dermatitis and how to avoid developing it whilst carrying out colouring and lightening services

 Diversion See Chapter 11, Unit GH17 Colour hair using a variety of techniques preventing dermatitis p. 263.

EKU *statement*

GH18 (eku12) The safety considerations which must be taken into account when carrying out colour correction services

Remember

 Salon cleanliness is of paramount importance the work area should be clean and free from clutter or waste items. Any used materials should be disposed of not left out on the side, which

● is unprofessional

● presents a health hazard to others of cross-infection.

What do you do if you think you have dermatitis?

Dermatitis is an occupational health hazard for hairdressers it is avoided by wearing non-latex disposable gloves for all processes or services that involve contact with chemicals. If you think you are suffering from dermatitis, then you should visit your doctor for advice and treatment. If you believe it has been caused or made worse by your work as a hairdresser, then you should mention this to your doctor and you must also tell your employer as employers are required by law to report a case of work-related dermatitis amongst their staff.

Colour correction preparation checklist

✔	Find the client's treatment record/or prepare a new one
✔	Make sure that the styling section and chair is clean, safe and ready to receive clients
✔	Make sure that the client is well protected with a clean fresh gown a colouring towel and cape
✔	Make sure you comb or brush the hair thoroughly before you start to remove tangles, see if all product can be removed and check for cuts or abrasions on the scalp
✔	Carry out your consultation to find out what needs to be done
✔	Look for contra-indications
✔	Conduct your tests based on the contra-indications found
✔	Record the responses to your questions (and update the treatment history)
✔	Note: if you need to do a skin test then no further action can be taken until the results of the tests are available
✔	If work has to be deferred, is a deposit required?
✔	Do any specialist materials need to be ordered such as colour strippers, treatments etc.?
✔	Make sure that you have your tools and products prepared and close at hand
✔	Make sure that you have checked the equipment that you need to use and it is ready and safe

GH18.2 Determine the problem

Colour correction considerations

Colour correction is proving to be the largest growing area of the hair colouring market and much of this is because:

- more people are having colouring services
- more people are experimenting with home colouring products
- our clients expect more, therefore pushing the boundaries of safe, guaranteed practice to the limits.

There are far more people having colour now than ever before. This growing market is looking for change and when they arrive in the salon, they want:

- modification of what they have had before
- something totally new or
- their dark roots lightened to match the over-processed, lightened ends, which are the result of one set after another of highlighting services.

These increasing salon colouring services will inevitably result in colour correction sooner rather than later and is therefore an essential part of level 3 work.

People experiment at home! Colour after colour is applied with the attitude 'this is easy anyway and it saves a fortune'. We all know what happens in the end. The biggest

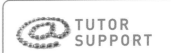

TUTOR SUPPORT

Project 12.1: Potential problems that could occur during colouring services

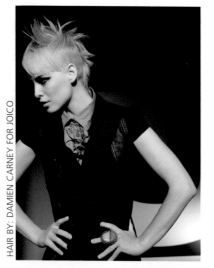

HAIR BY: DAMIEN CARNEY FOR JOICO

HAIR: RICHARD WARD, PHOTOGRAPHY: DANIELE CIPRIANI

problem for hairdressers is getting an honest historic account of what has taken place, when and with what!

We can't complain though, it's good business. (For those who can sort it out!)

Another reason for the increase in the number of people having colour correction is the unrealistic expectations of many clients.

Highlights/lowlights are a very attractive option for professional colouring. However, they do create some serious long-term problems if they are not carried out with the long term in mind from the outset. That might sound strange, but it's true. It is to do with the success of the service really.

Highlights are almost *addictive*; that is to say that when a new client is introduced to this form of colouring, they are compelled, by the colour's benefits to keep it up and keep coming back.

They are a great way for:

- cleverly and subtly covering grey hair
- introducing clients to colour
- personalising colour to individuals
- advertising your colouring skills
- enhancing the features of a hairstyle.

However, hair grows and it's the regrowth that creates the problem, at least initially. As the client's hair grows they become more conscious of the demarcation between the coloured hair and the natural roots. At the point where the hair has grown 2.5 cm a natural parting will show 5 cm of regrowth, a further colouring application would now be necessary. But will it be satisfactory to just highlight/lowlight the roots? In most cases not, particularly if several colours have been introduced to the hair. Even if the hair was only lightened, general shampooing, drying and weathering will have modified the colour on the ends, to the extent where newly introduced colour at the root will have little effect. So what do you do? In most situations, faced with the pressure of replicating what you did last time, you redo the service. This reintroduces colour to hair that has already been processed, even if it is to be taken through to the ends for the last few minutes. And now you have hair that will continue to change in porosity and condition creating a more difficult task for the future; that is, until you and your client agree to sort out the problem with colour correction.

Consultation for colour correction

The hardest part of colour correction work is establishing what has happened and how you are going to correct it.

You must look at the current state of the hair and from this and before you do any tests, ask the client questions to get a true picture of what has happened.

Example questions that need to be answered and recorded

Question to ask:	Reason for asking:
1. How long has the hair had this problem?	This will tell you if you have a worsening problem that could be linked to: 1 gradual deterioration from product fading over time or, 2 swift product failure where there has been a sharp degradation/deterioration

Question to ask:	Reason for asking:
2. What products do you normally use on the hair?	This will tell you if you have a product usage problem that could be linked to: 1 something that has been bought by the client and incorrectly/inappropriately used 2 poor or lack of home care advice
3. Have you tried to correct the problem yourself?	This will tell you if something has been bought and inappropriately used
4. How do you style your hair?	This will indicate whether the handling, styling or equipment has played any part in the problem
5. What sort of style do you want?	This will give you an idea of how much they are prepared to have cut and give you an idea of how much of the problem is going to be removed by cutting alone
6. Would you be prepared to have a different style?	If they haven't indicated that they want a different look; it at least addresses the point in very clear terms
7. What sort of colour effect are you trying to achieve	The main question that you need to ask. you will need to show examples and get a clear idea of what they want their hair to look like

At this point (although you haven't conducted any tests,) you should already have enough basic information to know whether the request is:

A achievable   B desirable   C realistic

Activity
Colour problems
Consider the following problems and then write your answers in your portfolio:
What could be the reasons for:

1 Permanent colour fading on the ends of long hair?

2 Permanent colour not taking properly on the roots?

3 Grey/white hair resisting semi-permanent colour?

4 Permanent copper red colour not taking on mid-brown hair?

5 Mid blonde hair looking ashen or green?

TUTOR SUPPORT

Discussion 12.1: Potential mistakes that could result in an unsatisfactory colour

Remember/Health and safety

Before using permanent or any long-lasting colours, you must always perform a skin (sensitivity) test. If there is any reaction, you cannot carry out the colouring. To do so could result in an allergic reaction and a possible personal injury claim.

What other factors are relevant?

Later in your consultation you should consider the following points:	
1. Age and lifestyle	Do these factors have any bearing on your decision? If so why?
2. Job or role	Will the result compliment what they do?
3. Fashion, look or image	Will it suit the client when it's finished?
4. Natural hair colour and skin tones	
5. Hair's texture, condition and porosity	Is the colour effect going to work?
6. Colour and technique you choose	Are your choices correct for the desired effect? Is what they want realistically achievable? Can the hair condition stand the clients wishes/expectations?
7. Time and costs involved	Be thorough and accurate, work out the time and costs. Is it still OK?

When you have taken these points into consideration, you should be able to determine which hair colours and processes you need to use.

Remember

Don't rush the consultation; you need to have a clear idea of what is needed. If you are unsure ask for a second opinion.

Diversion Colour tests are covered in more depth in Unit GH17 Colour hair using a variety of techniques (see pp. 266–268)

EKU *statement*

GH18 (eku24) The types and purposes of tests in the range
GH18 (eku27) How the results of tests can influence the colour correction service

Colour tests

There are a number of tests that must be considered before you carry out any colour correction work:

- *strand/test cutting* – carried out before attempting to colour the full head
- *skin test* – to assess the client's sensitivity to the colour
- *porosity test* – to assess the smoothness or roughness of the cuticle
- *elasticity test* – to determine the hair's state or condition
- *incompatibility test* – if metallic chemicals are present
- *development strand/colour test* – to check the process of colouring.

Essential knowledge look-up table: The following listed EKU are addressed in Unit GH17 Colour hair using a variety of techniques		**See pages**
TESTS AND TESTING		
GH18 (eku25)	The importance of following manufacturers' instructions for skin testing	268
GH18 (eku26)	When and how tests should be carried out and the expected results	268
GH18 (eku28)	The potential consequences of failing to carry out tests	266
GH18 (eku29)	The courses of action to take in the event of adverse reactions to tests and the contra-indications in the range (ie when to encourage the client to seek medical advice, when to explain the service is not possible, when a modification to the service will be necessary)	266
GH18 (eku30)	Why it is important to record test results	266

Record the details of your consultation

Every aspect of the work you undertake must be detailed accurately and this includes the responses to the questions that you ask during consultation.

Diversion See Unit GH17 Colour hair using a variety of services on pp. 268–269 for more information.

Activity

Complete the missing information in the table below. Keep a record of the correct test table within your portfolio.

Test	When is this test done?	Why is this test done?	How is this test done?
Strand test			
Skin test			
Porosity test			
Elasticity test			
Incompatibility test			
Colour development test			

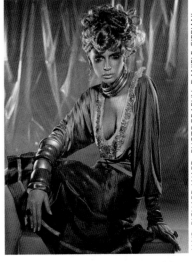

HAIR: RICHARD WARD, PHOTOGRAPHY: DANIELE CIPRIANI

Consultation checklist

✔ Look at the client's treatment history

✔ Identify any contra-indications by asking questions and looking through the hair for visible signs

✔ Find out what the client wants – use visual aids to establish requirements

✔ Assess suitability and achievability of the desired look

✔ Look for colouring problems or pre-service requirements

✔ Conduct any tests – check the results of hair tests against planned services

✔ Avoid confusing technical jargon; always clarify in simple terms what you mean

✔ Agree on a suitable course of action and give an idea of service timings and costs

✔ Summarise the main points of the consultation and get ready to start

✔ Whilst the service is being done, give the client some advice on how to maintain their hair at home and recommend those products that are suitable to use and those that are not

✔ Give them an idea of how long the effect will last (and prompt them to re-book their next appointment before they leave)

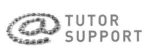

TUTOR SUPPORT

Discussion 12.2: Dealing with colour problems

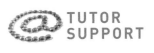

TUTOR SUPPORT

Discussion 12.3: Consultation for colour problems

Activity

The purpose of this activity is to look at the patterns of colour business over a period of time.

With permission from your salon supervisor, conduct a study over a three-month period to monitor the salon's colouring services. Keep a record in your portfolio for future reference.

You will need to create a system that will record the following numerical information:

- *simple root (retouch) application*
- *full-head colour*
- *partial colouring*
- *highlights and lowlights*

Then after collecting the data: what conclusions can you draw from your findings?

1) How many services for each of the above were carried out over the period?

2) Is there any pattern for the type of business occurring?

3) What percentage of business does retouch and full head colour contribute to the total colour business?

4) What percentage of business does high lights and partial colour contribute to the total colour business?

5) What amount of the colouring business incorporates colour correction techniques as part of the total service?

The following essential knowledge and understanding statements can be found in Chapter 11, Unit GH17 Colour hair using a variety of techniques.

Essential knowledge look-up table: The following listed EKUs are addressed in Unit GH17 Colour hair using a variety of techniques		See pages
COLOUR PRINCIPLES AND SCIENCE		
GH18 (eku31)	The principles of colour selection, including the International Colour Chart (ICC)	256
GH18 (eku33)	How the type and distribution of melanin creates natural hair colour	253
GH18 (eku34)	The effects of light and artificial lighting on the appearance of hair colour	265
GH18 (eku35)	The effects on the hair of different colour correction products	256
GH18 (eku36)	What is meant by the term 'oxidation'	279
GH18 (eku38)	How the different strengths of hydrogen peroxide affect colouring and lightening	259
GH18 (eku39)	The reasons for pre-softening and pre-pigmenting hair	271
GH18 (eku40)	Effects of temperature on the application and development of colour correction products	272
GH18 (eku41)	How to dilute hydrogen peroxide to form different strengths of solutions	260
GH18 (eku42)	The pH values of differing colouring products and lighteners	279
GH18 (eku43)	The importance of restoring the hair's pH balance after the colour correction process	272
GH18 (eku45)	Why it is important to leave the hair and scalp free of colour correction products	281
GH18 (eku46)	How and why the contra-indications in the range can affect the delivery of the colour correction service	264

Essential knowledge look-up table: The following listed EKUs are addressed in Unit GH17 Colour hair using a variety of techniques		See pages
PRODUCTS EQUIPMENT AND THEIR USE		
GH18 (eku47)	The types of tools, materials and equipment used for colour correction and how and when to use them	269
GH18 (eku48)	The different types of colour correction products available and when to use them	256
GH18 (eku50)	The importance of following manufacturers' instructions when measuring and mixing colour correction products	270
GH18 (eku51)	How to accurately measure and mix colour correction products to meet manufacturers' instructions	270
GH18 (eku52)	How and why pre and post treatments should be used when carrying out colour correction procedures	272
GH18 (eku53)	The importance of using products economically	270

GH18.3 — Plan and agree a course of action to correct colour

With the consultation done you will have a good idea of what you need to do, but now you have to explain this to the client.

Many people (and hairdressers too!) consider colour correction to be a simple task of repainting the walls with a different colour. You need to make sure that this is not the case and that any work that you undertake is both appreciated and looked after for the future.

Colour perfection?

Sometimes a perfect solution is unachievable; if this is the case you need to make this clear now. If you feel that you can get close to the required result; tell them, explain the reasons why perfection is not an option today. Make sure that you give them the advice on how the colour can be safeguarded and looked after to maximise its lasting benefits. Also make a point to tell them about the things that they need to avoid; some products or styling routines will work against your plan so make this known from the outset.

Finally, before starting, don't forget to give them a full run down on what the costs will be and how long it all will take. Any senior stylist knows that correction work is difficult to quantify in terms of timings, but think about it thoroughly as you don't want to end up trying to rush it.

Pre-pigmentation

In the majority of colour correction situations you will find that the client has lightened hair. If they want to change this back to their darker natural tones you will have to carry out pre-pigmentation before you can apply the target shade. This is the vital, *nightmare* colour process that if left out gives all those lovely shades of *green*!

TUTOR SUPPORT

Project 12.2: Risk assessment to cover colour correction services

EKU statement

GH18 (eku32) The principles of colour correction

GH18 (eku37) How oxidation agents affect the natural and artificial colour pigments

GH18 (eku39) The reasons for pre-softening and pre-pigmenting hair

GH18 (eku49) How and why the factors in the range can influence your choice of product and application techniques

GH18 (eku55) Methods of pre-softening and pre-pigmenting hair (see Chapter 11 and GH17 for pre-softening hair)

GH18 (eku56) Methods of applying and removing colour correction products

EKU *statement*

GH18 (eku59) How to recolour hair previously treated with lighteners using pre-pigmentation and permanent colour

GH18 (eku62) How the application and removal of lightener should be adapted to minimise scalp sensitivity and hair damage (see also GH17 for removal of lightening products)

GH18 (eku63) The types and causes of colour correction problems that may occur during processing and how to rectify them (e.g. over- and under-processing, skin staining, deterioration of hair condition, scalp sensitivity and product seepage)

GH18 (eku64) The potential problems of using colour correction products on previously chemically treated hair

Remember

👉 **The colour wheel**
Unwanted yellow tones are lessened by violet tones, green tones are lessened by introducing red (warmth), orange tones are lessened by blue.

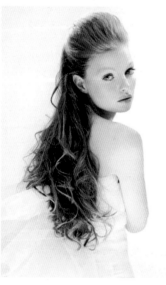

HAIR: MICHAEL BARNES FOR GOLDWELL

If natural depth say, base 5 is applied to pre-lightened hair with 3 per cent – 10 vol hydrogen peroxide it will look a khaki colour when it is dry. This happens because the hair is missing the essential larger, warm pigments. In any hair colour that involves colouring back, pre-pigmentation should be done first using a para-dye of around base 8 with a tonal quality of gold/red, i.e. Majirel 8.34.

Colouring back: Reintroducing colour into bleached hair

As more clients are willing to experiment with colour at home and want to change the appearance of their hair more frequently, the colour correction service is a growing market within the salon.

When recolouring (colouring back) bleached hair back to its original or a darker colour, you need to consider the condition of the hair – how porous it might be, and, in particular, whether there is sufficient colour pigment left in the hair for the hair to retain new pigment. Think back to how permanent colours work within the hair. Synthetic para-dyes, for example, work within the cortex of the hair, bonding into the hair's structure where the natural pigments are. Conversely, bleaching products simply remove all natural pigment from the hair and weaken the hair's internal structure.

So, if the hair's internal structure has been impaired then there will be less structure for reintroduced pigments to bond to. This fundamental aspect, if ignored, will have a major impact upon the visual effect of the hair.

However, this problem can be resolved by pre-pigmentation. During bleaching most of the natural pigments are removed. When these pigments are dissolved they create colourless, air-filled spaces a bit like the inside of a natural sponge. These gaps are not uniform in shape and when synthetic pigments are put back into the hair, not all will fit in the spaces they occupy. Some will come away during washing, leaving a very uneven and unattractive result.

So, to avoid green hair and to ensure that recolouring is successful, it is usual to pre-pigment (colour-fill) the hair. This is done by applying red or warm shades to the hair, before the final shade is applied. (If this is not done the hair may fade, become patchy or appear greenish.)

Decolouring

Synthetic (para-dyes) permanent hair colour can only be removed with a decolour treatment. All of the main colour manufacturers produce at least one. The decolouring process is also known as colour stripping and colour reducing and these products are quite different to bleaching products.

If a client's hair has been previously permanently coloured and the client wishes for the colour to be removed or to be changed, in order to go to a lighter shade, then only a colour remover (decolour) may be used. The chemical formulation of a colour reducer is very different from powder and emulsion bleach, hence, the colour reducer is specially developed to seek out and remove (dissolve) only the synthetic pigments within the hair.

Process preparation

EKU *statement*

GH18 (eku54) The importance of sectioning hair accurately for the colour correction service (see also colour selection principles in Unit GH17)

Always make sure that you protect your client before undertaking any permanent colouring operation. The removal of hair colour becomes more problematic in proportion to the length of hair: the longer the hair, the more difficult the task and the easier it is for spillages to occur. Clients waiting for colours to process often have to wait for long periods of time. Make sure that they are regularly attended to. And not just for checking development, check also for clothing protection placement of towels capes and especially for poorly secured hair and product drips!

Activity

Hydrogen peroxide strengths

Complete the table below by finding as many reasons as you can for the uses of the following hydrogen peroxide strengths.

Keep a record of your results in your portfolio.

Hydrogen peroxide strength	For what purposes would this strength be used?
3%	
6%	
9%	
12%	

Applying depth/tone into previously bleached hair (pale yellow blonde base 10)

Target depth	Amount of bleached lengths	Pre-pigment shade and development	Secondary processing and development
7–9	7.5 cm (approx. 3 inches)	Use a golden/red /3 or /34 shade of same depth (7, 8 or 9) mixed with water Apply from visible roots to ends 12–15 mins without heat	After washing, conditioning and drying, apply target depth 7, 8 or 9 and, if required, tonal ranges /30 or /34 or /03. from visible roots to ends with 3 per cent (10 vol.). Develop without heat for 20 mins
7–9	Over 7.5 cm (3 inches +)	Use a golden/red /3 or /34 shade of same depth (7, 8 or 9) mixed with water Apply to mid lengths and ends for 10 mins then apply to remaining light hair for a further 10–15 mins, without heat	After washing, conditioning and drying, apply target depth 7, 8 or 9, and if required, tonal ranges /30 or /34 or /03 mixed with 3 per cent hydrogen peroxide on mid lengths and ends first. Allow to develop for 10 mins Then apply to remaining hair for further 10–15 mins

Target depth	Amount of bleached lengths	Pre-pigment shade and development	Secondary processing and development
5–6	7.5 cm (approx 3 inches)	Use a red/copper of depth 8,43 or 7,43 mixed with water Apply from visible roots to ends Develop for 15 mins without heat	After washing, conditioning and drying, apply target depth 5 or 6, and, if required, tonal ranges /30 or /34 /03 or /4. from visible roots to ends with 3 per cent (10 vol.). Develop without heat for 20 mins
5–6	Over 7.5 cm (3 inches +)	Use a red/copper of depth 8,43 or, 7,43 mixed with water. Apply to mid lengths and ends for 10 mins then apply to remaining hair for a further 10–15 mins without heat	After washing, conditioning and drying, apply target depth 5 or 6, and if required, tonal ranges /3, /34, /03 or /4 mixed with 3 per cent hydrogen peroxide on mid lengths and ends first. Allow to develop for 10 mins. Then apply to remaining hair for further 10–15 mins
4	7.5 cm (approx 3 inches)	Use 7,44 mixed with water. Apply from roots to ends with water for 15 mins. After washing and conditioning dry the hair to check that tone is strong enough to receive secondary colour. If not repeat again.	After washing, conditioning and drying, apply base 4 mixed with 3 per cent roots to ends. Allow to develop for 10–15 mins
4	Over 7.5 cm (3 inches +)	Not recommended	
I.	Note: colours used within this table refer to L'Oréal Majirel shade chart (see p. 331)		
II.	Ashen tones, violet browns and violet reds should not be applied to pre-pigmented hair		

Note: colours used within this table refer to L'Oréal Majirel shade chart (see p. 331)

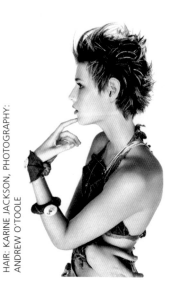

EKU *statement*

GH18 (eku60) How to recolour hair that has had artificial colour removed

Reapplying to natural depth

The removal of synthetic hair colour is usually only a part of a larger technical operation. More likely than not, it will be the client's wishes to return to her natural colour. Clients who merely want to change their hair colour to a different, darker, new shade would not normally have to go through the process of colour reduction first.

The reapplication of base shade follows the removal of the synthetic tones. However, hair that has undergone the reduction process does now respond to the application of new colour in a different way. This new state of the hair is called double processed hair. This degree of treatment will make the hair respond to reintroduced colour more readily. Therefore the porosity levels are increased, which means that the hair becomes more absorbent.

In these situations there are certain rules that should be observed.

- Do a colour test on the hair first mixed only with water.
- Try using a liquid-based quasi-permanent colour (e.g. Diacolour) as these are easier to apply evenly and more quickly.
- Choose a colour one shade lighter than the expected target shade to avoid *colour grab*.
- Check development every few minutes (scrape colour off the hair and rub between fingers to see the colour development clearly).

Removal of permanent, synthetic hair dyes

Checklist	Special attention
• Client expectation/ target colour	What is the purpose for removing the permanent hair dye, is it to: 1 Recolour back to natural depth and tone? 2 Recolour to a lighter shade? 3 Remove unwanted/discoloured tonal effects from the hair?
• Treatment history	If you have no previous history available for the client and you want to undertake the technical operation you must undertake a skin test and take a test cutting for incompatible chemicals and ability to achieve target shades before conducting any chemical process.
• Condition	What are the existing hair condition attributes (elasticity, porosity and strength)? Will these limit the effectiveness of the treatment?
• Hair length	The longer the hair, the more difficulty will be encountered in stabilising the evenness of the lightening.
• Natural hair colour	Do you know what the natural hair colour is? 1 If the natural hair colour is darker than the resultant, permanent hair colour, can the target colour be achieved without removing previous colour? 2 If the natural hair colour is lighter than the resultant permanent colour, how many levels of lift are required and is this feasible? (Reducing synthetic hair dye above four levels of lift is not recommended.)
• Uneven, permanent hair colour	Where worn lengths have produced an uneven colour effect the darker bands/areas must be lightened to match the other lighter areas first.
• Work method	Always follow the manufacturer's instructions when mixing and applying the product. Start on the darkest areas first, then on to lighter areas.* Often the consistency of colour reducers makes it more difficult to work with on pre-coloured hair, so make sure that the product is applied evenly.
• Development	Slow development is easier to control, so develop without thermal acceleration. Ensure adequate air circulation do not paste hair flat; lift sections and separate the hair to assist an even lifting process.
• Removal of product	Always follow the manufacturer's instructions and remove the product with suitable shampoo and tepid water. After conditioning, dry the hair before further processing.

* It is normally not necessary to apply to mid lengths and ends first, as worn hair colour tends to lighten on the ends anyway.

Activity

This activity covers some of the common colouring problems encountered everyday with the salon.

You are asked to help someone else with their consultation and you encounter the following problems.

Fill in the table with the missing information for what you think has occurred and how it can be rectified.

Colour problem	What is the likely reason for this?	How can it be resolved?
Colour not taking on white hair		
Hair appears green or khaki in certain lights		
Hair colour has faded a lot at the ends but has stayed on target nearer the root area		
Hair colour should be a natural base tone throughout, but appears redder near the roots		

EKU *statement*

GH18 (eku58) How to remove bands of colour

Banded hair colour

Sometimes colour correction is undertaken to counteract partial colouring defects. These types of technical problems can seem quite daunting, particularly when we are used to applying colour in either a 'blanket' operation or by sectioning and covering in foil. These problems can be overcome and usually require a change of mind set in their execution. There is something particularly different in tackling this type of situation though.

Horizontally banded hair colour will occur from one of the following:

- poor home product application
- poor home product reapplication and subsequent recolouring
- poor salon product application
- excessive heat/'hot spots' occurring during development
- uneven porosity of the hair (possibly from masking where conditioning treatments have bonded to different sites upon the surface of the hair unevenly).

Horizontally banded hair colour usually appears on long hair at, or near, one length. If the hair is to be restyled or layered it is worth cutting and drying first to see if the problem still exists.

If decolouring is still necessary in these areas, it would be advisable to apply the product by the following methods:

- use a thicker consistency: this will allow you to 'spot colour', applying freehand to the central areas of 'patchiness'.
- apply with the natural fall of the hair so that any natural light shadowing can easily be seen

Remember

Banded hair colour and gradation

Normally, when colour is applied to hair people tend to liken the process to painting. This is not a good comparison. Imagine painting emulsion on a dining room wall. We paint the wall white and the saturation of the paint covers where we pass the brush. On finishing the wall, say we want to change an area in the middle and we paint a blue horizontal stripe, wherever we apply the brush the saturation of the paint again will provide cover and change it to blue.

Banded hair colour, in contrast, often tends to a type of gradation of colour and this is particularly noticeable at the patchy edges. Part of the effect can be the result of how light reflects off the hair's surface, so when dealing with this situation look at the hair in different lighting backgrounds (ideally, natural daylight, white halogen light and somewhere away from bright lighting in more normally lit interiors).

- later, during development, extend the product to the edges of the gradated patches
- remove occasionally with warm water, then dry smoothly to see when the development is complete
- reapply to those areas requiring further development
- finally remove at the backwash with suitable shampoo and condition the hair with an anti-oxidising treatment.

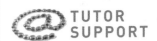

TUTOR SUPPORT

Project 12.4: Proprietary colour removers

Gradated colour

Gradated colour or gradation of colour is where the hue changes with the levels of saturation. For example, black and white mixed together create grey and, depending how much white or black is added, the colour either deepens or lightens, moving from shade to shade seamlessly.

This merging of colour occurs in hair naturally after colouring and it is difficult to remedy. It occurs partly by colour fade, i.e. the natural wear and tear and weathering. However, this subtle colour fading is far easier to tackle than the gradated banding that occurs after incorrect colouring. Imagine what happens when a dark colour, say base 5, is applied to natural hair base 7. As the hair grows, the regrowth becomes more obvious. Initially, this appears as a solid line of demarcation. But hair doesn't all grow at the same rate, and this becomes more apparent the further away from the roots the hair grows. The inconsistent growth blurs the edge of demarcation creating a gradated effect. In this scenario the recolouring is simple: just retouch with base 5. However, if the hair were to be colour stripped, then the complexity would be increased because of the uneven edge of colour to be removed.

EKU *statement*

GH18 (eku61) How to correct highlights and lowlights whilst retaining a highlight and lowlight effect

Discoloured highlights/lowlights and partial applications

Historically, we used the term 'discoloured hair' as a description for hair that has resulted from the presence of incompatible chemicals i.e. metallic salts. As cases of this happening are few and far between the term is now more usually applied in a different context. Partial colouring techniques are extremely popular and remain firmly as the 'professional only' route to achieving exciting colour effects. So, therefore, with ever increasing expectations by clients for partial colouring techniques, it is no surprise to find that much of the colour correction work undertaken within the salon is a result of previous highlighting and/or lowlighting services. Problems will tend to occur in the following instances:

- on longer hair over a period of time following several, subsequent treatments
- on hair that involves two or more newly introduced colours on an uneven background colour
- poorly executed application or removal of product/s
- over-porous hair
- hair subjected to excessive sunlight, UV or chlorinated swimming pools.

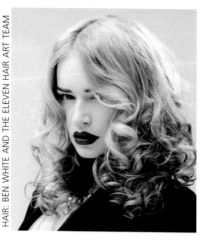

Remember

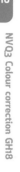

Colour stability
The stability of a synthetic colour within the hair is directly affected by the condition of the hair. The better the condition the more able the hair to retain the pigments. Conversely, the poorer the condition the less able the hair to retain the pigments.

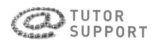

TUTOR SUPPORT

Discussion 12.4: Colour correction during applications of colour

Longer highlighted hair

Longer hair that has had several highlighting and/or lowlighting services is the most frequent reason for discoloured hair. Let's look at a typical example: a regular client has shoulder length hair of base 6 (dark blonde). The client has her first colouring service which involves two colours:

1 a lightener/bleach with 9 per cent

2 a beige mid-tone to harmonise the final effect.

After 6–8 weeks with regular washing and blow-drying the mid-tones fade off. Some pigments are washed away and some are absorbed into the more porous lightened hair, discolouring the original highlights. At the 12-week stage the client returns for a **T section highlights** (recolouring of the roots at the parting and sides). What do you do? You are unable to do a reapplication of the midtone just at the roots as the ends have faded off and similarly you may not be able to locate the initial bleached highlights! Most stylists will in this situation end up recolouring the hair with both colours again just within the T section but roots to ends.

The client is happy once again. However, a longer-term problem will start to develop. Much of the surface hair is now double processed (it has had two applications of the same chemicals). Double processed hair is more porous and this impaired condition leaves the client's hair in a state less able to retain colour pigments. So again a fade off occurs. This problem is compounded by the fact that the ends will now be predominantly lighter. The new roots will be darker and the hair in between will be lighter than the roots but not as light as the ends.

This colour state has now created an uneven background colour. A gradation from dark at the roots to light at the ends. Before any further partial colouring takes place this must be taken into consideration. At the point where this client wishes to once again have the same colours applied, a colour correction of the discoloured, background hair will have to be undertaken. This is done at the same time as the highlighting service. When the meshes of coloured hair are secured in their packets/foils, the remainder hair is coloured back to the natural shade. (However, this may make the problem far worse. If this newly introduced colour leaches out into the lightened hair all of the hair will be discoloured and the problem will be compounded further.)

Newly introduced colours

A similar problem occurs when newly introduced colours are applied to an uneven background. If the unevenness of the background colour is not corrected during the service the impact of the newly applied colour will be greatly devalued.

The hardest choice to make in this type of colour correction is whether to colour back the uneven background colour first, or to attempt the correction at the same time as the application of the new colours. If the hair needs pre-pigmentation you would be better advised to complete the task in two separate phases:

1 pre-pigment and then colour back the hair to natural base, then

2 carry out the partial colouring technique.

However, remember that hair that has been coloured back will be more porous and less able to sustain further colouring operations. This is particularly problematic if you intend to lighten portions of the hair. (It just won't work satisfactorily!) If you intend to lighten as well reintroduce colour to the background, you are better off conducting the process in a single phase. In other words, re-colour back the remaining hair that is not part of the partial colouring effect.

Over-porous hair

EKU *statement*

GH18 (eku44) Why it is important to avoid disturbing areas still processing when removing products from developed areas

GH18 (eku57) How to remove artificial colour

The condition of the hair dictates what should and can be done. Never ignore the obvious. As we have already stated, clients want more and this pressure by the client should not override common sense. If you believe that a treatment cannot be undertaken or is unachievable, it is your duty to tell the client your assessment of the situation. By all means get another opinion from a colleague, but if they agree, you must refuse the service:

Removing artificial colour

Make sure that when the colouring product is removed from the hair you rinse it without massaging, using only tepid or warm water. For example, the removal of a bleach lightener can be far more problematic than that of colour reducer (colour stripper) and this has more to do with the colouring technique that has been used. If different coloured highlights have been done with Easy Meche, foil, wraps, etc. these need to be removed carefully and individually as one colour may affect another.

Although the client's scalp has not been subjected to chemicals, it still might be sensitive from the colouring technique; again, the cooling action of the rinsing will stop the lightening process and make the client more comfortable. Afterwards the hair can be shampooed with a mild colour shampoo and conditioned with a pH-balancing anti-oxidising treatment.

Poor removal of colour products

As partial colour techniques become more involved the complexity of processes and procedures increases too. This is all too apparent in poorly removed colour products. When two or more colours are applied in the same operation, particular care must be taken in how they are removed. For example, let's take a client who has lightened highlights with vibrant copper lowlights on a reintroduced background of base 6.

In this example three separate colour combinations exist.

1 the highlight   2 the lowlight   3 the background.

Imagine what would happen in the following scenarios:

A Highlight packets are removed and shampooed at the same time as the low-light packets!

B Highlight packets are removed and rinsed with the background colour!

C All packets are removed and collectively shampooed at the same time!

Potentially, the effects created by clever techniques and artistic application can be totally wiped out if, during removal, the individual colour combinations aren't removed one by one.

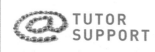

Activity

Complete the table below to indicate which and what amounts of pigments are present within each scenario.

Natural hair colour	What colour pigments are present within the hair?
Black hair	
Brown 'chestnut' hair	
'Celtic' red hair	
Blonde hair	
White hair	

GH18.4 Correct colour

@ TUTOR SUPPORT

Project 12.3: Manufacturer's instructions to find out their recommendations on the use of the colour for colour correction

Step-by-steps

Sorting out a common DIY disaster

Correcting (home applied) full head lightener by re-introducing natural tone and introducing highlights at the same time

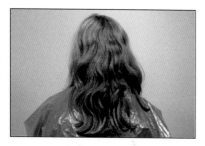

Step 1 Before

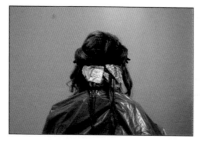

Step 2 Start the highlights at the lower nape

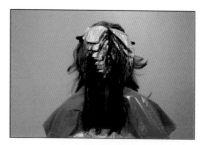

Step 3 Work up the back to the crown

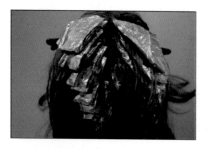

Step 4 Apply the natural base on to the interleave hair

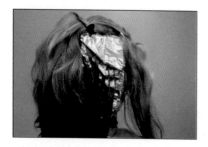

Step 5 Work through the sides

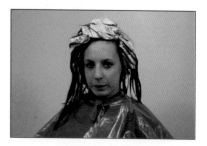

Step 6 Apply the natural base to the rest of the hair hair

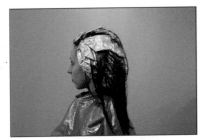

Step 7 Leave until the colour has developed

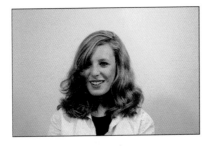

Step 8 Final effect

Highlight colour correction

Due to the imbalance of light and dark hair, these highlights have lost all definition. This is a common problem which occurs daily in hairdressing salons. When highlighting fine hair, it is all too easy to overdo it. This technique will correct the light-dark balance problem while redefining the definition with two harmonising colours.

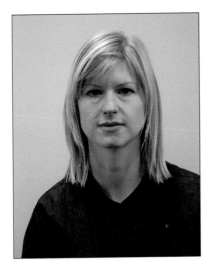

Step 1 Before

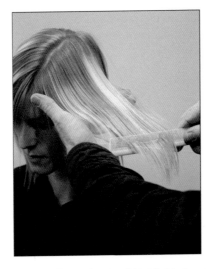

Step 2 Several sets of highlights have created over-bleached ends while the roots remain dark

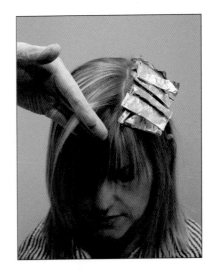

Step 3 Carefully select highlights from the previously lightened areas

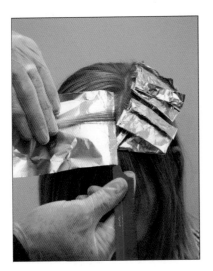

Step 4 Position the foil carefully below the individual sections of hair. Only paste the lightener on at the roots as the ends are already light enough

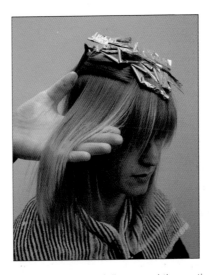

Step 5 Once the foils around the parting are in place, the ends can be coloured back in one easy step

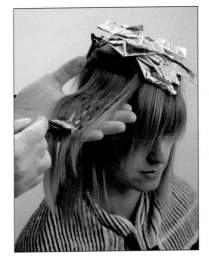

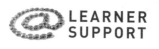

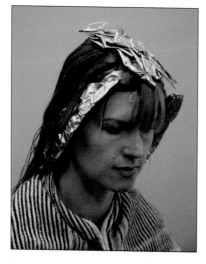

Step 6 When the colour has been applied to the lengths of the hair, a strip of foil can be placed so that it keeps the colour away from the skin while it develops

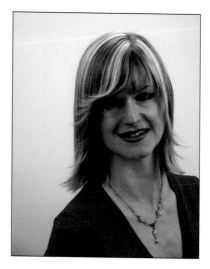

Step 7 The final effect

Colour correction (two-step process – pre-pigmentation and re-colouring)

This is a common problem with any length of hair. In this scenario the hair has been bleached and the client wants to return to her natural colour. However, the hair has too little yellow pigment present and the hair has to be pre-pigmented with red/gold pigment before natural depth can be achieved or the hair will go green! Although the client wishes to return to her natural depth, experience says that many clients find that type of dramatic change too much to handle. Here is a new, exciting alternative to re-colouring. Flat, single dark colours only look good if the hair has lots of shine. Unfortunately, shine doesn't last very long so the best course of action here would be to introduce a variety of tones into the hair. This way the hair 'comes alive' with texture, dimension and a head-turning excitement!

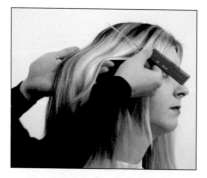

Step 1 Before

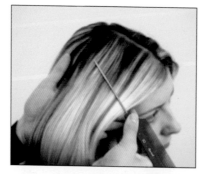

Step 2 The previously bleached hair is too light for single step processing; the lightened hair must be pre-pigmented first

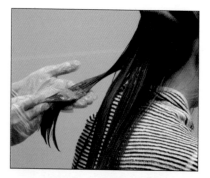

Step 3 Apply a red/gold (Majirel 7.43 + 3 per cent developer) to the dry hair first

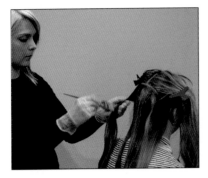

Step 4 Start at the lower nape and work up through the back of the head until all of the hair is coloured with the pre-pigmenter

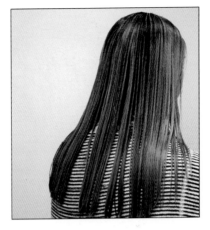

Step 5 Comb through to ensure the application is even

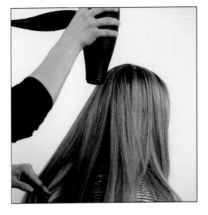

Step 6 After 30 minutes' development, shampoo away the colour and re-dry the hair ready for the next step of the process

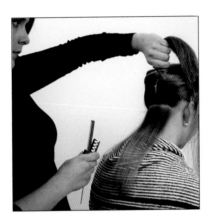

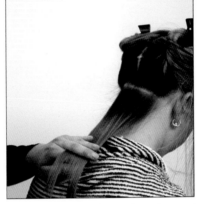

Step 7 A technique of naturalised highlighting is chosen as the preferred way of introducing depth and tone back into the hair. Section the hair ready for woven highlights

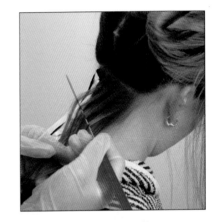

Step 8 Introduce the two different highlights to the hair

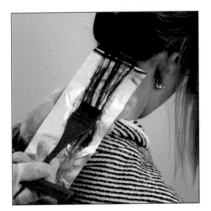

Step 9 Apply the colour to the foils

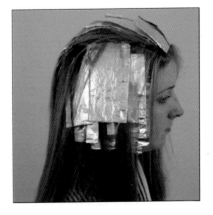

Step 10 With all the highlights in place, mix the interleave tone ready for application

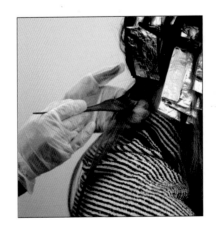

Step 11 Apply a mix Dark Brown Dia Colour and 3 per cent developer to all the hair between the foils

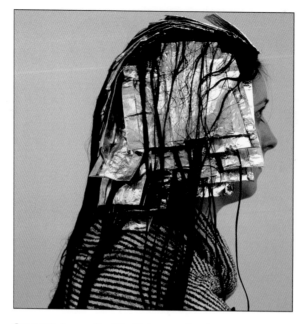

Step 12 Leave the Dia Colour to develop for maximum saturation, then carefully remove the colours at the basin and dry the hair into style

GH18.5 Provide aftercare advice

EKU *statement*

GH18 (eku65) How to give clear instructions to those with less technical knowledge and experience than yourself

GH18 (eku66) How to give effective advice and recommendations to clients

GH18 (eku67) How to maintain hair colour and condition

GH18 (eku68) Products for home use that will benefit the client and those to avoid and why

GH18 (eku69) How lifestyle can affect the colour correction result (e.g. active sports, career and job requirements)

GH18 (eku70) How the continual use of heated equipment can damage the hair

GH18 (eku71) The recommended time intervals between colouring and other services.

The corrective service doesn't end with the salon processing; the condition of the client's hair will be impaired and you need the client to help you maintain the colour's ability to last and the condition during routine daily handling.

'Diagnosing a course of action is one thing, but it should be followed by prescription too.'

You should tell them what sorts of products that they could use that would make their colour last and reduce the risk of fading. Also make a point of telling them what they should avoid, as some products will reduce the effects of your colouring causing it to fade prematurely or lose its intensity or vibrancy.

Explain the benefits of maintaining their hair in good condition: hair in good condition is easier to manage, it looks better and is noticeable to everyone else as well.

Lifestyle

Normal everyday wear and tear is a major reason for colouring problems and colouring problems often lead to colour correction. Lifestyle has the biggest impact upon hair condition and client expectation. Busy work schedules, social lives and the search for the sun all have a major impact.

For example: how many time have you recommended a shampoo/conditioner to a client, and the client to have gone away and used it, only to come back and say that it was great for a while, but then it didn't seem to have the same effect? So she went back to using her own particular favourite (probably because it smells nicer or is advertised by a celebrity icon).

The truth of the matter is that what you recommended actually did its job. The client has forgotten the original problem and now focuses on a new one – to her it seems that the product has stopped working because her needs have now changed. This constantly changing situation is difficult to master particularly when the client arrives in the salon and somehow seems to expect you, in the few minutes she is there, to guess what will happen to her hair if:

1 she goes on an exercise binge and swims at the local pool every day

2 spends two weeks in the Caribbean

3 spills paint on her hair during redecorations at home or

4 gets talked into trying a home colour because a friend found it to be a great winner!

Home- and aftercare checklist

✔	Talk through the colour effect as you work; tell them how they can maintain their hair by optimising both the look and the condition of their hair
✔	Explain how lifestyle factors can effect their hair colour and ways that they can combat these factors
✔	Show and recommend the products/equipment that you use so that the client gets the right things to enable them to get the same effects
✔	Tell the client how long the effect can be expected to last and when they need to return for re-colouring
✔	Warn them about the products that will have a detrimental effect on the colour by telling them what these products would do
✔	Warn the client about how incorrect handling or styling may reduce the length of time that the new effect will last

Remember

You need to make sure that you provide the correct advice so that your client can make the most out of her colour correction. Recommending the right products and ways in which they should style and manage their hair is essential to a long-lasting effect.

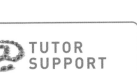

TUTOR SUPPORT

Short answer test

Checkerboard

I know how to prepare clients before undertaking any chemical service ☐	**I know how to prepare the equipment and materials before they are used upon the client** ☐	**I can carry out colour consultation and understand the colour correction process** ☐
I know and understand the science in respect to colouring and lightening ☐	**I always carry out tests prior to any new colour correction service** ☐	**I know and understand the health, safety and hygiene risks that clients are exposed to in chemical work** ☐
I know and understand the effects that colouring and lightening products have upon the hair ☐	**I know how to recognise simple colouring problems** ☐	**I know how to implement colour correction procedures** ☐
I know how to carry out a variety of full head and partial colour correction techniques on a variety of hair lengths ☐	**I always carry out working practices according to the salon's health and safety policy** ☐	

Additional items:

I know and understand the potential problems and risks of not testing hair before chemicals are introduced ☐

I know and understand the ways of diluting hydrogen peroxide to make other strengths ☐

Assessment of knowledge and understanding

Revision questions

Quick quiz: A selection of different types of questions to check your knowledge.

Q1   A _____ /test cutting is carried out before colour to assess what colour can be achieved.   Fill in the blank

Q2   A bleach lightener lasts longer than the effects of a high lift colour.   True or false

Q3   Which of the following are definite contra-indications to a colour correction service?   Multi selection

Sensitive skin	☐	1
Damaged hair	☐	2
Poor elasticity	☐	3
Bleached ends	☐	4
Banded hair colour	☐	5
Gradated colour	☐	6

Q4   Decolouring requires pre-pigmentation.   True or false

Q5   Which of the following tests is carried out during colour/lightening services?   Multi choice

Skin test	○	a
Incompatibility test	○	b
Porosity test	○	c
Development	○	d

Q6   Lighteners alter the pigmentation of hair within the cuticle.   True or false

Q7   Which of the following affect the development of colouring?   Multi selection

Heat	☐	1
Poor application	☐	2
Time	☐	3
Sectioning	☐	4
Combing	☐	5
Peroxide strength	☐	6

Q8   Yellow tones within hair are neutralised by adding _____ tones.   Fill in the blank

Q9   Which of the following could produce a green effect if not done correctly?   Multi choice

Lightening hair	○	a
Colouring back	○	b
Decolouring	○	c
Root retouch	○	d

Q10 Lightened hair that appears too gold can be neutralised by adding mauve.   True or false

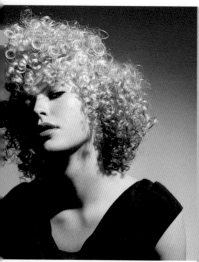

GH22

| GH22.1 |
| GH22.2 |
| GH22.3 |
| GH22.4 |

CREDIT VALUE
FOR UNIT GH22

8 Credits

More information About contra-indications, tests, consultation and customer care

See Unit G21 Provide hairdressing consultation services

Diversion Your responsibilities under COSHH regulations GH22 (eku6) and Electricity at Work GH22 (eku7)

See Unit G22 Monitor procedures to safely control work operations

Your responsibilities for customer records under Data Protection Act GH22 (eku5)

see Appendix 4

Chapter**thirteen**
Perming hair

Creative perming: quick overview

Unit title

GH22 Create a variety of permed effects

This is an **optional** unit for hairdressing and barbering at level 3, it is made up of four main outcomes

Main outcomes

GH22.1 Maintain effective and safe methods of working when perming hair

GH22.2 Prepare for perming

GH22.3 Create a variety of permed effects

GH22.4 Provide aftercare advice

What do I need to do for GH22.1?

- Make sure that the client is adequately covered, protected and prepared for the service
- Make sure that the working position is comfortable and safe for both you and the client
- Keep the work area clean and tidy and that waste materials are disposed of properly
- Work without causing risks to you or your client's health and safety
- Work efficiently and effectively
- Provide clear instructions to those assisting you
- Accurately maintain the client's treatment records

What do I need to do for GH22.2?

- Identify any contra-indications to perming the client's hair
- Carry out tests and record the outcomes
- Prepare the tools, products and equipment ready for use

What do I need to do for GH22.3?

- Use visual aids to explore different effects and looks for your client
- Apply products safely, accurately, efficiently and in line with manufacturers' instructions
- Use a variety of creative winding techniques to achieve the desired result
- Straighten hair by using large curlers or combing through
- Monitor and check the desired movement
- Ensure that the hair is neutralised correctly after development
- Identify and resolve problems as and when they occur
- Finish the effect so that it compliments the client's features and image
- Confirm the finished effect with the client

What do I need to do for GH22.4?

- Give accurate constructive aftercare advice on how the client can maintain their hair and perm

What aspects do I need to cover for GH22.1, GH22.2, GH22.3 and GH22.4?

- A variety of perming products and equipment
- A variety of contra-indications to perming services
- A range of factors that affect or influence perming
- A variety of hair tests
- Different types of creative winding techniques

What aspects do I need to know for GH22.1, GH22.2, GH22.3 and GH22.4?

- Your salon's requirements for preparation, timings and expected standards of service
- How to work safely, effectively and hygienically when perming hair
- The different factors that can affect or influence successful perming (and neutralising services carried out by others)
- The tests that need to be done prior to and during the perming services and the records that you must make
- The science of perming and neutralising and the effects of the different perming chemicals upon the hair
- A range of different perming and neutralising products; how they work and when they are used

Keywords

Pre- and post-perming treatments
These are special products that can even out the porosity before perming enabling the hair to take at the same rate and will return the hair back to a natural pH 5.5 after neutralising to maintain a good condition

Piggy back wind
A technique of winding curlers/rods into hair to create a multi-textured effect that has curls/movement of differing diameters

Spiral wind
A technique of winding longer hair from root to point, instead of point to root, which produces a curl diameter that is even throughout the length of the hair

Weave wind
A technique of winding rods into the hair so that part of the mesh taken leaves hair out providing a multi-textured effect that has some waved and some straight hair

Double wind
An extension of a weave wind where the hair left out of the rod is wound on another rod with a different diameter

Root perm
A technique for winding rods near the roots of the hair whilst leaving the remaining lengths out. The effect produces lift at the roots whilst maintaining the natural lie of the hair at the ends

A Straightener

An ammonium-based lotion similar to perms that can be used to remove wave in hair

Information covered in this chapter

- The preparations that you must make before carrying out any perming and straightening service

- The tools and equipment used during perming, straightening and neutralising, their maintenance and the preparations that you should make

- The factors that influence successful results in perming and neutralising services

- A range of perming techniques on different hair lengths

- The aftercare advice that you should give

- The effects of timing and temperature upon hair during processing

- How pH is restored after perming and why this is important

- The aftercare advice and recommendations that you should give to clients

Introduction

Perming and colouring are arguably the most complex aspects of contemporary hair-dressing. The combination of client's expectations, reality and ability to maintain their hair carefully and competently between salon visits is crucial. These factors have made perming a very problematic technical procedure. As we strive to obtain softer, kinder, longer-lasting results on longer-length hair, a division, based upon technical ability, experience and confidence, now exists between professional hairdressers and it is still growing. These stylists now fall into the following groups:

- those technicians who can
- hairdressers who can but won't and
- others who cannot.

Foreword

By now you will have experienced all sorts of clients and all the different hair types and textures too. One common thing though that will have had a huge impact on your day-to-day work is the client's hair condition and how that factor has either helped or hampered you in what you were trying to achieve.

Moisture is the key. If the hair retains its natural moisture levels after perming, the signs of healthy hair are obvious: shine, easy 'comb-ability' and great flexibility. Together these features indicate a style that is easily managed.

Lose these qualities and the hair will be dull, lifeless, tangled and difficult to manage. So after giving away the big secret, let's see how you get everything else right too.

Note

If you have recently completed your NVQ level 2 you will already be familiar with the underpinning principles and knowledge for perming, neutralising and straightening hair.

If you want to refresh your memory for this topic continue from this point onwards; alternatively, jump forwards to:

GH22 (eku 1) Maintain effective and safe methods of working when perming hair
GH22 (eku 2) Prepare for perming
GH22 (eku 3) Create a variety of permed effects
GH22 (eku 4) Provide aftercare advice

How perms work

EKU *statement*

GH22 (eku32) The effects of perming products and neutralisers on the molecular structure of the hair

Hair Science

The chemical changes that take place within the hair

'Perming' is the term given to the physical and chemical processing of hair, usually changing it into waves or curls. Unlike the movement and curl or smoothness produced by blow-drying or setting, the adding of movement to hair produced by perming is permanent: the hair does not return to its previous state when it is dampened. However, hair continues to grow and the new hair retains its natural shape. So, the waves and curls produced by perming gradually get further and further away from the scalp as the hair grows. To keep the same style the hair will, at some point, need to be permed again.

Because perming really does make a permanent change to the hair, you cannot easily correct mistakes (as you can with blow-styling, for example). The process also involves a variety of chemicals and chemical changes. It is therefore important that you make sure you understand what you are doing.

Diversion Before going ahead with this section, refer to 'the chemical properties of hair' in Chapter 1 Unit G21 Provide hairdressing consultation services (p. 16).

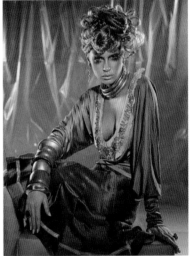

HAIR: RICHARD WARD

Changing the keratin

Of the cross-links between the polypeptide chains of hair keratin, the disulphide bonds or bridges give hair its shape. Each disulphide bridge is a chemical bond linking two sulphur atoms, between two polypeptide chains lying alongside each other. During perming (and straightening) some of these links or bridges are chemically broken, making the hair softer and more pliable, allowing it to be moved into a new position of wave or curl. Only 10–30 per cent (depending on lotion strength) of the disulphide bridges are broken during the action of perming. If too many are broken, the hair will be damaged beyond repair. You need to keep a check on the progress of the perm to ensure that:

- the desired curl shape or strength is achieved
- the chemical action is stopped at the right time.

You do this by rinsing away the perm lotion and neutralising the hair.

During neutralising, pairs of broken links are joined up again at different sites along the hair. The newly formed cross-links (disulphide links) hold the permed hair firmly into its new shape.

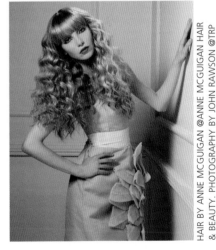

HAIR BY ANNE MCGUIGAN @ANNE MCGUIGAN HAIR & BEAUTY. PHOTOGRAPHY BY JOHN RAWSON @TRP

Changing the position of the bonds

The hair is first wound with tension on to some kind of former, such as a curler or rod. This is the *moulding* stage. Then you apply perm lotion to the hair, which makes it swell. The lotion flows under the cuticle and into the cortex. Here it reacts with the keratin, breaking some of the disulphide bonds between the polypeptide chains. This *softening* stage allows the tensioned hair to take up the shape of the former: you then rinse away the perm lotion and neutralise the hair. This fixing stage permanently rearranges the *disulphide bonds* into the new shape.

This process can also be described in chemical terms. The softening part that breaks some of the cross-links is a process of *reduction*. The disulphide bridges are split by the addition of hydrogen from the perm lotion. (The chemical in the perm lotion that supplies the hydrogen is called a 'reducing agent'.) The keratin is now stretched: it is in a beta-keratin state.

EKU *statement*

GH22 (eku39) The importance and effects of restoring the hair's pH balance after the perming process; see also pre- and post-perm treatments

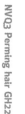
EKU *statement*

GH22 (eku1) Your salon's requirements for client preparation

GH22 (eku2) Your salon's expected service times for basic perming and neutralising

GH22 (eku8) Your salon's image and expected standards of service

GH22 (eku10) The range of protective clothing and products that should be available for clients

GH22 (eku11) The type of personal protective equipment that should be available and used by yourself

GH22 (eku12) Why it is important to use personal protective equipment

The final part of the process, the *fixing* stage, re-creates bonds at different positions between polypeptide chains. It occurs by an oxidation reaction. New disulphide bridges form and these rearranged links hold the hair in a different shape. The hydrogen reacts with the oxygen in the neutraliser, forming water. (The chemical in the neutraliser that supplies the oxygen is called an 'oxidising agent' or 'oxidiser'.) The keratin is now in a new, un-stretched form: it is alpha-keratin state again.

Acidity and alkalinity: the pH scale

The pH scale measures acidity or alkalinity. It ranges from pH 1 to pH 14. **Acids** have pH values from 1–6, whereas **alkalis** have values ranging from pH 8–14. Substances that are neither acid or alkaline, i.e. neutral, have a pH value of 7. The higher the pH number, the more alkaline is the substance; the lower the pH number, the more acid the substance.

The normal pH of the skin's surface is 5–6, referred to as the skin's acid mantle. This acidity is due in part to the sebum, the natural oil produced by the skin. The levels of pH can be measured using pH universal indicator and Litmus papers will indicate whether something is acid, alkaline or neutral.

If hairs are placed in alkaline solution they swell and the cuticle lifts. In slightly acid solutions the hair contracts and the cuticle is smooth. However, stronger acidic or alkaline solutions will impair the hair's structure, causing it to break down.

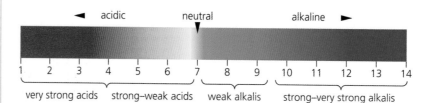

The pH scale

EKU *statement*

GH22 (eku13) How the position of your client and yourself can affect the desired outcome and reduce fatigue and the risk of injury

GH22 (eku14) Why it is important to position your tools and equipment for ease of use

GH22 (eku15) Why it is important to use personal protective equipment

GH22 (eku16) The safety considerations which must be taken into account when achieving the permed effects

GH22.1 Maintain effective and safe methods of working when perming hair

Protecting the client and yourself

Gowning the client

Perms are generally applied to hair – by the *post-damping* method (where the lotion is applied and easily absorbed into previously wound sections of hair) – and the solutions tend to be very watery and mobile. This, potentially, could be a hazard to the client unless you take adequate precautions. The majority of perm lotions are alkaline. If they drip or soak into textiles they will be held against the skin like a poultice. This is potentially very dangerous as it could cause irritation, swelling and even cause burns! This is also a problem if it does go onto the client's clothes as it may even discolour the fabrics to.

Make sure that you protect your client well so that this never happens. Put on a chemical-proof gown and secure into place, a clean, fresh towel around their shoulders. On top of this you should fix a plastic cape, ensuring that it is comfortable around the neck.

Barrier cream

After gowning, you can now apply the barrier cream to the hairline.

Remember

For clients – barrier cream provides a resistant layer to the skin, helping to prevent the action of chemicals upon their skin.
For you – wearing disposable vinyl gloves provides a barrier from chemicals having any contact with your skin.

Protecting yourself

Your salon must provide all the personal protective equipment (PPE) that you may need in routine daily practices. Perming involves the handling and application of chemicals, so this is one of those occasions where you must protect yourself from their harmful effects. Always read the manufacturer's instructions and follow the methods of practice that they specify. You are obliged to wear and use the PPE provided for you, these being disposable vinyl gloves, a waterproof apron and barrier cream.

The Control of Substances Hazardous to Health Regulations (COSHH) 2003 lay out the potential risks that hairdressing chemicals can have. You need to make yourself aware of the information provided by the manufacturers about their handling, storage and safe disposal. Generally, perm solutions should be stored in an upright position, in a cool, dry place away from strong sunlight. When they are used they should be applied in a well-ventilated area and if there is any waste (materials that cannot be saved and used another time) it should be disposed of by flushing down the basin with plenty of cold water.

Remember

Disposable gloves
Your salon will be providing disposable vinyl gloves for your personal safety when you are handling any chemicals in the workplace.
Make sure that others are using them too when they carry out any duties involving the handling of chemicals.

Working effectively

Experienced hairdressers work in a way that makes the most out of the time available: they optimise the way in which they work. You need to learn the ways in which you can optimise your time and effort so that your work is both productive and effective. There are a number of ways that you can make this happen:

Minimise waste Get into the habit of eliminating waste. All the resources that you use cost money and affect the businesses profitability, you can be more effective by maximising your time and efforts whilst minimising the cost of carrying out your work.

EKU statement

GH22 (eku17) Why it is important to keep your work area clean and tidy

GH22 (eku18) Methods of working safely and hygienically and which minimise the risk of cross-infection and cross-infestation

GH22 (eku19) The importance of using products economically

GH22 (eku20) The importance of personal hygiene

GH22 (eku21) How and why it is important to check electrical equipment used to aid the perming process

GH22 (eku22) Methods of cleaning, disinfecting and/or sterilisation used in salons

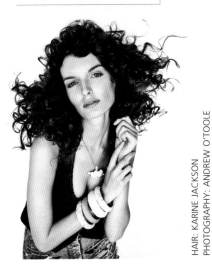

HAIR: KARINE JACKSON
PHOTOGRAPHY: ANDREW O'TOOLE

EKU statement

GH22 (eku6) Your own responsibilities under the current Control of Substances Hazardous to Health Regulations in relation to the use of perming products

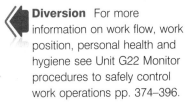

Diversion For more information on work flow, work position, personal health and hygiene see Unit G22 Monitor procedures to safely control work operations pp. 374–396.

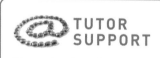 326

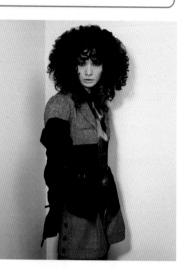 NVQ3 Perming hair GH22

HAIR BY: MELANIE TUDOR@ EN ROUTE HAIR AND BEAUTY, WAKEFIELD PHOTOGRAPHY BY: JOHN RAWSON@ TRP

EKU statement

GH22 (eku4) Your salon's and legal requirements for disposal of waste materials

TUTOR SUPPORT

Project 13.3: Risk assessment for perming services

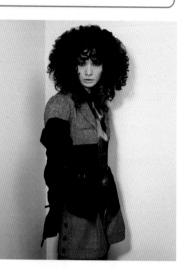

EKU statement

GH22 (eku9) What contact dermatitis is and how to avoid developing it whilst carrying out perming services; See Unit G22 p. 393

TUTOR SUPPORT

Discussion 13.1: Equipment needed to protect the client

Remember

Dermatitis is an occupational hazard for hairdressers; you reduce the risk by wearing disposable vinyl gloves when using chemicals, they provide you with a guaranteed barrier against the action of harsh chemicals upon the skin.

Remember

Remove and dispose of waste items as soon as possible; don't leave used cotton neck wool, plastic caps etc. around at the basins. Put them into a covered bin.
Wash, dry and replace perm curlers/equipment in the trays as soon as possible. Check perm rubbers for chemical damage and replace worn, split or broken ones.

Remember

Cold wave lotions
Making the most out of the salon's resources should be second nature. Don't throw away what's left in the perm bottle after application (provided it has not been dispensed into another applicator bottle). You can use the cold wave type perms another time.

Maximise your time Always make good use of your time. There are always things to do in a hairdressing salon and most of them relate to preparation.

- Prepare the salon by organising work areas so that it is ready to receive the clients.
- Prepare the materials, look out for stock shortages and record them.
- Prepare the equipment, organise the cleaning and washing of combs, rods flexible foam and rigid curlers.
- Prepare client records, and get things ready for when they arrive.
- Prepare the trolleys, get the right materials organised and ready.

Activity

This activity will help you to review the preparations that you should make before carrying out any perm service. Complete the table below and keep a copy in your portfolio for future reference.

Essential aspect	Why should you do this?
Wear PPE	
Prepare the work area	
Check the equipment	
Look for contra-indications	
Record test details	
Prepare the client	

Diversion For more information on dermatitis see Unit G22 pp. 485

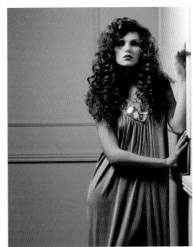

NVQ3 Perming hair GH22

HAIR BY: ANNE MCGUIGAN @ ANNE MCGUIGAN HAIR AND BEAUTY, LEIGHTON BUZZARD, PHOTOGRAPHY BY: JOHN RAWSON@TRP

Types of perm

For the client a perm is a major step – they will have to live with the result for several months. They may not be familiar with the range of perming solutions available so you will need to explain what the differences are and what is involved in each.

- Cold, permanent wave solutions, such as L'Oréal's Dulcia, or Synchrone, are mild alkaline perms. These types of perm are widely available and simplest to use with applications for all hair types and most conditions. These solutions tend to have a pH at around 9.5 so they are a fairly strong alkali that will swell the hair and affect around 20 per cent of the disulphide bridges. They reduce the natural moisture levels within the hair and are therefore better on normal to greasy hair types. They are particularly good for achieving strong, pronounced movement and curl and therefore create lasting effects that can withstand the high maintenance of regular blow-drying, setting etc.

- Acid wave solutions – such as Zotos's Acclaim – provide alternatives for perming when the hair is sensitised and needs to retain higher moisture levels or requires softer, gentler movement. They have lower pH values at around 6–7 and are therefore much gentler in the way that they work. They are suited to drier, more porous hair types too. Acid perms are two-part solutions and require the components to be mixed together just before application so that the perm is self-activated. Any residual lotion left over after application will not last and must be discarded.

- Exothermic perming systems – such as Zotos's Warm and Gentle – tend to be similar to acid waves in their chemical composition and therefore can have similar benefits. The only difference is that these perms need heat to be activated and will self-generate this when the two chemical parts (reagents) are added together, without the need for accelerators or hood dryers.

GH22.2 Prepare for perming

Remember

Contra-indications for perming
The following list indicates situations when perming should *not be undertaken:*

- When the hair is particularly porous (possibly over-bleached) having varying levels of porosity throughout the lengths (poorly coloured or lightened).
- When the scalp has abrasions or sensitive areas.
- When the hair is weakened, broken or damaged.
- When the hair is inelastic (does not have any ability to stretch and return to same length).
- When incompatible chemicals have been used on the hair (Just for Men, Grecian 2000, compound henna etc.).
- When there is any evidence of physical or chemical changes on the hair or scalp and the client is unable to provide you with a full, satisfactory account of what actions have been taken.
- Any evidence of scalp disease or disorder.

EKU *statement*

GH22 (eku41) The types and purpose of equipment used during the perm development process

GH22 (eku44) The manufacturers' instructions for the specific perming and neutralising products in your salon

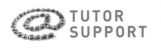

TUTOR SUPPORT

Project 13.1: Contra-indications indicating that a perm service should not be given

Remember

Most acid and all exothermic perms require the mixing of parts A and B together before the perms are applied to the curlers. This starts a chemical reaction, enabling the perm to work on the hair. Make sure that you protect yourself and your client by wearing disposable gloves and an apron and applying barrier cream and moistened cotton wool around the client's hairline, so that any drips do not cause any irritation or burning of the skin. It is advisable to check that the client is comfortable during processing and, if necessary, change the cotton wool again with more moistened cotton wool.

Note. If a perm requires parts A and B to be mixed together, you will have to dispose of any residual, unused lotion after the perm. It will not keep.

EKU *statement*

GH22 (eku23) The importance of questioning clients to establish any contra-indications to perming services

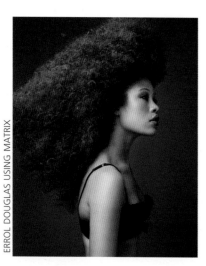

Activity

Consultation is an essential part of any hairdressing service and perming has its own particular aspects and considerations.

Complete the table below to identify how you would find out about the following information.

Keep a record of this information within your portfolio.

Contra-indications	How would you identify this?
Skin sensitivity	
Allergic reaction	
Skin disorder	
Incompatible products	
Damaged hair	

Consultation

Find out your client's requirements – what they expect from perming – and determine whether this is the best solution bearing in mind the added maintenance, care and attention needed to achieve the desired effect.

- Consider the style and cut, together with your client's age and lifestyle.
- Examine the hair and scalp closely. If there are signs of inflammation, disease or cut or grazed skin, do not carry out a perm. If there is excessive grease or a coating of chemicals or lacquer you will need to remove these by washing with a pre-perm shampoo first. Previously treated hair will need special consideration.
- Analyse the hair texture, condition and porosity.
- Carry out the necessary tests to select the correct perm lotion.
- Always read manufacturer's instructions carefully.
- Determine the types of curl needed to achieve the chosen style.
- If this is a regular client, refer to the records for details of previous work done on their hair.
- Advise your client of the time and costs involved. Summarise what has been decided, to be sure there aren't any misunderstandings.
- Minimise combing and brushing, to avoid scratching the scalp before the perm.
- Update the client's treatment records for future reference.

Match the perm to the needs of the hair

It is important to make sure you choose the most suitable perm lotion, the correct processing time and the right type of curl for the chosen style. Consider the following factors.

1 *Hair texture* – For hair of medium texture, use perm lotion of normal strength. Fine hair curls more easily and requires weaker lotion; coarser hair can often be more difficult to wave and may require a stronger lotion for resistant hair. (Although this is not true for oriental hair types.)

2 *Hair porosity* – The porosity of the hair determines how quickly the perm lotion is absorbed. Porous hair in poor condition is likely to process more quickly than would hair with a resistant, smooth cuticle. See the section on pre-perming treatments later in this chapter.

3 *Previous treatment history* – 'Virgin' hair – hair that has not previously been treated with chemicals – could be more resistant to perming than hair that has been treated. It would therefore require a stronger lotion and possibly a longer processing time.

4 *Length and density of hair* – Longer heavier hair requires a tighter curl than shorter hair because the hair's weight will cause it to stretch. Short, fine hair may become too tightly curled if given the normal processing time.

5 *Style* – Does the style you have chosen require firm curls or soft, loose waves? Do you simply wish to add body and bounce?

6 *Size of rod, curler or other former* – Larger rods produce larger curls or waves; smaller rods produce tighter curls. Longer hair generally requires larger rods. If you use very small rods in fine, easy-to-perm hair, the hair may frizz; if you use rods that are too large you may not add enough curl.

7 *Incompatibility* – Perm lotions and other chemicals used on the hair may react with chemicals that have already been used – for example, in home-use products. Hair that looks dull may have been treated with such chemicals. Ask your client what products are used at home, and test for incompatibility.

Remember

Clients that have been taking health supplements such as cod liver oil over long periods of time will notice that they affect the way that the perm takes in the hair. (When cod liver oil supplements are taken, increased levels of moisture are deposited into the hair which, ultimately, overloads the hair and results in limp curls.)

 Diversion To check, make a test curl before you start (see hair tests p. 331).

Remember

Always record the details of the consultation/service for future reference.

Remember

Some medical conditions affect the way that hair responds. For example, clients with thyroid problems may find that perms don't seem to take properly or last.

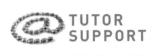 **TUTOR SUPPORT**

Discussion 13.2: Consultation for perm service

EKU statement

GH22 (eku45) How and why the factors in the range can affect your choice of perming products

What should you find out before you start?

First of all	Things to consider
Does the client know of any reasons that would affect your choice of service?	Ask the client about their hair to find out if there are any known reasons why the service cannot continue – are there any contra-indications?
What type of perm would be best to suit their needs?	Should you be using a cold wave, acid or exothermic?
How can the desired effect be best achieved?	What type of wind should you use, conventional, brick directional? What size curlers should you use, what curl or movement is required? How long does it need to develop?
How long will it last?	Is perming suitable for the hair type, condition and texture?
How much will it cost?	Is perming a cost-effective solution for the client?
How long will the process take?	Is there enough time to complete the effect? Has anything changed as a result of the consultation? Would this service now need to be rebooked or do you have the time to complete it still?

First of all	Things to consider
How will it affect the hair?	Will the long-term effects be what the client expects?
Is the hair suitable for perming?	Have you tested the hair and skin beforehand to see if there are any contra-indications or hair condition issues that will affect the result?

Now consider	
What are the client's expectations?	How will the perm enhance or support the style and the hair? What are the benefits for them?
What are the results of your tests?	Examine the hair: does it present any limitations for what you intend to do?
What is the hair condition like?	Are there any factors that will change the way in which perming will work on the hair?
	What previous information is available?
What do the client's records say?	Does this information influence the choice and perm process?
How will you show the effect to the client?	Have you got any illustrations of the finished effect?

What contra-indications are you looking for?

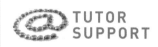

TUTOR SUPPORT

Discussion 13.3: Influencing factors affecting perm solutions and techniques

EKU *statement*

GH22 (eku26) The types and purposes of tests

GH22 (eku27) When and how tests should be carried out and the expected results

GH22 (eku28) How the results of tests can influence the perming service

GH22 (eku29) Potential consequences of failing to test

GH22 (eku30) The courses of action to take in the event of adverse reactions to tests (e.g. the type of reactions you need to report to another, more senior person)

GH22 (eku31) Why it is important to record test results

Contra-indications are	How could you find out?	How else would you know?
Skin sensitivity	By asking the client if they have ever had a reaction to hair or skin products in the past	Patch test/sensitivity test
Allergic reaction	By asking the client if they have ever had a reaction to hair or skin products in the past	Patch test/sensitivity test
Skin disorder	Ask the client if they know about any current skin disorders	Examine the scalp to see if there are any physical signs of skin abrasions, discolouration, swellings, infestation or infections
Incompatible products	If you see the results of any previous colour ask what type it was, how was it done?	Look for discoloration or unnatural colour effects on the hair. Test for incompatibles
Medical reasons	Ask the client if they know of any current medical reasons that they have that could affect a perming service	Examine the hair; look for signs of healthy active growth. If there are signs of weakened, damaged, broken or missing hair; ask for more information. Test for elasticity and porosity
Damaged hair	Ask the client if they are any current known reasons why the hair is in its current state/condition?	Examine the hair; look for signs of healthy active growth. If there are signs of weakened, damaged, broken or missing hair; ask for more information. Test for elasticity and porosity

Hair tests

Elasticity test This tests the tensile strength of the hair. Hair in good condition has the ability to stretch and return to its original length, whereas hair in poor or damaged condition will stretch and will not return to original length.

Porosity test The purpose of this test is to find out how well protected the inner cortex is by the cuticle layers. Porous hair has a damaged cuticle layer and readily absorbs moisture; this presents a problem when drying, as this hair takes longer to dry and often lacks an ability to hold a style well. This can be done by taking a small section of hair and sliding from the root, through to the points, between your fingertips. From this you can feel how rough or smooth it is. Rougher hair (as opposed to coarse hair) is likely to be more porous, and will therefore process more quickly.

Incompatibility test Professional hairdressing products are based upon organic chemistry formulations. These are incompatible with inorganic chemistry compositions and will cause damage to the client's hair. This test will identify whether metallic salts are present within the hair, a clear contra-indication that the perm may be carried out. Protect your hands by wearing disposable gloves. Place a small cutting of hair in a mixture of hydrogen peroxide and ammonium hydroxide. Watch for signs of bubbling, heating or discolouration: these indicate that the hair already contains incompatible chemicals. The hair should not be permed, nor should it be coloured or bleached. Perming treatment might discolour or break the hair, and might burn the skin.

Pre-perm test curl If you are unsure about how your client's hair will react under processing you could conduct a pre-perm test curl. Sometimes this can be done on the head and in other situations where there isn't sufficient time etc. you will need to cut your sample for testing. Wind, process and neutralise one or more small sections of hair. The results will be a guide to the optimum rod size, the processing time and the strength of lotion to be used. Remember, though, that the hair will not all be of the same porosity.

Development test curl This test is always carried out after the hair has been damped with perm solution and during the processing time. It will determine the stage of curl development so that the processing is not allowed to continue beyond the optimum. Unwind – and then rewind – rods during processing, to see how the curl is developing. If the salon is very hot or cold this will affect the progress of the perm: heat will accelerate it, cold will slow it down. When you have achieved the 'S' shape you want, stop the perm by rinsing and then neutralising the hair.

Record the results

Make sure that you record the details of any test that you conduct. Update the client's record card in full and immediately after you have done the test. Don't leave it until later, you might forget! These records are essential information that will be needed again and help to show that a competent service has been provided at that time.

This would be vitally important if there was a problem at some later stage, particularly if it involved any legal action taken against the salon.

Pre-perm and post-perm treatments

Matching the correct perm lotion to hair type is an essential part of the hair analysis. However, many perming solutions come in only a coloured, normal or resistant formula and this alone will not cater for all hair conditions. Dry, porous hair will absorb perming

EKU statement

GH22 (eku3) When and how to complete client records

GH22 (eku24) Why it is important to record client responses to questioning

GH22 (eku25) The legal significance of client questioning and the recording of clients' responses to questioning

GH22 (eku31) Why it is important to record test results

Remember

Record the results
After any treatment or tests have been carried out always update the client's records immediately. These tests and the findings are critical to the client's well being and the salon's good name. You should record the:

- date
- the test carried out
- development times
- results
- recommended home care or follow-up advice given.

Remember

Record the client's responses to your questions and the comments about how the results of any tests affected their hair and skin.

Remember

Temperature has a major impact on perming. This could be general salon temperature or by added heat from a hood dryer. In either case remember that processing times will be reduced considerably.

EKU *statement*

GH22 (eku36) The effect of pre-perm and post-perm treatments on the hair structure

EKU *statement*

GH22 (eku33) How hair that has been sensitised from previous treatments and heat damage reacts to the application of perming products

GH22 (eku34) When to use different types and strengths of perming products

GH22 (eku35) How the chemical composition of perming products varies and how this affects your choice for use on different hair types

GH22 (eku38) Why heat should not be used on sensitised hair

GH22 (eku49) How and why it is necessary to adapt your working methods and choice of perming products to suit sensitised hair

EKU *statement*

GH22 (eku42) The different types of perming products and how they are used to create curled and straightened effects

EKU *statement*

GH22 (eku45) How and why the factors listed in the range can affect your choice of perming products

GH22 (eku50) Methods of applying perming products when using the winding techniques in the range

solutions more readily; therefore special attention needs to be given in these situations. Pre-perming treatments are a way to combat these conditioning issues. Porous hair that is suitable for perming will have an uneven porosity throughout the lengths. Hair that is nearer the root will have a different porosity level to that at mid-length hair or that of the ends. Therefore the hair's porosity levels will need to be evened out, i.e. balanced before the perm lotion is applied. This enables the hair to absorb perm lotion at the same rate, evening out the development process and ensuring that the perm doesn't over-process in certain areas. A pre-perming treatment is applied before winding on damp hair and combed through to the ends. Any excess is removed and the hair is wound as normal.

After perming and neutralising it is also necessary to rebalance the hair's pH value back to that of 5.5. Post-perm treatments do this by removing any traces of residual oxygen from the neutralising process.

Sensitised hair

It is unlikely that you will find female clients without some sort of previous processing on their hair (although male clients with virgin hair are the norm). Women often have had previous services, such as highlights, lowlights and full and partial head colouring, and this creates its own particular problems.

Any previous chemical processing on the client's hair is going to be a critical factor in:

- deciding whether perming is suitable
- and if it is suitable; selecting products that will do the job satisfactorily without causing any further damage.

Previous processing is not necessarily a contra-indication, but it is a major issue for retaining or re-establishing a good condition. Dry hair loses one of the key indicators of hair in good condition and that is shine.

If you glance back at the chapter foreword you will see a reference to moisture and its essential aspects for keeping hair in good condition.

The hair's natural 'background' moisture is important for the following reasons:

- it provides shine and lustre on the hair
- it stops the hair looking dry or porous
- it helps to provide flexibility and therefore the hair's elasticity.

As you now see, moisture is directly linked with the key indicators of good condition and without it one or more of those features are diminished.

Sensitised hair lacks this natural moisture and is therefore more susceptible to over-processing during perming. During processing the curl/movement develops more quickly (as with any porous hair) and is generally a weaker/limper result than on unprocessed hair. This doesn't mean that it is resistant to perming; on the contrary it soaks up the lotion far more readily.

If during your consultation you find these signs on your client's hair; then make sure that you initially protect the hair with a pre-perm treatment to assist in evening out the porosity and then select a solution that is developed for the type of hair you are working with.

For example, if you are considering a perm on highlighted hair you must use a lotion that is developed for hair with varying degrees of porosity on the *same* head, such as an acid-balanced perm ZOTOS Acclaim. A general cold wave lotion will *fry* the hair and you will have a ball of frizz to contend with!

Likewise if you are perming coloured hair then, again, you need to match the requirements of the hair to the product you want to use.

Hair can become sensitised from the misuse of heated styling equipment too. Excess heat will raise the hair's cuticle and make it act in a similar way to that of chemically treated hair. It isn't a case of the lesser of two evils; both processes have a long-lasting and detrimental effect on the hair and should be handled and considered just the same.

Activity

Hair tests

Complete this activity by filling in the missing information in the spaces provided

Type of test	What is the purpose of the test?	How is the test carried out?
Elasticity		
Porosity		
Incompatibility		
Development test curl		
Pre-perm test curl		

EKU *statement*

GH22 (eku47) The different perming effects that can be created by the use of the sectioning and winding techniques in the range

Perming techniques: quick reference guide

Perm technique	Final effect	Ideal length	Lotion type	Equipment
Root	Lift and body at root area only	Layered hair or graduated hair 100–150 mm long	Acid or alkaline, often used as thick cream or paste	Conventional rods, often used with non-porous end papers
Directional	Lift and body with definite forced movement	Layered hair or graduated hair 100–150 mm long	Acid or alkaline	Conventional or oval rods
Weaving	Textured soft and stronger movement at ends	Layered hair or graduated hair over 75 mm long	Acid or alkaline	Conventional or oval rods
Piggyback (double wind)	Textured curl with varying curl diameters	Layered hair or graduated hair over 75 mm long	Acid or alkaline	Conventional rods
Stack wind	No root lift but strong end movement/curl	Graduated hair 150 mm down to 70 mm	Acid or alkaline	Conventional rods

Perm technique	Final effect	Ideal length	Lotion type	Equipment
Zigzag	Strong geometric, angular movement	One length or long layered hair 250 mm	Alkaline	Perming chopsticks/u-stick rods
Spiral	Vertical cascade curls with uniform diameter	Long layered hair or one length over 250 mm	Alkaline	Spiral rods or foam covered flexible wavers

GH22.3 Create a variety of permed effects

Perming is a straightforward procedure – the more organised you are, the simpler and more successful it will be. Once you have consulted your client and made the necessary tests, you are ready to start.

Checklist : The basics

✔	Prepare your materials, trolley, curlers lotions etc.
✔	Protect your client and clothes as necessary with a gown, towel and cape
✔	Refer to records and your consultation to identify any special requirement
✔	Shampoo the hair to remove product build up, grease etc.
✔	Towel-dry the hair (excess water would dilute the perm lotion, but if the hair is too dry the perm lotion won't spread thoroughly through the hair)
✔	If the client requires a pre-perm treatment, apply it now. Make sure you have read the instructions carefully
✔	If you are pre-damping (if the styling requirements dictate this) as opposed to post-damping apply your lotion evenly and carefully (see below)

Remember

Wear disposable non-latex gloves from the beginning. It is inconvenient to have to put them on later.

Activity
Perming techniques
Complete this activity by filling in the missing information.

What effects do these perming techniques achieve?

Technique	How is this technique done?	What effects does it achieve?
Spiral wind		
Double wind		
Weave wind		
Root perm		

Perming tools and equipment

- The pin-tail comb is useful for directing small pieces of hair onto the curler. The pin-tail comb is narrower than a plastic tail comb so you can guide the wound hair around the wound section to make sure that all the hair has an even tension.
- Fibre end papers or wraps are specially made for winding perms. Very few hairdressers would consider winding without them as they ensure control of the hair when it is wound. Fold them neatly over the hair points (never bundle them). The wrap overlaps the hair points and prevents fish-hooks. For smaller or shorter sections of hair, half an end wrap is sufficient – a full one would cause unevenness. Other types of tissue may absorb the perm lotion and interfere with processing, and these are best avoided.

Many kinds of curler are suitable for perm winding. Plastic, wood and PVC foam are amongst the commonest materials used. The manufacturer uses different colours to indicate size. The greater the diameter or the fatter the curler, the bigger the wave or curl produced. The smallest curlers are used for short nape hair or for producing tight curls. Most curlers are of smaller diameter at the centre: this enables the thinner, gathered hair points to fill the concave part evenly and neatly as the hair is wound, widening out to the shoulder of the curler as you wind closer to the head.

Basic sectioning

The first part of the process is to divide the hair into sections that will be easy to manage and wind. Done properly, sectioning makes the rest of the process simpler and quicker. If it's not done well though, you will have to resection the hair during the perm and this may spoil the overall result.

Cold perm sectioning

1 Following shampooing and towel-drying, comb the hair to remove any tangles.
2 Make sure you have the tools you will need, including a curler to check the section size.
3 Now divide the hair into six sections, as follows, using clips to secure the hair as you work:
   - divide the hair at or near the crown into a horizontal mesh, no wider than a perm rod, secure the top hair out of the way
   - divide the back hair into a vertical, yet parallel section down into the nape, secure in sectioning clip(s)
   - divide the front hair approximately above both mid-eyebrows to create a central parallel section meeting the first division at the crown; secure in sectioning clip(s)
   - divide the sides into two equally wide sections, one continuing down into the nape and the other terminating above the ears
   - divide the opposite side likewise to give two equal width sections.

Basic wind

The basic wind is a classic technique for producing an even amount of movement from points to roots all over the head. Although this technique is lacking in imagination the

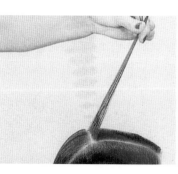

Winding: taking a hair section

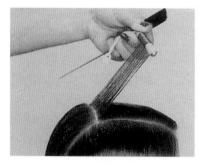

Winding the section onto the curler

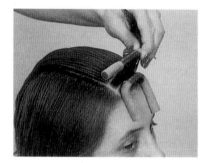

Winding: securing the curler

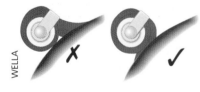

Winding: depth of section

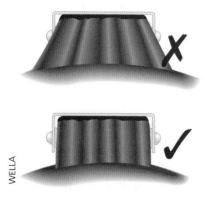

Winding: width of section

basic principles of winding with a firm and even tension (but without stretching the hair) underpins all the other alternative techniques (see also 'Alternative winding techniques' pp. 339–340.).

Basic method

1 Divide off a section of hair of a length and thickness to match the curler being used.

2 Comb the hair firmly, directly away from the head. Keep the hair together, so that it doesn't slip.

3 Place the hair points at the centre of the curler. Make sure the hair isn't bunched at one side and loose at the other, or twisted.

4 Hold the hair directly away from the head. If you let the hair slope downwards, the curler won't sit centrally on the base section: hair will overlap and the curler will rest on the skin.

5 Before winding, make sure the curler is at an angle suited to the part of the head against which it will rest when wound.

6 Hold the hair points with the finger and thumb of one hand. The thumb should be uppermost.

7 Direct the hair points round and under the curler. Turn your wrist to achieve this. The aim is to lock the points under the curler and against the main body of hair. If they don't lock, they may become buckled or fish-hooked. Don't turn the thumb too far round or the hair will be pushed away from the curler and won't lock the points.

8 After making the first turn of the curler, pass it to the other hand to make the next turn. The hands need to be in complete control: uncontrolled movement or rocking from side to side may cause the ends to slip, the hair to bunch, or the firmness to slacken.

9 After two or three turns the points will be securely locked. Wind the curler down to the head in a steady and even pressure, keeping the curler horizontal. (If it slips, wobbles or bunches the curl result will be uneven.)

10 At the end the curler should be in the centre of the section. If it isn't it will need to be rewound.

11 Secure the curler. Don't let the rubber band pinch or press the hair as it may cause damage or cause 'pull burns'.

Acid and alkaline perming solutions

The systems we currently use to perm hair rely on alkaline- or acid-based solutions. Their benefits and suitability for use are listed here.

Alkaline

- Effective on strong, coarse, resistant hair which is difficult to wave.
- Alkaline lotion, up to pH 9, is suitable for different hair textures.
- The lotion swells the hair, lifts the cuticle and penetrates to the cortex.
- Less winding tension is required.
- Suitable for all winding techniques.
- The test curl forms a stronger, sharper shape.
- The hair must be neutralised.

- The higher the pH and the stronger the lotions, the more potential there is for damage.
- No additional heat is required.

Acid

- Suitable for fine, delicate, porous and previously chemically processed hair.
- Shrinks hair and smoothes cuticle.
- Some require additional heat to be applied: climazone, rollerball, accelerator or infra-red dryer.
- Make sure that the reagents are activated by mixing the solutions correctly: check with the manufacturer's instructions.
- The test curl forms a softer, looser shape – a crisp, snappy test curl could result in overprocessing.
- Needs a longer processing time than alkaline perms.
- Pre-damp or post-damp – more often post-damp.

Processing and development

Perm lotion may be applied by:

- *Pre-damping method* – this is more useful when winding long hair and lotion penetration from the outside of the curler to the inner centre is more problematic when the rods/curl formers have been wound. (Follow the manufacturer's instructions.)
- *Post-damping method* – which is generally more convenient and you can wind the hair without wearing gloves and the time taken in winding doesn't affect the overall processing time.

Applying the perm lotion

Most modern perming systems come in individually packed perm lotions, ready for application. Others may need to be dispensed from a litre-size bottle to a bowl, before applying to the wound head using cotton wool, a sponge or a brush.

- Underlying hair is often more resistant to perming (e.g. at the nape of the neck), so you could apply lotion to those areas first.
- Keep lotion away from the scalp. Apply it to the hair section, about 12 mm from the roots.
- If post-damping, apply a small amount of the perm lotion to each rod; do not oversaturate as the lotion will flood onto the scalp and will drip on to the client, possibly causing either irritation or burning on the scalp or skin.
- It is better to apply the lotion again once the first application has started to absorb into the hair.
- Don't overload the applicator, and apply the lotion gently. You will be less likely then to splash your client.
- If you do splash the skin, quickly rinse the lotion away with water.

Processing time

Processing begins as soon as the perm lotion is in contact with the hair. The time needed for processing is critical. Processing time is affected by the hair texture and condition, the salon

Remember

Pull burns
This happens when perming curlers/rods are wound in and fastened too tightly; causing the follicle to be pulled open and perm solution collecting in the rim causing a burn.

Remember

Always read the instructions carefully before applying products.

EKU *statement*

GH22 (eku40) Why the accurate timing and thorough rinsing of products is necessary

Remember

Health and safety
Don't pack curlers with dry cotton wool. This absorbs the perm lotion; it also keeps it in direct contact with the skin, causing irritation.

Remember to use a barrier cream across the hairline. Don't let barrier cream get on the hair, however, as it will prevent the lotion from penetrating into the hair.

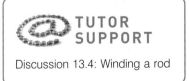

TUTOR SUPPORT

Discussion 13.4: Winding a rod

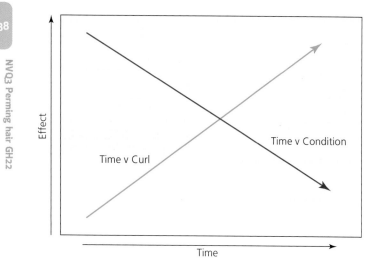

The effects of perm whilst processing

temperature and whether heat is applied, the size and number of curlers used and the type of winding used.

The perm needs to be checked during the development so that over-processing is avoided. The optimum processing ensures that the curl is maximised whilst there is no detrimental effect to the hair condition.

The table below shows two intersecting lines; both have a time element, but each one has a different resultant effect.

The green line is an increase in curl development over time, where the red line is a decrease in hair condition/damage over time. Ideally, where the two lines cross; it will denote the optimum perm processing. At this point a curl development check will show a good 'S' movement without loss of essential hair moisture and subsequent impaired condition.

Hair texture and condition Fine hair processes more quickly than coarse hair and dry hair than greasy hair. Hair that has been processed previously will perm faster than virgin hair.

Temperature A warm salon cuts down processing time; in a cold salon it will take longer. Even a draught will affect the time required. Usually the heat from the head itself is enough to activate perming systems. Wrap your client's head with plastic cap to keep in the heat. Don't wrap the hair in towels: these will absorb the lotion, slow down the processing or create an uneven, patchy result.

Some perm lotions require additional heat from computerised accelerators, roller balls or dryers. Don't apply heat unless the manufacturer's instructions tell you to – you might damage both the hair and the scalp. And don't apply heat unless the hair is wrapped; the heat could evaporate the lotion or speed up the processing too much.

Curlers Processing will be quicker with a lot of small sections on small curlers than with large sections on large curlers. (The large sections will also give looser results.)

Winding The type of winding used, and the tension applied, can also affect processing time. Hair wound firmly processes faster than hair wound slackly – in fact, if the winding is too slack it will not process at all. Hair wound too tightly may break close to the scalp. The optimum is a firm winding without tension.

Development test curl This involves testing the curl during processing. As processing time is so critical, you need to use a timer. You also need to check the perm at intervals to see how it's progressing. If you used the pre-damping technique, check the first and last curlers that you wound. If you applied the lotion after winding, check curlers from the front, sides, crown and nape.

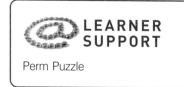

Perm Puzzle

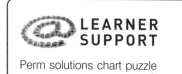

Perm solutions chart puzzle

Checking standard or round curlers, bendy curlers

- Unwind the hair from a curl former. Is the 'S' shape produced correct for the size of curler used?
- If the curl is too loose, rewind the hair and allow more processing time. (But if the test curl is too loose because the curler was too large, extra processing time will damage the hair and won't make the curl tighter.)

If the curl is correct, stop the processing by rinsing.

Checking other perming systems

If you have used another perming system, such as U sticks, where a bend is not so easy to see, you will need to use your judgement by slightly unravelling the former from the hair to assess the degree of movement achieved. With alternative systems more accents are put upon development timing rather than curl checks (This is also true for straightening processes where no curl is evident.)

Alternative/creative winding techniques

Basic sectioning and winding techniques create lateral waves and curl that are in the horizontal plane to the head: this is not the only curl placement option.

Spiral (vertical) curl movement

Selecting the size and position of the curls The spiral curl is dependent on the length of the client's hair. If the hair is less than 10 cm long it will be difficult, and perhaps impossible, to form spiral shapes of any size. Hair longer than 10 cm will permit reasonable spiral formations: longer hair will enable fuller, thicker and longer curls to be shaped.

The position that these spiral curls take and the overall effect they produce must be discussed with your clients: you must ensure that they understand what is being done. Because the handling and maintenance of this type of perm is quite different to traditional methods, it is important that they know how to maintain the effects before they leave the salon.

Spiral curls may be formed all over the head, length permitting, or they may be formed and positioned to make a cascade in the nape. Alternatively, bunches of spiral curls may be positioned asymmetrically. The degree of the spiral curl shape and the effect finally produced is for you and your client to determine jointly at the outset.

Starting the wind The spiral wind can be started at the root end of the hair or from the hair points. If you use a curl former that is of the same thickness overall, the curl you produce will be even throughout. If you use a former that tapers or is concave, the results will be uneven.

For the resultant curl to be even, springy and smooth, your winding must be firm without undue tension, wrapped cleanly over the former and secured without indenting or marking the wound hair.

If you apply uneven tension to your winding, the spiral formation will be inconsistent – the loops and turns will not follow on and there may be gaps in the shape.

Securing the wind When you secure the hair formers, be careful not to cut into the wound hair. Breakage could result if you did. Follow the recommendations of the makers of the curl former that you are using. You must also ensure that the formers are secured firmly: if they are loose, the hair may drop or unwind.

Monitoring the perm process Once you have completed your winding and secured the formers, you must monitor the perm process. If the perm lotion is applied to the hair before winding – a technique called pre-damping – the winding must be carried out without delay. Alternatively, the lotion can be applied after the winding is complete – post-damping. Perm processing is always timed from the moment the lotion is applied.

You will need to check the development of the perm process. You can achieve this by taking a test curl. By gently unwinding the hair part-way you can check the development

Remember

Health and safety
Take care not to splash your client's face while rinsing. Even dilute perm lotion can irritate the skin. If perm lotion enters the client's eye, flush out immediately with cold running water. Ensure the water drains downwards away from the face. Seek help from a qualified first aider.

EKU statement

GH22 (eku46) The sectioning and winding techniques in the range that are suitable for different types of hair

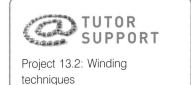

TUTOR SUPPORT

Project 13.2: Winding techniques

of the S shape. If the shape is loose then further development may be required. If the shape is well formed, begin neutralising straightaway: the perm is said to have 'taken'. As well as monitoring the timing carefully you must check the following:

- ensure your client's comfort
- keep excess lotion off the skin to avoid skin irritation
- remove damp cotton wool (used to protect the skin) when it has absorbed the lotion or scalp 'burns' will occur
- continually reassure the client so that she never feels she has been forgotten
- use a timer which makes an audible noise when the time has elapsed.

Typical problems

These are some typical problems when producing spiral curls:	
The root end is straight	You can avoid this by securing the former firmly at the root end of the hair. The helical loops of hair will be too loose if they are not firmly wound and in close contact with the former.
Hair flicks out	Ensure that the hair is not twisted when you form the spiral curl. After each turn, the hair should be repositioned. If you allow the hair to twist, an irregular spiral will be formed: this could cause the hair to stick out from the head. It is difficult to remedy this afterwards.
The spiral curl is too loose	Provided that the hair condition permits it, the hair may be reprocessed. You must take special care if you do this as the hair will be far more receptive to the perm lotion and could easily become over-processed.

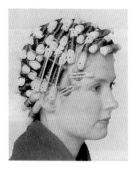

Directional winding

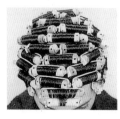

Staggered or brick winding

Perming hair of different lengths

Short lengths of hair (less than 10 cm) are not suitable for permanent spiral curls because it is impossible to form the helical shape on the curl former.

Medium hair lengths (10–15 cm) do allow spiral formations. These are likely to be short and narrow.

Longer lengths of hair (15 cm and longer) are the most suitable. Here there is sufficient hair to produce a variety of full, long, springy shapes. Greater lengths allow the hair to be placed onto the former more easily and a wider variety of curl formers may be used.

Direction and degree of movement

The direction of perm movement is determined by the angle that you wind and position the curlers or rods. If a forward direction of the fringe area is required, the wound curlers must be positioned accordingly.

The degree of perm movement is the 'tightness' or 'looseness' of the wave or curl. This is determined by:

- size of curlers, rods or formers used
- time for which the hair is processed
- amount of tension used
- hair texture and its condition
- perm lotion strength
- type of winding used.

Directional winding

The hair is wound in the direction in which it is to be finally worn. This technique is suitable for enhancing well-cut shapes. The hair can be wound in any direction required and the technique is ideal for shorter hairstyles.

Staggered winding or brick winding

The wound curlers are placed in a pattern resembling brickwork. By staggering the partings of the curlers, you avoid obvious gaps in the hair. It is suitable for short hairstyles.

Weave winding

The normal size section is divided into two and then the hair is woven. A large curler is used to wind the upper subsection and a smaller one is used for the lower subsection. This produces two different curl sizes, giving volume without tight curls. Alternatively, one sub-section is wound and the other left unwound. With short hair this produces spiky effects.

Double winding

This technique consists of winding a section of hair halfway down on a large curler, then placing a smaller curler underneath and winding both curlers down to the head. This produces a varied curl effect.

Piggyback winding

This is winding using a small and a large curler. The normal size section is wound from the middle onto a large curler, down to the head. The ends are then wound from the points onto a smaller curler, which is placed on top of the large curler. This produces softly waved roots and curly points. Alternatively this technique can be used to produce root movement only by not winding the point ends.

Stack winding

This is used where fullness of long hair is required, with little curl movement on top – it is ideal for bobbed hair lengths. The sections are wound close to the head in the lower parts; the upper sections are part wound only at the points. This allows the curlers to stack one upon another.

Other types of perm which give volume support

Root perms This type of perm creates movement at the lower root end of the hair. The hair is wound at the root ends only: the point ends are left out and not processed. This allows the hair to produce fullness and volume. Reperming must be kept strictly to the regrown root ends.

Body perms The root and middle hair lengths can be processed to give added body to the hair.

Roller perms, semi- or demi-perms These involve the application of a weaker form of perm lotion, which lasts for six to eight weeks. Reprocessing can take place through the hair lengths after this time has elapsed. These are not intended to be permanent, but to produce body fullness.

Other types of perming equipment

Foam rollers and formers

1 Take a small rectangular section of hair.
2 Secure the hair points in an end paper.

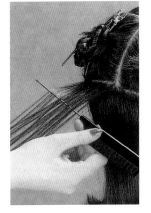

Weave winding

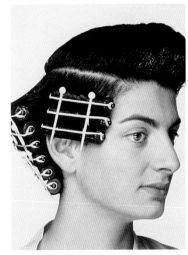

Stack winding

EKU *statement*

GH22 (eku48) The types of tools that can be used to achieve the perming effects in the range (e.g. chopsticks, spiral rods, U stick rods, foam rollers, formers)

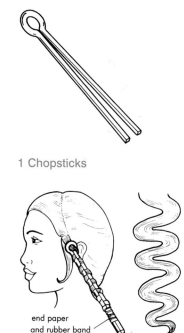

1 Chopsticks

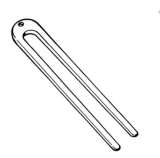

end paper
and rubber band

2 Position on the
head

3 The
expected curl

1 U-stick rods

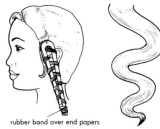

rubber band over end papers

2 Position on the
head

3 The
expected curl

3 Wind the hair around the foam roller.

4 Secure the roller in position by bending over the ends.

5 Repeat steps 1–4 to complete the entire head.

Chopsticks

1 Take a small square section of hair and protect it with one or more end papers.

2 Place the hair section through the loop and hold it securely.

3 Separate the chopstick legs and wind in a figure of eight.

4 Secure the end paper on to the chopsticks using a rubber band.

5 Repeat steps 1–4 to complete the entire head.

U-stick rods

1 Take a small square section and pull it through the middle of the u-stick.

2 Wind the hair in a figure-of-eight movement around the u-stick.

3 Protect the ends with one or more end papers.

4 Secure the end papers on the u-stick with a rubber band.

5 Repeat steps 1–4 to complete the whole head.

Straightening hair

Straightening or relaxing processes have always, in one form or another, been applied to hair because people with very tightly curled hair have wanted less curly or smoother looks. Most early relaxing processes were physically based and temporary in their effects, but today's chemical techniques can produce effective and permanent results.

Hair Science

Straightening hair
Two-step process
The chemistry of hair relaxing with a thioglycollate derivative is a two-step process, similar to permanent waving. The disulphide bridges in the cystine links between the keratin chains of the hair are reduced (broken) by the action of the ammonium thioglycollate in the relaxing cream/gel/lotion. This softens the hair, which can then be moulded into its new relaxed shape. This is followed by neutralisation, which is an oxidation process (a reaction with oxygen). Cysteine groups pair up again to form cystines, and the disulphide bridges reform in new positions. (See the section on neutralising in this chapter.)

Preparation

In addition to carrying out the normal preparation of your client (see the beginning of this chapter) and covering their hair, as well as ensuring you have all the tools/materials required, you should double-check the following for this service:

Preparation: Points to consider

✔	client's needs
✔	your client's hair type (curly or wavy) and hair texture (fine, medium or coarse)
✔	whether your client's hair is 'virgin' (chemically untreated) hair; if so, it may be more resistant to relaxing
✔	the condition of the hair if it has previously been chemically treated e.g. coloured
✔	the hair and scalp for signs of poor condition, sensitivity or disease
✔	contra-indications are present, then refer to your seniors so a decision can be made
✔	with your client, exactly what is to be done, about how long it will take and what it will cost
✔	that the client is comfortable and that they remain so throughout the service.

Test the hair

Always make tests on your client's hair to ensure that it is in a suitable state for relaxing, particularly when dryness, brittleness or breakage of the hair are evident. The following tests are recommended (see p. 331 on testing hair):

- a test cutting, to check the likely result of the intended process
- elasticity check, to determine the hair condition
- porosity check, to determine the rate of absorption
- testing a strand, to check on process development
- incompatibility test, to detect the presence of metallic compounds.

Factors affecting product choice and application

Product knowledge is essential. Whatever you decide to use, you must be familiar with it. You must study the manufacturer's instructions for use before your client arrives or before you attempt to apply the product. (This also applies to your tools and equipment.) You should only decide on the most suitable strength of chemical product after doing the following:

- The consultation with your client and making sure you know exactly what your client requires.
- Checking to determine whether your client is taking any prescribed medication, and if they have any allergies.
- Examining the hair and scalp condition.
- Finding out the results of the relevant tests.
- Checking with a salon senior or specialist (proceed only after agreement is reached).
- Ensuring products are in stock to avoid disappointing your client.
- Deciding whether the hair is fine, medium, coarse, thick, thin, porous or resistant (coarse hair requires the longest processing time and fine hair the shortest; grease or heavy chemical build-up on hair can block the relaxer product; hair that has been previously bleached, permed, straightened or relaxed can be very receptive and may process very fast).
- Noting any other helpful information.

Remember

Always remember to wear protective gloves when handling chemicals.

EKU statement

GH22 (eku53) How to check the degree of straightness achieved

Remember

Most of the methods of curling hair can be used to relax hair. 'Straightening' is the term given to describe curl and wave reduction. As with curling, straightening hair may be temporary or permanent.

You can begin the straightening process once you have considered the following factors:

- Whether the hair is in a suitable condition for processing (for instance, a rough cuticle could indicate uneven porosity; which would be likely to affect the result).
- The salon temperature – a hot salon could speed processing, a cold one could delay it.
- The hairstyle required after the hair has been straightened, taking into account your client's head and face shape and hair growth patterns. If the client's hair is to change from very curly to very straight, they may need guidance from you about managing it afterwards and about home maintenance products.

A straightening method

The following method uses ammonium thioglycolate i.e. perm lotion to straighten hair, *but this should not be used in place of the manufacturer's instructions*.

- Section the hair into four: centrally, from forehead to nape, and laterally, from ear to ear.
- Apply the basing product.
- Subdivide the nape sections into smaller ones.
- Apply the cream, gel or lotion, avoiding the skin. Do not go closer than 12 mm from the scalp.
- Comb the hair gently. Use a comb with widely spaced teeth. Some manufacturers advise you to wait till the hair has softened before combing.
- Do not continually comb the hair when it is soft. Treat it gently at this stage – it can easily break. Leave the hair as straight as the client requires.
- Processing time depends on the product and the hair. Softly curled hair relaxes quickly. Tighter, curled hair takes longer. It is safest to monitor continuously throughout the process. Do not exceed the manufacturer's recommended time for processing.
- When processing is complete, you may apply neutralisers. Neutralisers vary; some are based on hydrogen peroxide. Whichever product is used, it must thoroughly cover the area treated.
- After final rinsing and conditioning with moisturisers or other products, the hair may be styled.

Neutralising

Introduction

The successful outcome of a perm is dependant on the correct processing and the way the hair is rebalanced during the action of neutralising.

In this section we will look at:

- the principles of neutralising perms
- how neutralising works
- choosing a neutraliser
- neutralising techniques
- what to do after perming.

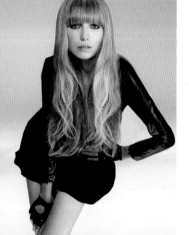

SHARON PEAKE @ ETHOS, MANCHESTER, PHOTOGRAPHY BY JOHN RAWSON @ TRP

EKU *statement*

GH22 (eku43) The different types and uses of neutralising agents

GH22 (eku51) Methods of applying neutraliser to suit the different winding techniques in the range

Rebalancing the hair

Neutralising is the process of fixing the curl or movement into the hair, whilst returning the hair back to a balanced chemical state. An industry term, 'neutralising' is a little misleading. In chemistry, a 'neutral' chemical condition is neither acidic nor alkaline (pH 7.0).

Conversely, during the hairdressing treatment of 'neutralising', the previously processed hair is returned to the skin's healthy, slightly acidic natural state of pH 4.5–5.5. Rebalancing the pH value of the hair is essential for maintaining hair in good condition, if the hair is not rebalanced the hair will be dry, porous and the perm will be very difficult to manage afterwards.

How neutralising works

As described earlier, perm lotion acts on the keratin in the hair. The strongest bonds between the polypeptides are the disulphide bridges. Perm lotion breaks some of these, allowing the keratin to take up a new shape. This is how new curls can form.

What neutralising does is to make new disulphide bridges. If you didn't neutralise the hair it would be weak and likely to break, and the new curls would soon fall out. Neutralising is an oxidation process – a process that uses oxidising agents such as hydrogen peroxide, sodium bromate and sodium perborate.

Choosing a neutraliser

Manufacturers of perm lotions usually produce matching neutralisers. These are designed to work together. Always use the neutraliser that matches the perm lotion you've used. As most perms are individually packed you will find a perm lotion and its matched neutraliser in the box.

Remember

Read labels and check contents of boxes before use.

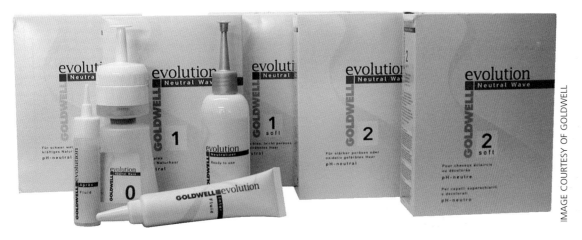

IMAGE COURTESY OF GOLDWELL

Neutraliser

A neutraliser may be supplied as an emulsion cream, a foam or a liquid. Always follow the manufacturer's instructions. Some can be applied directly from the container, others are applied with a sponge or a brush.

Neutralising technique

Neutralising follows directly on from perming. Imagine that you have shampooed, dried and wound the hair. The hair is now perming, and you are timing the perm carefully and making tests to check whether it is complete. You will also be reassuring the client that they have not been forgotten! As soon as the perm is finished, you need to be ready to stop the process immediately.

Preparation

1 Gather together the materials you will need.

2 Make sure there is a back basin free. (This makes it easier for you to keep chemicals away from the client's eyes.)

First rinsing

1 As soon as the perm is complete, move your client immediately to the back wash. Make sure they are comfortable.

2 Carefully remove the cap. The hair is in a soft and weak stage at this point, so don't put unnecessary tension on it. Leave the curlers in place.

3 Run the water. You need an even supply of warm water. The water must be neither hot nor cold as this will be uncomfortable for the client. Hot water will also irritate the scalp and could burn. Check the pressure and temperature against the back of your hand. Remember that your client's head may be sensitive after the perming process.

4 Rinse the hair thoroughly with the warm water. This may take about five minutes or longer if the hair is long. It is this rinsing that stops the perm process – until you rinse away the lotion, the hair will still be processing. Direct the water away from the eyes and the face. Make sure you rinse *all* the hair, including the nape curlers. If a curler slips out, gently wind the hair back onto it immediately.

Applying neutraliser

1 Make sure your client is in a comfortable sitting position.

2 Blot the hair thoroughly; using a towel (you may need more than one). It may help if you pack the curlers with cotton wool.

3 When no surplus water remains, apply the neutraliser. Follow the manufacturer's instructions. These may tell you to pour the neutraliser through the hair, or apply it with a brush or sponge, or use the spiked applicator bottle. Some foam neutralisers need to be pushed briskly into the hair. Make sure that neutraliser comes into contact with all of the hair on the curlers.

4 When all the hair has been covered, time the process according to the instructions. The usual time is five to ten minutes. You may wrap the hair in a towel or leave it open to the air – follow the manufacturer's instructions.

5 Gently and carefully remove the curlers. Don't pull or stretch the hair. It may still be soft, especially towards the ends, and you don't want to disturb the curl formation.

6 Apply the neutraliser to the hair again, covering all the hair. Arrange the hair so that the neutraliser does not run over the face. Leave for the time recommended, perhaps another five to ten minutes.

Second rinsing

1 Run the water, again checking temperature and pressure.

2 Rinse the hair thoroughly to remove the neutraliser.

Remember

When applying a conditioner apply to the palms of the hands first and gently work the conditioner through the hair. Do not massage the scalp or pull or comb the hair as it may soften the newly formed curl.

3 You can now treat the hair with an after-perm (anti-oxidant) or conditioner. Use the one recommended by the manufacturer of the perm and neutraliser, to be sure that the chemicals are compatible.

Perm aids or conditioner and balanced conditioners (anti-oxidants) help neutralise the effect of the chemical process by helping to restore the pH balance of the hair to pH 4.4–5.5 and smooth down the hair cuticle improving the hair's look, feel, comb-ability and handling.

Step-by-step: Neutralising

1 First rinse; rinse each curler to remove perming lotion.

2 Towel dry; blot dry each curler to remove excess moisture.

3 First application of neutraliser; carefully apply neutraliser to each curler – leave for 5 minutes.

4 Remove curlers; carefully unwind curlers and remove end papers.

5 Second application of neutraliser; apply more neutraliser to ends of hair and leave for 3–5 minutes before final rinsing with warm water.

At the end of the neutralising process, you will have returned the hair to a normal, stable state.

- The reduction and oxidation processes will have been completed.
- The hair will now be slightly weaker – fewer bonds will have formed than were broken by the perm.
- Record any hair or perm faults on the client's record card. Correct faults as appropriate.
- *Under-neutralising* – not leaving neutraliser on for long enough – results in a slack curls or waves.
- *Over-oxidising* – leaving the neutraliser on too long or using oxidants that are too strong – results in weak hair and poor curl

The hair should be ready for shaping, blow-drying or setting.

EKU statement

GH22 (eku54) Types and causes of problems that can occur during the perming and neutralising processes for the hair type on which you are working and how to rectify them

EKU statement

GH22 (eku55) Products for home use that will benefit the client and those to avoid and why

GH22 (eku56) How the continual use of heated equipment can affect permed hair

GH22 (eku57) Recommended time intervals between perming and other services

GH22 (eku58) How lifestyle factors can affect the hair (e.g. swimming, time necessary for hair maintenance)

GH22 (eku59) How perming can affect other services (e.g. the need for regular cutting, effect on colour services)

GH22 (eku60) How to maintain the permed effect achieved

GH22 (eku61) The need for the client to avoid tension on the hair

GH22 (eku62) How to give effective advice and recommendations to clients

GH22 (eku63) How to give clear instructions to those with less technical knowledge and experience than yourself

TUTOR SUPPORT

Short answer test 1

TUTOR SUPPORT

Short answer test 2

LEARNER SUPPORT

Perm test puzzle

TUTOR SUPPORT

Discussion 13.5: Perming faults

After the perm

Check the results of perming.

- Has the scalp been irritated by the perm lotion?
- Is the hair in good condition?
- Is the curl even?

Dry the hair into style.

- Depending on the effect you want, you may now use finger-drying, hood drying or blow-drying.
- Treat the hair gently as the hair may take a few washes to settle in. If you handle it too firmly the perm may relax again.

Advise the client on how to manage the perm at home.

- The hair should not be shampooed for a day or two.
- The manufacturer of the perm lotion may have supplied information to be passed to the client
- Discuss general hair care with your client.

Clean all tools thoroughly so that they are ready for the next client.

Complete the client's record card.

- Note details of the type of perm, the strength of the lotion, the processing time, the curler sizes and the winding technique.
- Record any problems you have had. This information will be useful if the hair is permed again.

Perming problems and solutions

	Possible cause	Immediate action	Future action
Hair/scalp damage Breakage	Too much tension or bands on curlers too tight. Hair over-processed – chemicals far too strong	Apply restructurant or deep-action conditioner to remainder of hair	Use less tension. Review choice of lotion, timing, etc.
Pull burn	Perm lotion allowed to enter follicle. Tension on hair excessive. Poor rinsing of surplus perm lotion	Apply soothing moisturiser to affected area. If condition serious, refer to doctor	Use less tension. Take smaller meshes
Sore hairline, skin irritation	Chemicals allowed to come into contact with skin. Poor scalp ventilation	Consult regarding allergies, then apply soothing moisturiser to affected area. If condition serious refer to doctor	Curlers to rest on hair not skin. Keep lotion away from scalp. Renew cotton wool after damping
Straight frizz	Lotion too strong for hair. Excessive winding tension. Hair over-processed	Cut ends to reduce frizz Apply restructurant or penetrating conditioner	Ensure appropriate lotion is used in future. Wind with less tension. Time carefully
Perm result/effect Too curly	Curlers too small. Lotion too strong	If hair condition allows, reduce curl amount by relaxing	Ensure appropriate curlers and lotion are used

	Possible cause	Immediate action	Future action
No result	Lotion too weak or not enough used. Curlers too large. Poor neutralising. Hair under-processed	If hair condition allows, reperm hair with suitable lotion*	Use appropriate lotion and rods. Process perm and neutraliser in line with manufacturer's instructions
Fish-hooks	Hair points not wrapped properly. No end papers	Remove ends by cutting	Check points of hair are wrapped correctly. Use end papers
Perm weakens	Poor neutralising. Hair stretched excessively while drying	If hair condition allows, reperm hair*	Check method and timing of neutraliser. Do not overstretch while drying hair
Good result when wet, poor when dry	Hair stretched while drying. Ineffective neutralising. Over-processed	If hair condition good, reperm.* Apply conditioning agents to moisturise hair	Check method and timing of neutraliser. Avoid stretching while drying
Uneven curl	Uneven winding technique. Uneven tension. Uneven lotion application. Ineffective neutralising	If hair condition allows, reperm affected areas*	Check wound curlers before applying perm lotion or neutraliser
Straight pieces	Lotion not applied evenly Rods too large	If hair condition allows, reperm affected area**	Ensure even lotion application

* Don't re-perm the hair unless its condition is suitable. For example, you should not re-perm if the hair is over-processed. Conditioning treatments and/or cutting may help. Discuss the problem with a senior or your trainer.

** Before attempting to correct this fault make sure that the hair is not over-processed. Dampen the hair to see how much perm there is.

GH22.4 Provide aftercare advice

Clients need your help to look after their hair at home. You must give them the right advice so that they can make the most of their new perm and style between visits.

You should tell them what sorts of products that they could use that would benefit the condition and manageability of their hair. You should also make a point of telling them what they should avoid, as some products will work against the new perm.

Explain the benefits of maintaining their hair in good condition: hair in good condition is easier to manage, it lasts longer, looks better and is noticeable to everyone else as well.

Home- and aftercare checklist

✔	Talk through the permed or straightened effect as you work; tell them how they can maintain their hair by recreating the look and maintaining the condition of their hair
✔	Explain how delicate the hair is after perming and how excessive stretching during styling will reduce the life of the perm
✔	Explain how lifestyle factors can effect their hair colour and ways that they can combat these factors
✔	Show and recommend the products/equipment that you use so that the client gets the right things to enable them to get the same effects

Remember

Remember to tell them how a new perm needs particular care in the way that it is handled and that stretching during styling will weaken the result and could even cause the perm to fail prematurely.

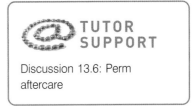

TUTOR SUPPORT

Discussion 13.6: Perm aftercare

Diversion For more information on advice and the recommendations that you should give to clients following a chemical service see Unit GH18, Provide aftercare advice section p. 316 and Unit GH17. Provide aftercare advice section p. 287.

✔	Tell the client how long the effect can be expected to last and when they need to return for re-perming or straightening
✔	Warn them about the products that will have a detrimental effect on their hair by telling them what these products would do
✔	Warn the client about how incorrect handling or heated styling may reduce the length of time that the new effect will last

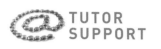

TUTOR SUPPORT

Discussion 13.7: Product recommendation to maintain curl and style

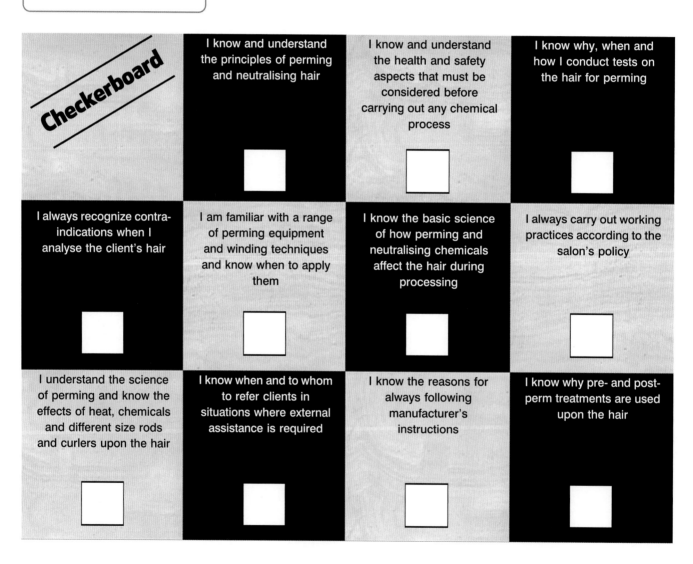

Checkerboard

I know and understand the principles of perming and neutralising hair ☐

I know and understand the health and safety aspects that must be considered before carrying out any chemical process ☐

I know why, when and how I conduct tests on the hair for perming ☐

I always recognize contra-indications when I analyse the client's hair ☐

I am familiar with a range of perming equipment and winding techniques and know when to apply them ☐

I know the basic science of how perming and neutralising chemicals affect the hair during processing ☐

I always carry out working practices according to the salon's policy ☐

I understand the science of perming and know the effects of heat, chemicals and different size rods and curlers upon the hair ☐

I know when and to whom to refer clients in situations where external assistance is required ☐

I know the reasons for always following manufacturer's instructions ☐

I know why pre- and post-perm treatments are used upon the hair ☐

seeing. For an example of how you and the client might see different things, see Unit G21, p36.

This is the fundamental part of consultation and probably the hardest thing to do.

However, in the promotional sense we are trying to create exactly those types of effect. We use all the aspects of; accessories, make-up and clothes to enhance the total look and it is always the total look that stimulates the audience.

Remember

Keep all the source material in your originating portfolio so that you can provide your team with a 'story board' of the elements that create your final designs.

Remember

Working with designs
In looking for material to add to your portfolio, you are more likely to find aspects or elements of images that you want to use within larger designs or images. It is unlikely that you will find complete, finished compositions of work to show the team and without these finished effects you can't expect a warm, enthusiastic response from clients.

Activity

Building a portfolio of ideas and themes
This section explores the aspects of design and looks at the possible sources for gaining and developing a working portfolio that you could use and continue to build upon when you are working with clients in the barber shop/salon.

Use the information covered within this chapter to create you own portfolio of work. How you choose to display this information depends upon your skill and artistic abilities. Whether you want to collect examples of work you find, or sketches from ideas, or pictures of your own work, it's all up to you.

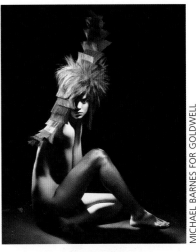

MICHAEL BARNES FOR GOLDWELL

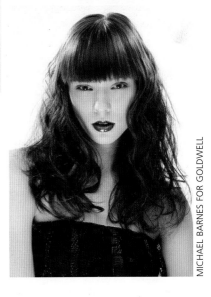

MICHAEL BARNES FOR GOLDWELL

Thinking about creative design

Creative style design is a process of logical analysis which sets out to achieve a 'personalised' overall appearance or image. This is rather like following a recipe. We use, mix, add and blend various essential ingredients, which together combine to take on a new form that is completely different from what we started with. If the recipe is followed carefully, the result can be guaranteed. If it is not, a disaster may occur.

A creative stylist can imagine the final effect and then work out the components needed to create that particular look. Working at this level of expertise is what separates the creative/artistic stylist, from the average 'all-rounder'.

Analysing the essential components

If you look at the style design components in isolation, as building blocks, you will be able to approach creativity for demonstration, competition or photography in a logical and systematic way.

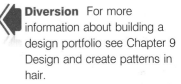

Diversion For more information about building a design portfolio see Chapter 9 Design and create patterns in hair.

EKU *statement*

GH21 (eku6) Basic principles of design, scale and proportion when creating an image

GH21 (eku7) How to identify and develop a theme as a basis for a hairdressing design image

GH21 (eku8) Ways of visually presenting your design image effectively to others

GH21 (eku9) Ways in which additional media can be used to complement the overall design image

GH21 (eku10) The importance of presenting your final results in a professional way

Design aspects:

- shape and form
- lines and angles
- textures
- movement and direction
- balance and imbalance
- less is more.

Other hair aspects:

- dimensions, distribution abundance
- colour depth and tone
- condition
- hair type
- work method
- specialised techniques
- moulding, forming and shaping
- products.

Design aspects

Shape and form

- Look at images: in life, in the media, from history, on the internet.
- Your design's underlying theme can be derived from almost anything.

In a design context The starting point or design basis is fundamental to the finished effect. It may sound obvious, but this is where most of the work in researching ideas is done. Spend a lot of time thinking about this as you don't want to lose sight of your theme later in the process, as this will de-rail your total concept.

In a hair context The overall effect is created by the structure of the underlying parts of the hair. This image is carefully composed of shape, form, direction and dimension. As a stylist, you must mentally interpret what you see. Often a picture will provide the initial idea for creating a theme. You must imagine a three-dimensional effect from a two-dimensional illustration. Getting this right, and relaying the information to others in a way that is easy to understand, is half the battle. This is an essential part of style composition and evaluation.

Before going any further with planning, see if you can create a mock up of your ideas on a practice block. If you need to use other materials such as plastics, wood, paper or card then this is the chance to see if the overall concept actually works.

Having analysed these overall aspects you can dissect the style further into its component parts.

Lines and angles

- How does the line, the direction in which the hair will be positioned, flow?
- Do you want to create straight, linear effects with sharp angles or softer flowing lines with curves?

In a design context Attention to detail is key to the success of any design plan. Look at the theme and see how you are going to get around the problems of lines, corners and angles. Regardless what you choose – stronger or softer looks – remember that this needs to be continued throughout the whole image.

In a hair context The perimeter of the hairstyle is formed by the outside line of the hair. The distance of this line from the scalp forms the depth of the shape. The lines and angles of the hair inside the perimeter affect the finished shape of the style. The hair

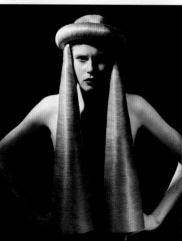

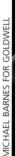

outline forms semicircles which may be seen from the front, sides and back. The lines within this may be vertical, horizontal or crossing diagonally. These features help to create the visual effect.

Textures

- How will you achieve the finished effects?
- How will this impact the style you create?

In a design context In design, the textures that you see and want to copy are often easily redrawn, or enhanced by computer graphics. However, in hair design work the effects are much harder to achieve as you are working in 3D.

For example, think about waves that you see in water or the folds created by silk; how do you create the same effect within hair?

In a hair context Hair can be styled and finished with a variety of techniques. Each has its own specific principles, allowing hair to be crafted and positioned in different ways. You can create a range of different effects by using any one or a combination of blow-drying, scrunch-drying, finger- or hand-drying, stretching or straightening, back-brushing, backcombing, teasing, wet or dry setting and tonging. These techniques can be used to lift, smooth, bend or flatten hair. Individually or collectively, they contribute to the inner and outer style structure and directions in which the hair moves.

Movement and direction

- What movement and direction will the final effect have?
- Are the final effects a flowing shape or disjointed random texture?

In a design context If you look at any good design there are certain rules that apply and if these rules are broken a less than satisfactory affect results. True, you can always push boundaries with non-conformist, rebellious effects. But you need to have clear objectives of what/who you are trying to achieve/impress.

An art critic will say that the purpose of art is to create a reaction of some sort.

So, if you are demonstrating to a live audience then the purpose is to gain clients, isn't it? Or do you just want to be talked about?

In competition work the effects are designed to cause reactions, so a lot more creative freedom is expected.

In a hair context The direction that the hairs take, individually and collectively, affects the overall style. The position and line of the hair gives direction to the style. The variation of this line produces direction within the style: the more varied the line direction, the more movement will be seen, showing as texture, wave or curl. A fluid or flowing line gives a softer effect, whereas broken lines of movement create a harder visual impact. The more breaks within the style continuity, the greater the contrasts and usually the more jarring the results too!

Balance and imbalance

- Does balance relate to symmetry?
- Does imbalance relate to asymmetry?
- If balance and symmetry convey harmony, do imbalance and asymmetry convey discord?

A design concept The vast majority of commercial work undertaken in salons today leads us, as hairdressers, to ensure that both sides of the haircut are of an even length,

Remember

In competitions the judges will look very closely for inaccurate flow. Crossed hairs, disconnected flow and poor execution usually amount to fewer points.

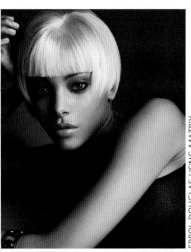

ERROL DOUGLAS USING MATRIX

that weight is proportionally distributed, that degrees of curl or straightness are maintained throughout the hairstyle. What we are required to do by the majority of clients is to produce a finished effect that may have originated from a picture; that is modified to suit the client and become the perfect example of symmetry. This may be a nice style, but does it still have the same impact as the original picture? Why not? (Well, we had to take the fringe shorter so the client could see out, or we needed to calm down the volume so that it would be suitable for work, etc.)

What is often happening with the best fashion images is that we automatically convert an impactive, dynamic, asymmetrical image into a recessive, passive, symmetrical style. If you have never considered this before, start analysing your favourite style images.

Going back to the questions: Does balance relate to symmetry? And does imbalance relate to asymmetry? The truth is that the best images, which are often asymmetrical in appearance, contain a visually excellent *artistic balance*.

The diagrams try to explain further this unlikely concept. In the first figure we have a 'seesaw' with equal masses on each of the opposing ends. As these masses are of equal weight we arrive at equilibrium, an apparent balance which is symmetrical and harmonised. In the second figure we have a seesaw which has a weight on one end and another heavier weight counterbalanced across the pivotal point. We now arrive at another form of equilibrium or balance that is asymmetrical and discordant. Looking at the two figures in turn, which one catches your eye more readily? This is the attention span afforded by your potential clients when looking through magazines and that brief opportunity that both PR and marketing have in which to sell an idea!

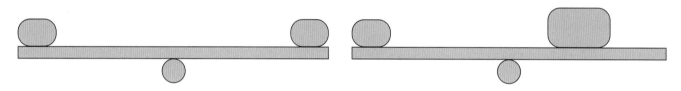

Aesthetic balance

Less is more: A design cliché

You may already have found that; the most impactive, designs involve less visual information. So why is that? The whole idea of marketing is to pass a message from the company to a potential buyer and in order for that message to be understood a smaller or reduced amount of information is conveyed, as there is less time for the message to be received.

This can be proven in a design context by corporate logos. These are usually reduced to a few colours, a particular type font and perhaps a simple graphic thrown in too.

For example, think of L'Oréal's logo – what could be simpler? Or Wella with the flowing hair logo? Some of the world's best-known names have the simplest of detail. Think about the Nike tick.

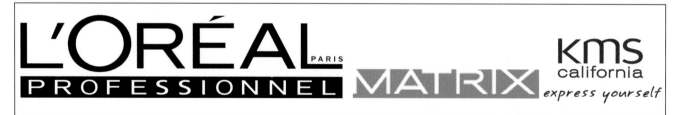

Sample logos

Minimalism is a fashion, it just happens to be having a long and successful run.

Activity
Brands and logos

Use the internet to search through hair product websites.
Find as many company logos that you can and a sample of say two or three product ranges that they manufacture.

Now for each one:

1 complete the product manufacturer's name

2 draw a colour sketch of their corporate logo

3 give examples of some of their product brands

4 provide your comments on what you think that either the logo or brands say as a message to the consumer.

Product manufacturer	Corporate logo	Brands	Comments about logo/brands

Please note

The following essential knowledge relates to technical skills found elsewhere in this book

GH21 (eku30) Current techniques for creatively styling, dressing and finishing hair

GH21 (eku31) The types of products, tools and equipment available for the techniques in the range and the effects they can create

GH21 (eku32) How added hair can be used to enhance and support a design image

GH21 (eku33) The design and styling limitations of different types of added hair

GH21 (eku34) The types of non-conventional items that may be used when styling hair and the effects they can create

GH21 (eku35) The manufacturers' instructions for the specific products, tools and equipment you intend to use

Other hair aspects

Dimension, distribution and abundance

- What are the style dimensions height, depth, etc.?
- What is the natural distribution of the hair?

The dimensions of a style are formed by the height at which the hair is positioned, the width of the bulk of the hair and the depth of the style. The length of the hair gives the visual effects of perimeter line and internal style structure.

NVQ3 Develop your creativity GH21

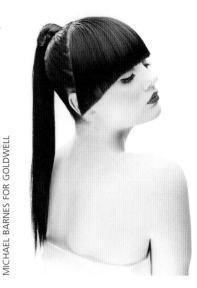

MICHAEL BARNES FOR GOLDWELL

The hair's natural abundance and distribution pattern are also important. Height can make round faces look longer; width can broaden a thin face; hair can be angled away from or towards extreme features to make them look bigger or smaller. However, it is essential to remember that there is a limit to what can be done.

The number of actively growing hairs on a client's head is a basic element in deciding on style and shape, as well as taking into consideration texture, length, hair type and patterns of growth.

If you have a particular model in mind, will they have enough hair to create the look that you want? Would you be better off using added hair or hair extensions?

Colour depth and tone

- How light or dark are the effects going to be?
- How light or dark can you take the hair that you will be working with?
- What tonal quality does the hair have?
- Can it be changed to another tonal range?

The colours, hues and tones that you visualise in your concept may not be actually achievable on real hair. Therefore will you be better off using synthetic, artificial hair or some other material? Would photography enhance the colours better in a studio lighting set-up? Will your colour combinations be able to be seen by your audience?

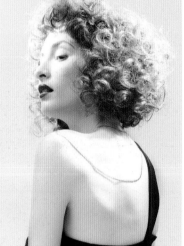

BEN WHITE AND THE ELEVEN HAIR ART TEAM

Condition

- What is the condition of the hair?
- Can it be improved?

The condition of the hair – its state of health – affects most of the other style components. It directly affects all aspects of style choice and also the durability and manageability of the hairstyle to be created. Avoid poor-conditioned hair in photography and any external events at all costs. Or at least try to improve the look of the model's hair by a course of reconditioning treatments.

Remember

Regardless of the quality of styling, poor condition will always show through. Avoid using models with unsuitable hair.

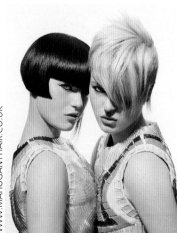

MAHOGANY HAIRDRESSING SALONS AND ACADEMY
WWW.MAHOGANYHAIR.CO.UK

Hair type

- What type of hair are you working with?

Imagine the limitations that some types of hair over others. For example, Oriental hair possesses certain properties and qualities that European hair does not.

Choose the right types of hair to portray your design concepts in their best possible ways.

Work method

- Plan the sequence of events which achieve the desired result.
- Always consider safety first.
- Follow manufacturer's instructions.

Methods of creating different style effects vary and there is usually more than one route to achieving the required effect. If you apply your chosen method systematically, it can be repeated if and when required again. The same goes for the team too; if you are planning a demonstration then you will need to inform others about what they should be doing and when they should be doing it too.

Specialised techniques

- Decide which effects you want to create before you start.
- Is there any special equipment needed to achieve the desired effect?

Hair moulding, shaping, finger waving, curling, plaiting, pleating, twisting and weaving can all be used to create special styling effects. Rollers, velcro rollers, flexible foam-covered rollers, spiral rollers, pins and clips are the tools of hair shaping. You must decide which effects are required before you apply these tools. These are the mechanical aids to hair styling and are additional to the chemical tools and techniques now available.

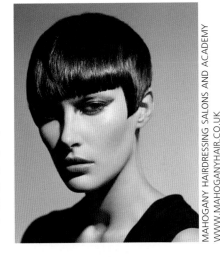

MAHOGANY HAIRDRESSING SALONS AND ACADEMY
WWW.MAHOGANYHAIR.CO.UK

Moulding, forming and shaping

- Shaping and forming – cutting and moulding.
- Hair symmetry/asymmetry should balance the final effect.

Some types of hair can now be styled in ways which were previously impossible. Unruly hair can now be tamed and difficult hair can achieve realistic shapes. To shape and form hair is to cut and mould – to create. This involves the distribution of portions of hair into fitting outlines and positions. Proportioning the hair means arranging and fitting it to the underlying head and face foundation. The outline shape or silhouette can be viewed from different directions and the balanced symmetry of the hair shape should generally be pleasing and harmonious.

Products

- Select the styling product to achieve the desired effect.
- Select the finishing product to achieve the desired effect.

Products play an immense roll in creating the effects that you want to portray. You need to work with and test the products that are going to be needed during the event. Never leave anything undetermined, your design plan must provide a product brief so that you can:

- build it into the overall budget
- get everyone else to achieve the same results for using the right products
- get your audience to see the benefits of using these products.

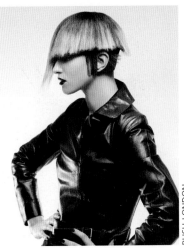

RUSH LONDON

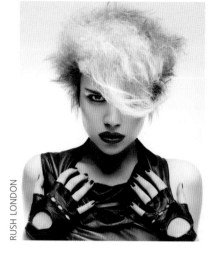

RUSH LONDON

Remember

Products will have a huge impact on the finished results. Use finishing products sparingly as you can always add to the effect, but you can't do anything about overloaded hair, you will have to start again (if there is time)!

Creating the plan and its components

For more information on the detailed planning aspects for external events:

- initial preparation
- working to a budget
- setting your objectives
- pitching your idea to management
- informing involved parties
- health and safety considerations.

Diversion See Chapter 17 Planning promotional activities – Unit H32 Contribute to the planning and implementation of promotional activities pp. 423–439.

Remember

Create a plan

Identify the objectives. What is the purpose of the demonstration? Is it, for example, staff training or salon promotion?

Prepare the resources. What resources do you need? How many people do you expect to attend?

GH21.2 Produce a range of creative images

Diversion For more information on external demonstration and health and safety considerations see Chapter 17 Contribute to the planning and implementation of promotional activities, Hairdressing demonstration p. 431.

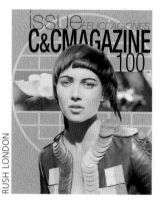

RUSH LONDON

Photography and photo sessions

Why do it?

The power of a good photograph is undeniable. It instantly says more about your work and the image you want to project than any free editorial or paid for advertising. However, while fun, photo sessions are not easy. They can be time consuming, expensive and sometimes disappointing if not properly coordinated. So how do you go about things? First, ask yourself why the salon would want to invest in an expensive photo session:

- To attract more clients into the salon through coverage in the consumer press?
- To raise your industry profile via the trade press?
- For salon advertising?

You can make a start by researching the magazines and newspapers in which you hope to have your salon's work published and check the sort of photographs they use. Individual titles will have a distinctive house style: the type of work published in *Hair* and *Elle* is very different from that in teenage magazines, and a world apart from local newspapers.

Remember

Art direction

Define your look. Questions to consider are:

- Will the look be classic, fashionable, avant garde or themed?
- Will the finished effect be the result of a process, say a colouring, cutting or other technique, or created by specific products?
- Will the look have more impact in black and white or colour?
- What clothes and accessories are best suited to the look?
- What image effect are you trying to create – natural, classic, dramatic or romantic?
- Should the photographer have free rein in the creative aspects of lighting, props, camera angles, backdrops and effects?

Putting it together

Once you've decided on the look you're going to go for, start to create your photographic team.

The model

Picking a suitable model can be a tricky task. A common mistake is to choose a pretty girl with unsuitable hair or vice versa; ideally she should have a combination of both. Remember that a conventionally pretty face isn't always photogenic, so study each model's photographic portfolio carefully:

- Look for regular features and bright, clear eyes. Avoid prominent chins and noses, over-full lips or dark circles under the eyes. The skin should be clear (even the most skilful of make-up artists won't be able to disguise completely obvious blemishes), and she should have a long, slim, unlined neck and a good profile to give the photographer maximum scope.
- Ensure the hair suits the type of work you plan to do.
- Tell your model what you have in mind, if you are planning a total change in hair length or colour let them know.
- Your model must also have the right features to fit your look – a sweet face is no good if you want an aggressive punk image.

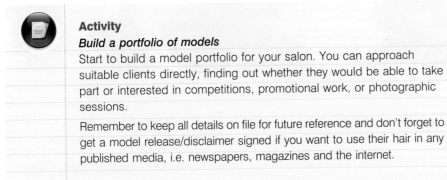

Activity

Build a portfolio of models

Start to build a model portfolio for your salon. You can approach suitable clients directly, finding out whether they would be able to take part or interested in competitions, promotional work, or photographic sessions.

Remember to keep all details on file for future reference and don't forget to get a model release/disclaimer signed if you want to use their hair in any published media, i.e. newspapers, magazines and the internet.

EKU *statement*

GH21 (eku1) The importance of effective communication

GH21 (eku2) The importance of confidentiality and what might happen if this is not maintained

GH21 (eku3) How and when to participate in discussions and move them forward

GH21 (eku4) How to make openings in conversations to encourage people to speak

GH21 (eku5) The importance of confirming your understanding of what has been said to you

EKU *statement*

GH21 (eku15) The potential hazards you must consider when working at any venue

GH21 (eku16) The steps that should be taken to minimise risks when working at any venue

GH21 (eku17) How and if local bye-laws and legislation may limit your use of tools and equipment

GH21 (eku18) Health and safety procedures applicable to any venue you use

GH21 (eku19) The safe and effective working methods for the techniques in the range

GH21 (eku20) The potential hazards that may be present as a result of using additional media in your design image and the precautions you should take to reduce risks to health and safety

EKU *statement*

GH21 (eku29) The common problems associated with photographic shoots, hair shows and competitions (e.g. staffing, tools and equipment breakdowns and time overruns, etc.) and how to resolve them

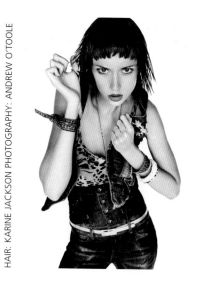

HAIR: KARINE JACKSON PHOTOGRAPHY: ANDREW O'TOOLE

The photographer

Always opt for someone who specialises in hair, beauty or fashion photography. See as many as you can, with portfolios, to check their ideas are in tune with yours. Confirm the booking in writing and brief him/her in detail on the image and 'feeling' you are aiming for.

Don't be afraid to shop around; get quotes for work. If you have set the budget for the photography, let the photographer know. If they are aware that the costings are capped they will work with you in achieving that aim.

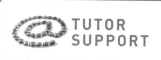

TUTOR SUPPORT

Project 14.1: Designing three different styles

The make-up artist

A good make-up artist is vital. Bad make-up will ruin a shot. If you can afford it, always use a professional, but don't ask for the impossible. A make-up artist, however good, can't completely change a model's face. Research and brief a make-up artist as you would a photographer.

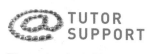

TUTOR SUPPORT

Discussion 14.1: Diverse images

Always ask your make-up artist how much time they will need and build this into your running schedule (see Chapter 17 Make a time schedule p. 432).

You can't rush them once they have started so why not test the effects well before the day?

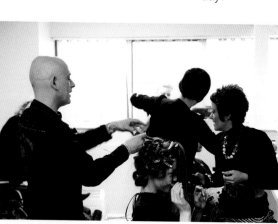

HAIR: NHF INSPIRE, PHOTOGRAPHY: SIMON POWELL

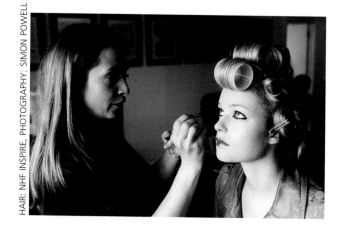

HAIR: NHF INSPIRE, PHOTOGRAPHY: SIMON POWELL

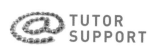

TUTOR SUPPORT

Project 14.2: Aspects of organising the event

Clothes and accessories

Decide on the time of year you hope to have the photographs published and bear in mind that most monthly magazines work three months ahead.

What type of clothes work best? Obviously this depends on the image you want to achieve and whether you are working with a professional stylist.

Where possible, use *trend forecasts* to give you forthcoming seasonal fashions, never wait until the clothes are in the shops (unless you are doing live demonstrations) as you don't want your shots to date too quickly. If you don't have access to agency samples or loaned stock, then go for neutral fashions that don't scream out a particular season. Necklines should be simple and jewellery effective, but don't overload – if in doubt, leave out.

Storyboard the plan

Think about the designs and put together a storyboard by cutting out images you like from magazines. Once you've decided on the styles, work out how you are going to achieve them. By creating a theme for your collection you'll have more chance of greater coverage.

Teamwork is the key to a successful photographic session, so let those involved know exactly what they will be doing.

Create your inclusion lists

Draw up a list of the equipment and products you'll need, and check them off when packing your session tool kit. The general rule is to take everything – and then add anything else that might come in handy.

On the day

Have a clear idea of the looks you want to create but have in mind several alternatives as back-up. Pay attention to detail and make sure you see a digital still of every style before the photographer starts.

Look closely at the results and pick up on faults not obvious to the naked eye; this isn't always easy. Faults to look out for include gaps in the style, stray or crossed hairs on clothes/face, rumpled clothes, pins showing or too much product/make-up.

Be decisive and don't settle for second best. If you're not completely happy with a shot, say so nicely. Always check through the camera; you'll be surprised how different something looks through the lens.

Backdrops and lighting

Keep backgrounds simple so as not to distract from the hair. Plain backdrops are the golden rule and should be slightly darker for blondes and lighter for darker hair so that the outline shape shows up more clearly.

Ideal backdrop colours:

- light blues for blonde hair and subtle harmonised effects
- white for dark hair and red hair for strong contrasting images that stand out
- reds for strong impactive contrasts on blonde or dark hair.

Make sure hair is well lit and the photographer isn't indulging in some fancy lighting effects that show off his artistry rather than yours. Regardless that photographers use

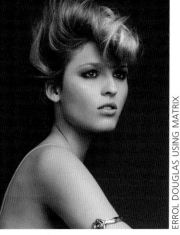

ERROL DOUGLAS USING MATRIX

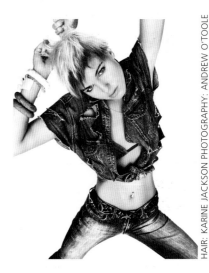

HAIR: KARINE JACKSON PHOTOGRAPHY: ANDREW O'TOOLE

Remember

Studio time is valuable and costly, do any major hair preparation work before the shoot.

studio flash to bring the most out of their photographs, they also use a background of studio lighting that is still very hot to work under. So try to do as little retouching in studio lighting as possible, since the model's make-up might start to run!

File format

Most professional photographers tend to work with digital photography rather than film as the benefits are plain to see:

- fast, instant results that can be viewed externally to a monitor
- easily transferable by memory stick on CD or DVD
- they can be sent with press releases, electronically, as attachments
- touch-ups and post-production editing are easier and far more cost-effective than a re-shoot!
- there are a variety of file formats for all sorts of published/printed options
- fast uploads to websites
- publishers and printers prefer to handle digital files rather than film as they incur fewer production costs

Magazine publishers and printers tend to accept digital files in the following formats:

- jPeg and   - tiff.

A *jPeg* file format is a compressed image format that all publishers seem happy to use and as a compressed format the images are optimised and made smaller. The reduction in file size makes the image more portable whilst maximising the information without losing too much quality.

A *tiff* file format is an uncompressed image, hence the images tend to be much larger and are unsuitable for email attachment. The quality is much better than jPeg, but very few publications reproduce images either large enough or well enough to make a difference anyway.

Remember

File formats
There are other file formats other than jPeg and tiff. Bitmap files are also popular as well as camera manufacturer file formats such as Nikon's RAW. A RAW file is an uncompressed digital file with similar quality to that of a tiff file.

For publication purposes the resolution of the files is far more important, so an image-editing program such as Adobe Photoshop or Adobe Fireworks is useful in resizing the image to the ideal output. Ideally an image should be a minimum of 300 dpi. That means that the digital image has a printed resolution of no smaller than 300 dots per inch.

The overall image dimensions are not so important, as the publishers will choose the size that they want to use. But with even mid-range professional cameras with optical resolutions of 6–12 million pixels, each digital image can range from 2.5 MB up to 12 MB, so a CD can hold hundreds of finished images.

If, however, the images are to be printed as posters for use in displays, then the higher the resolution the better. Hence a tiff is preferable by far as the source file as the image will be smoother as the overall poster is made larger.

Publishing to a website

If the images are to be used on a website, then the original images can be made much smaller, by optimisation, to enable fast download times. Typically, a digital image starting at 4.0 MB can be reduced to 40 KB a staggering 100 times smaller, for a very good, screen quality image.

Hairdressing competitions

Entering hairdressing competitions can be great fun and a great motivator for staff. It is however, very challenging and requires a lot of personal discipline, dedication and thorough practice in order to achieve the right look that will catch the eye of the adjudicators. Competitions vary enormously between local, regional and national and will also vary in the way that entrants partake.

For example, the *L'Oréal Colour Trophy* is a national competition. It is initially shortlisted at regional level by a photographic entry. Entry dossiers are sent out to participating salons early in the New Year. The closing date for finished dossiers is early March. After a preliminary judging, selected styling teams are invited to take part in the regional finals, where entrants have to demonstrate their work 'live' in front of a large audience and against the clock. Winners from each of the regions are then invited to take part in the grand final in a top London hotel in late spring.

Conversely, *NHF competitions* at regional levels allow all member salons and colleges to participate on the competition floor. Finalists from individual regions are then invited to take part at national level. The *British Hairdressing Awards* are again a national competition that is shortlisted by photographic entry. In this competition entrants take part in a variety of categories including Regional, Avant Garde, Artistic Team, London and British Hairdresser.

National competitions: UK Skills (www.ukskills.org.uk)

UK Skills, a not-for-profit organisation, manages the delivery of innovative, high-profile competitions and awards (Including hairdressing) which showcase excellence and demonstrate how exceptional performance improves individual and organisational success.

Established in 1990, UK Skills works to raise the profile of skills in the UK and oversee the UK's premier set of skills competitions, WorldSkills UK. UK Skills also manages the UK team entry to WorldSkills, the biggest skills competition in the world. Most recently UK Skills spearheaded the bid to bring WorldSkills to London in 2011. *WorldSkills London 2011* will be a truly global showcase for skills and young people from across the world.

UK Skills also manages the National Training Awards which celebrate exemplary training in the workplace; from coordinating the awards' famously robust judging processes to organising celebration events across the UK.

Remember

The Hairdressing and Beauty Industry Authority (Habia) have issued the following tips to help you get started before you step on to the competition floor.

- Watch the trade press for news about when and where competitions are taking place.
- Go along to competitions and watch what happens. See what type of work is successful in competitions and keep an eye on emerging trends and fashions.
- Ask trainers and tutors for advice. Also take advice from people who have entered or know about competitions.

TUTOR SUPPORT

Project 14.3: Hairdressing competition scene

Remember

Copyright
The photographer retains copyright to the finished works. Unless you have purchased that right from them, you are not able to use the material for any display purpose unless it has been cleared (preferably in writing) beforehand.

Remember

European and WorldSkills Competition (www.worldskillsuk.org)
WorldSkills UK is the UK's premier set of skills competitions for young people and adults. Their main aim is to help raise the standards of training and performance at work by strengthening the contribution of skills competitions to the UK economy.

WorldSkills UK is supported by government, participating countries and a host of other partners across business, industry and the world of education and training.

TUTOR SUPPORT

Project 14.4: Evaluating plans

- Read the rules carefully and know exactly what is required.
- Take time to find exactly the right model, one with the right type of hair, the right age and with looks that fit into the competition rules. A beautiful girl with good deportment helps considerably, but if her hairline is not up to scratch she may put you out of the competition.
- Understand that competition work is very different from salon work. Colouring in particular can often be a lot stronger on a competition floor than the salon floor.
- Regular competitors stress the importance of preparation.
- Check and prepare your equipment.
- Take time to find the right model, particularly if you are trying to express a specific image or theme.
- Product knowledge and application is imperative. Never attempt to style a model's hair without testing the product's effects on her hair beforehand.
- Practise, practise and practise.

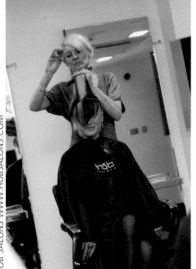

HOB SALONS WWW.HOBSALONS.COM

Many hairdressing organisations, colleges and major manufacturers run or sponsor competitions. If this is something that you would like your salon to be involved in, encourage your salon to run an in-house competition first. This is a good way of 'acclimatising' your staff to the pressures of competing.

Live competition (on the day)

You have prepared your model and you have practiced the look for hours. Now the day of the competition has arrived. Stage fright has struck. Keep calm, there is nothing to worry about. Everyone, including the 'great names', suffers from nerves at this time – not just the stylists but the models too.

The style you do must conform to the competition rules: for example, if a day style is required, don't go over the top with elaborate hair up or hair ornaments. If it's free style, a wider choice is allowed. Once you and your fellow competitors have finished your models, you'll be asked to leave the floor so the judges can take over.

They proceed to choose the most competently designed and dressed head of hair. Depending on the type of competition, the judges will award points covering all aspects of style ranging from technical detail, shape, movement, use of colour and artistic adaptation.

The British Hairdressing Awards

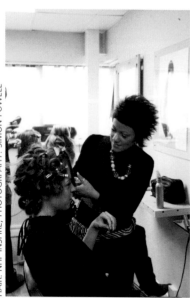

HAIR: NHF INSPIRE, PHOTOGRPAHY: SIMON POWELL

The British Hairdressing Awards were created in 1985 and have become hairdressing's most prestigious and high-profile competition. Almost every top salon in the nation enters these awards. For the winners it can be the highlight of – or indeed the launch pad for – a long and glittering career. In fact the awards have been the making of many of our top stylists, as well as raising the standard of hairdressing photographic work overall in this country. Since 1990 the British Hairdressing Awards have been owned and presented by *Hairdressers Journal* (previously the event belonged to its sister publication *Hair And Beauty* magazine). Schwarzkopf UK, however, has been the exclusive sponsor since the awards' inception.

How do they work? There are 16 awards categories: eight regional categories; six specialist categories (Newcomer and Artistic Team of the Year, plus Men's, Afro, Avant-Garde and Session Hairdresser of the Year); the more recent British Film Hairdresser of the Year; and the ultimate award, British Hairdresser of the Year. Entrants are judged primarily on photographic work – they are required to supply four prints for an initial judging session, then another four if they make it through to the finals – and on a resumé of the past year's show and seminar work they have conducted, plus trade and consumer press coverage they have obtained.

You can enter any category you like (so long as you meet the relevant requirements), except the British Film, Session and British categories. The winner of British Film is determined by experts within that particular field. Finalists in Session and British are nominated by a panel of trade and consumer hair and beauty experts. Session stylists are judged on their professional portfolio. British finalists are judged on their portfolio of eight photographic prints and, separately, on a resumé of their contribution to raising the profile of the British hairdressing industry over the past 12 months. On occasions, it has been the latter that has decided the overall winner.

There are two judging stages. First-round entries are judged by members of the British Hairdressing Awards Hall of Fame – hairdressers who have won an Award three times, plus honorary members, including Vidal Sassoon and Robert Lobetta. They have the invariably difficult task of whittling down each category to six finalists, examining each portfolio for technical expertise and commercial flair.

The second round judging takes place when finalists have submitted their additional four prints, and when nominees in the Session and British categories have submitted their portfolios and resumés. At this stage, the jury consists of around 30 prominent hair and beauty expert editors of consumer and trade magazines; for example, dignitaries from hairdressing associations and leading salon owners who have not participated in the awards themselves. Their scores determine the overall winner in each category.

Finally, bringing months of nail-biting tension to an end, the results are announced at the British Hairdressing Awards presentation ceremony at the end of November in a top West End hotel. This is the time when the hairdressing industry turns out in its most sumptuous and glittering force – national press and TV cameras now cover the event as a matter of course. For some of the finalists the evening will inevitably end in disappointment. For 16 others, however, it will mark the beginning of a year of celebration and widespread recognition.

How can I win? Ultimately, there is no recipe for guaranteed awards success – who can predict what will catch the eye of the judges? However, experience shows that following certain photographic guidelines could possibly increase your chances of winning.

- *Be professional* with your portfolio – use a professional photographer, make-up artist and, above all, professional models is a must. Gone are the days when you could get away with taking snapshots of your best clients with your salon reception as a location. (Admittedly, some salons still do – but they never make the finals.) The more successful awards entrants have long since wised up to the fact that an initial investment in people who will reflect their own hairdressing work to best effect usually reaps dividends later on down the line. 'It would never occur to me not to use a professional model,' says Trevor Sorbie, 'even though they can cost me an arm and a leg.' Has the principle paid off? Well, Trevor has won British Hairdresser of the Year no less than four times so far.

- *Work to a theme* There is a theory (and recent results would seem to bear it out) that a portfolio of pictures shot specifically for the awards stands a better chance of success than a random collection of prints culled from various shoots throughout the year. Certainly, judges seem to respond better to a set of pictures where there is an overall theme – all hair up, for example, or all black-and-white shots – as they tend to be easier on the eye and 'work' as a collection. Also, it shows you've really thought about your entry and how best to show off your talent.

LEARNER SUPPORT

Creative skills wordsearch

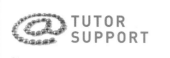

● *Don't go overboard* With the exception of the Avant-Garde category, it's a pretty safe bet that the judges will be looking not only for technical excellence but also commercial relevance. In other words, fantasy hairstyles will not win you marks. Instead, try to have your pictures reflect current hair trends, or at least display images that your clients could actually respond to. That means wearable styles, great colour, beautiful perms and good all-round suitability to current tastes and fashions.

GH21.3 Evaluate your results against the design plan objectives

EKU *statement*

GH21 (eku11) The purpose of evaluation activities

GH21 (eku12) The areas on which you should collect feedback

GH21 (eku13) Methods of gaining feedback from others

GH21 (eku14) The potential commercial benefits that can arise from creative hair design work

The important aspects of evaluation have been covered comprehensively elsewhere in this book. To review this content see H32.3 Participate in the evaluation of promotional activities in Chapter 17.

This covers the following information:

● evaluating the response

● collecting, collating and evaluating the response

● presenting an evaluation response

● other relevant information.

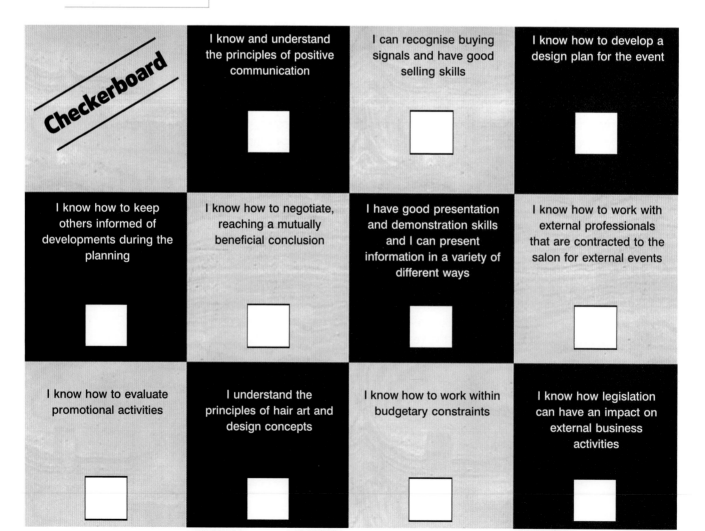

Checkerboard

I know and understand the principles of positive communication ☐	I can recognise buying signals and have good selling skills ☐	I know how to develop a design plan for the event ☐
I know how to keep others informed of developments during the planning ☐	I know how to negotiate, reaching a mutually beneficial conclusion ☐	I have good presentation and demonstration skills and I can present information in a variety of different ways ☐	I know how to work with external professionals that are contracted to the salon for external events ☐
I know how to evaluate promotional activities ☐	I understand the principles of hair art and design concepts ☐	I know how to work within budgetary constraints ☐	I know how legislation can have an impact on external business activities ☐

Assessment of knowledge and understanding

Revision questions

Quick quiz: a selection of different types of questions to check your knowledge.

Q1   An image is compressed by the process of _____.   Fill in the blank

Q2   Evaluation is an important part of any planning process.   True or false

Q3   Which of the following are *not* aspects of style design?   Multi selection

Shape	☐ 1
Form	☐ 2
Growth	☐ 3
Lines	☐ 4
Angles	☐ 5
Lifestyle	☐ 6

Q4   A jPeg is an uncompressed digital file format.   True or false

Q5   What is the smallest image resolution suitable for magazine reproduction?   Multi selection

100dpi	○ a
200dpi	○ b
300dpi	○ c
400dpi	○ d

Q6   You can publish images of models without their permission   True or false

Q7   What file formats will produce an image suitable for the printing a large display poster (1.2m × 1.8m)?   Multi selection

jPeg	☐ 1
RAW	☐ 2
Gif	☐ 3
Tiff	☐ 4
mPeg	☐ 5
Mov	☐ 6

Q8   The _____ run competitions at regional levels for salons and college students.   Fill in the blank

Q9   What colour backdrop would be best for a model with a very short, spiky dark hairstyle?   Multi choice

Black	○ a
Grey	○ b
Brown	○ c
White	○ d

Q10 Avant garde is a mode of classic fashion.   True or false

Part**three**
Supporting management

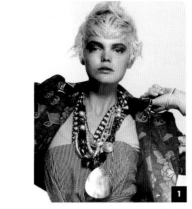

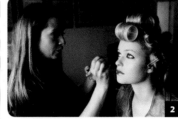

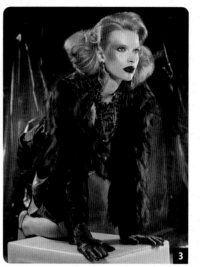

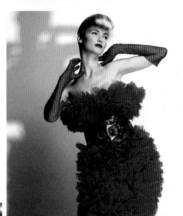

1 Hair by: Lewis Moore @ Francesco Group, Streetly Photography by: John Rawson @ trp **2** Hair: NHF Inspire, Photography: Simon Powell **3** Hair: Richard Ward, Photography: Daniele Cipriani **4** Hair by: Christopher Appleton @ George's Hair Salon, Leicester Photography by: John Rawson@trp **5** Hair by: Tim Lawton @ TPL Hairdressing, Nantwich Photography by: John Rawson @ trp **6** Hair by: The Artistic Team @ TPL Hairdressing Photography by: John Rawson @ trp **Left** Hair: NHF Inspire, photography: Simon Powell

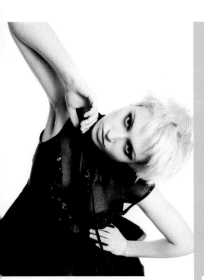

FELLOWSHIP FOR BRITISH
HAIRDRESSING
F.A.M.E. TEAM 2008

G22

G22.1

G22.2

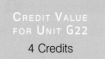

CREDIT VALUE
FOR UNIT G22

4 Credits

 More information Other
related information on:

- first aid and
- fire safety/prevention

can be found in
Appendix 2 of this book.

Health and safety: quick overview

Unit title

G22 Monitor procedures to safely control work operations

This is a **mandatory** unit for hairdressing and barbering at level 3, it is made up of two main outcomes

Main outcomes

G22.1 Check that health and safety instructions are followed

G22.2 Make sure that risks are controlled safely and effectively

What do I need to do for G22.1?

- Keep up to date with health and safety legislation
- Keep staff informed of health and safety developments
- Confirm that health and safety training for staff is up to date
- Respond promptly to breaches in safe working practices

What do I need to do for G22.2?

- Keep up-to-date accurate records of any identified or reported risks
- Report hazards to the appropriate people
- Confirm that adequate precautions have been taken
- Check that other people are aware of risks and that they know what action they should be taking within their responsibilities
- Monitor the workplace systems and controls set in place to control health and safety risks

What aspects do I need to cover for G22.1 and G22.2?

- The health and safety aspects of the working environment that cover; salon areas, storage and dispensing areas, staff and private areas, lavatories and washrooms

What things do I need to know for G22.1 and G22.2?

- The difference between a hazard and a risk

- Your expected, duties, legal responsibilities and personal standards in respect of maintaining a healthy and safe working environment

- Who are the responsible people to whom you report health and safety issues

- Why you should promptly deal with reported risks within the workplace

- Safe working practices and your salon health and safety policy and procedures

- Effective ways of monitoring others health and safety within the work environment

- The sources for reliable health and safety information

Introduction

Your role in health and safety within the salon at level 3 requires that you actively take part in the day-to-day monitoring of health and safety for everyone within the salon environment. Your responsibilities extend beyond the duty of care that you must show whilst you work, you now have the responsibility for:

- keeping abreast of health and safety developments

- making sure that the health and safety training needs of less experienced staff is identified and communicated to management

- that health and safety records are kept up to date and made available for those that need to have access to them.

This chapter follows looks at the current health and safety legislation and how you will be applying yourself in the workplace with particular reference to this information.

The process of monitoring workplace health and safety is a responsibility of all senior staff in a salon, not just that of the manager or proprietor. This responsibility extends beyond the salon's staff to all people entering the business e.g. clients, suppliers, contract cleaners, etc.

As a level 2 hairdresser/barber you had a duty of care to your employer for taking responsibility for your own actions in the ways that you worked. Now, as a level 3 student, you must now broaden your role in monitoring the workplace health and safety for everyone.

Keywords

Hazard
A hazard is something with a potential to cause harm

Risk
A risk is the likelihood of the harm occurring

Control
The ways in which risks identified are eliminated or reduced to an acceptable level

Monitoring
Somebody responsible for checking incorrect practices

Risk assessment
Is a careful examination of what could cause harm to people in the workplace

Information covered in this chapter

- Your responsibilities for health and safety within the working environment

- Safe, healthy and hygienic practices

- Controlling risks in the workplace

- Health and safety regulations

EKU statement

G22 (eku8) Why you should promptly deal with or report hazards and risks in the workplace

Although Unit G22 is focused upon your monitoring of the health and safety arrangements in your working environment, by definition, it assumes that you are up to date with the latest health and safety legislation and regulations.

Therefore as a supplement to those aspects, this chapter provides a summary of the main regulations affecting your place of work.

However, the duplication is intended as an *aide memoire* or refresher and provides you with a brief overview of the main considerations that affect you and the others that you are responsible for.

Activity

For this activity you will create a resource list for health and safety information for your own future use.

When completed the table below should cover a broad range of areas affected by health and safety regulation. You need to find out the missing information and then keep this reference table within your portfolio for future use.

The first one is completed for you.

Area of H and S	Applicable regulations	Website address	Associated leaflets	Other sources of information
Handling chemicals	COSHH	www.coshh-essentials.org.uk	*Control of substances hazardous to health. The Control of Substances Hazardous to Health Regulations 2002 (as amended).* HSE Books 2005 ISBN 0 7176 2981 3	HSE's InfoLine (tel: 0845 345 0055)

G22.1 Check that health and safety instructions are followed

What health and safety law requires

The basis of British health and safety law is the Health and Safety at Work Act 1974. This Act sets out the general duties which employers have towards employees and members of the public, and employees have to themselves and to each other.

These duties are qualified in the Act by the principle of 'so far as is reasonably practicable'. In other words, an employer does not have to take measures to avoid or reduce the risk if they are technically impossible or if the time, trouble or cost of the measures would be grossly disproportionate to the risk.

What the law requires here is what good management and common sense would lead employers to do anyway: that is, to look at what the risks are and take sensible measures to tackle them.

Your role is to assist your employer in fulfilling these duties.

The Management of Health and Safety at Work Regulations 1999 (the Management Regulations) generally make more explicit what employers are required to do to manage health and safety under the Health and Safety at Work Act. Like the Act, they apply to every work activity.

The main requirement on employers is to carry out a risk assessment. Employers with five or more employees need to record the significant findings of the risk assessment and this could be part of your role.

Risk assessment should be straightforward in a work environment such as a typical salon or barber's shop. (See undertaking risk assessment p. 381.)

Besides carrying out a risk assessment, employers also need to:

- make arrangements for implementing the health and safety measures identified as necessary by the risk assessment
- appoint competent people (this could be you) to help them to implement the arrangements
- set up emergency procedures
- provide clear information and training to employees
- work together with other employers sharing the same workplace.

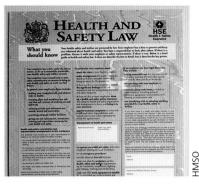
HMSO

Remember

Regulations
Regulations are law, approved by Parliament.

How regulations apply

Some regulations apply across all work locations, such as the Manual Handling Regulations, which apply wherever things are moved by hand or bodily force, and The Display Screen Equipment Regulations, which apply wherever VDUs are used.

Besides the Health and Safety at Work Act itself, the following apply across the full range of workplaces:

1 Management of Health and Safety at Work Regulations 1999: require employers to carry out risk assessments, make arrangements to implement necessary measures, appoint competent people and arrange for appropriate information and training.

2 Workplace (Health, Safety and Welfare) Regulations 1992: cover a wide range of basic health, safety and welfare issues such as ventilation, heating, lighting, workstations, seating and welfare facilities.

3 Health and Safety (Display Screen Equipment) Regulations 1992: set out requirements for work with visual display units (VDUs/computers).

4 Personal Protective Equipment at Work Regulations 1992: require employers to provide appropriate protective clothing and equipment for their employees.

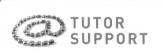
TUTOR SUPPORT

Project 15.1: How regulations determine what is carried out in the salon

5 Provision and Use of Work Equipment Regulations 1998: require that equipment provided for use at work, including machinery, is safe.

6 Manual Handling Operations Regulations 1992: cover the moving of objects by hand or bodily force.

7 Health and Safety (First Aid) Regulations 1981: cover requirements for first aid.

8 The Health and Safety Information for Employees Regulations 1989: require employers to display a poster telling employees what they need to know about health and safety.

9 Reporting of Injuries, Diseases and Dangerous Occurrences Regulations 1995 (RIDDOR): require employers to notify certain occupational injuries, diseases and dangerous events.

10 Noise at Work Regulations 1989: require employers to take action to protect employees from hearing damage.

11 Electricity at Work Regulations 1989: require people in control of electrical systems to ensure they are safe to use and maintained in a safe condition.

12 Control of Substances Hazardous to Health Regulations 2002 (COSHH): require employers to assess the risks from hazardous substances and take appropriate precautions.

Employees' responsibilities

The word responsible is used many times and in many ways at work. It may be something that you already used to and it may be something that you welcome. However, as we all have a role to play at work, the role of self-responsibility; shouldering the *weight* of our actions and the impact that it has on others really comes in to play. You play an important part in spotting potential hazards and preventing accidents and therefore helping your salon and colleagues to avoid any emergency situations arising.

In addition to your general employee responsibilities, with your experience, you also have the duty to help monitor the health and safety of others that you work with.

So what specifically will you be doing?

Communication is the first and most vital aspect of your role. You may be responsible for making the team aware of the health and safety aspects:

- by the information displayed around the work place, e.g. posters, leaflets, employer liability insurance, etc.
- by telling staff things that your employer wishes them to know, e.g. new developments, courses or health and safety training
- by seeing potential situations and telling others when unsafe working practices occur, e.g. clients or staff not wearing the provided PPE
- by seeing hazards and taking prompt action yourself, e.g. sweeping up clippings on the salon floor, removing equipment with loose plugs or unraveling coiled leads, clearing up spilt chemicals quickly and safely.

Record keeping

You may be required to complete and maintain records for:

- risk assessments made in the workplace by you or your employer, e.g. COSHH assessments, manual handling, contact dermatitis
- accidents that have occurred and the actions that were taken, e.g. maintaining the accident book
- periodic tests of equipment made by relevant, competent people, e.g. PAT tests, general equipment checks.

Health and safety training;

- identifying when team members have particular health and safety training needs and reporting that back to management, e.g. COSHH, manual handling, fire safety, emergency evacuation, PPE
- updating your own health and safety knowledge by using appropriate sources for information, e.g. www.hse.gov.uk, www.coshh-essentials.co.uk.

EKU statement

G22 (eku16) Reliable sources of health and safety information

Employer's responsibilities

The following list of regulations provides a summary of the main responsibilities that the employer has.

Management of Health and Safety at Work Regulations 1999

The main regulation requires the employer to appoint competent personnel to conduct risk assessments for the health and safety of all staff employed or otherwise and other visitors to the business premises. Staff must be adequately trained to take appropriate action, eliminate or minimise any risks. Other regulations cover the necessity to set up procedures for emergency situations, reviewing the risk assessment processes. In salons where five or more people are employed, there is the added obligation to set up a system for recording the findings of risk assessment, this could be written or on computer.

The main requirements for management of health and safety are as follows:

- identification of any potential hazards
- assessing the risks which could arise from these hazards
- identifying who is at risk
- eliminating or minimising the risks
- training staff to identify and control risks
- regular reviewing of the assessment processes.

Young workers at risk

There is also a requirement to carry out a risk assessment for young people. Any staff member who is under school leaving age must have a personalised risk assessment kept on file. This would be applicable for those on work experience or Saturday staff.

COSHH Risk Assessment

habia
standards • information • solutions

Staff member responsible: **Natasha Smith**   Date: **1st September 2005**   Review Dates: **10th January 2006**

Hazard	What is the risk?	Who is at risk?	Degree of risk high/med/low	Action to be taken to reduce/control risk
Aerosols (List aerosols used in your salon)	These can contain flammable gases and irritant chemicals. There is a risk of fire, explosion and intoxication.	Everyone in the salon, but in particular the user of the aerosol and the client.	Low	Look for aerosols with non-flammable gases if possible. Do not expose to temperatures above 50°C. Do not pierce or burn containers. Do not inhale.
Permanent wave neutraliser (List products used in your salon)	Irritant to the skin and eyes. Moderately toxic if swallowed or inhaled.	Stylists, juniors, trainees and clients.	Medium	Store in a cool place. Reseal after use. Do not use on damaged or sensitive skin. Avoid breathing in. Never place in an unlabelled container.

EXAMPLE

HSIP2a

©HABIA

COSHH Risk assessment

Activity
Conducting a risk assessment

Procedure for conducting risk assessment:

1   Take a walk around the salon looking for any hazards, i.e. anything with the potential to cause harm. By using a similar form to the example shown above, it will help to organise the necessary information.

2   Decide what the risk is and who could be harmed by those hazards. Broken tiles at the backwash may only affect the staff, whereas loose carpet in reception would affect all visitors.

3   For each of the listed hazards decide what level of risk exists, e.g. low, medium or high. Then looking at each entry, ask yourself if the risk can be eliminated or reduced.

4   Write down the findings of your risk assessment (salons with less than five employees do not have to record these findings). However, you may get a visit from Environmental Health and written records will prove that the assessments have been made.

5   Review your risk assessments at regular intervals. The introduction of new equipment, different product ranges or chemical processes will potentially create new hazards. Setting a review date within the assessment process will ensure that your salon is kept up to date in the future.

Workplace (Health, Safety and Welfare) Regulations 1992

These regulations superseded the Offices, Shops and Railway Premises Act 1963 (OSRPA) and cover the following workplace key points:

- maintenance of the workplace and the equipment in it
- ventilation, temperature and lighting
- cleanliness
- sanitary and washing facilities
- drinking water supply
- rest, eating and changing facilities
- storage of clothing
- glazing
- traffic routes (work thoroughfares)
- work space.

Amendments and additions in this Act provide new requirements for employers with particular attention for glazed areas such as windows and doors, etc. Any transparent and translucent partitions must be made of safe materials and if they could cause injury to anyone they should be appropriately marked. (Note narrow panes of glass up to 250 mm are excluded from this Act.)

Other amendments have particular rules for rest rooms and rest areas and suitable rest facilities to be provided for any person at work who is either pregnant or a nursing mother. OSRPA has slowly been phased out and been replaced by the Workplace (Health, Safety and Welfare) Regulations 1992.

Personal Protective Equipment at Work Regulations (PPE) 1992

The PPE Regulations 1992 require managers to make an assessment of the processes and activities carried out at work and to identify where and when special items of

Remember

 What are hazardous substances?
Hazardous substances include:

- substances used directly in work activities (e.g. adhesives, paints, cleaning agents)

- substances generated during work activities (e.g. fumes from soldering and welding)

- naturally occurring substances (e.g. grain dust)

- biological agents such as bacteria and other micro-organisms.

clothing should be worn. In hairdressing environments, the potential hazards and dangers revolve around the task of providing hairdressing services – that is, in general, the application of hairdressing treatments and associated products. (Many requirements under this Act will have been met in complying with COSHH regulations.)

Potentially hazardous substances used by hairdressers include:

- solutions like hydrogen peroxide in varying strengths
- caustic alkaline such as perming solutions of varying strengths
- flammable liquids, such as hair sprays which are often in pressurised containers
- vapours from chemical products
- colouring products.

All these items require correct handling and safe usage procedures and for several of them this includes the wearing of suitable items of protective equipment.

Control of Substances Hazardous to Health Regulations 1999 (COSHH)

The purpose of COSHH regulations is to make sure that people are working in the safest possible environment and conditions. A substance is considered to be hazardous if it can cause harm to the body. It only presents a risk if it is:

- in contact with the skin or eyes
- absorbed through the skin or via the eyes (either directly or from contact with contaminated surfaces or clothing)
- inhaled, i.e. breathing in substances in the atmosphere
- ingested via contaminated food or fingers
- injected
- introduced to the body via cuts and abrasions.

Hair products must comply with stringent UK cosmetics products safety regulations. The regulations detail how ingredients such as hydrogen peroxide, perming solutions and some hair dyes can be used. Under new legislation introduced in the EU manufacturers have to list on the label all the ingredients that are used in their products. Therefore employers must make an assessment to find out:

- what products are used
- what is the potential of a product for causing harm
- what is the chance of exposure
- how much people are exposed to, for how long and how often
- can the exposure be prevented and, if not, how is it adequately controlled.

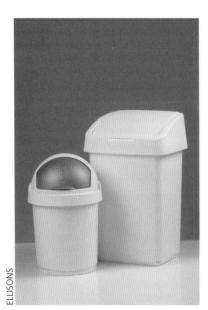

ELLISONS

Wherever safer products are available they should be used; where not, the exposure should be controlled. Exposure can be controlled by:

- providing good ventilation
- using the product only in recommended concentrations
- clearing up spillages or splashes immediately
- resealing containers immediately after use
- providing safe storage
- using personal protective equipment.

This information is taken from *COSHH Regulations – A Guide to Health and Safety of Salon Hair Products* – www.coshhessentials.org.uk

Further guidance for health and safety from Habia

The Hair and Beauty Industry Authority (Habia) produces and continually updates a comprehensive information guide for hairdressers.

The HABIA Health and Safety for Hairdressers Pack

This pack comprises of a strong, hard cover, four-ring binder with clearly defined sections. These cover all the necessary aspects of health and safety legislation, combined with ready to use checklists, policy documents and tailormade systems. Also included within the pack are a number of official documents, advisory leaflets and essential emergency signs. Habia recommended method for undertaking risk assessments is particularly useful and easy to follow, with pullout, ready-to-complete forms. The Good Practice information for undertaking COSHH risk assessment is based on their recommended system.

Main features of the pack:

- Official forms and notices for you to copy and use in your salon
- How to write and produce a health and safety policy with a blank version for you to personalise
- An accident book adhering to the new guidelines
- Health and Safety Risk Assessments, Fire Risk Assessments and COSHH Risk Assessments in example formats for guidance and as blank forms for you to complete
- Large print and a clear uncluttered layout make the information easy to read
- Fully up to date as of the date of purchase
- Fire exit signs

Activity
Health and safety

1 Read the instructions on the label of each chemical or product in your salon.

2 Further information for each individual type of product can be found in the Guide to Health and Safety in the Salon Booklet, or by using the manufacturer's data sheet.

3 If the product could cause harm, list it on the risk assessment form (see example risk assessment form on p. 380) together with the risk and who is at risk.

4 Using the information provided on the label, decide on the level of risk. (From your previous experience with the routine chemicals that you use at work, such as bleach, colour or perming solutions, you'll be able to decide the degree of risk.)

5 Decide how you could minimise and control the risk. Suggest a possible replacement for a high risk product with a lower risk product. If this is not possible, try to decide how you go on to control risk, remembering that personal protective equipment (PPE) is only to be used as a last resort.

6 In some cases your manager may need to replace certain products. See if you can find information, or source better personal protective equipment. This can be documented as an ongoing action plan, making sure that all relevant members of staff understand the actions that have been taken.

7 Discuss the completed risk assessment with staff and make sure that they are fully trained to use all products safely.

8 Remember to review your COSHH assessment on a regular basis and don't forget to add in any new products that have been introduced to the salon and keep all data sheets filed safely for future reference.

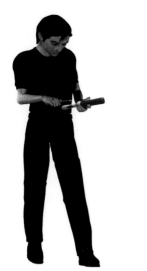

Electricity at Work Regulations 1989

The Electricity at Work Regulations 1989 cover the installation, maintenance and use of electrical equipment and systems in the workplace. Equipment must be checked by a qualified person on a yearly basis and if any maintenance is required this should be carried out by a qualified electrician.

An electrical testing record should be kept for each piece of equipment and should clearly show:

- electrician's/contractor's name, address, contact details
- itemised list of salon electrical equipment along with serial number (for individual identification)
- date of inspection
- date of purchase/disposal.

Health and Safety (First Aid) Regulations 1981

Diversion (See Appendix 2 and www.hse.gov.uk for more information on First Aid.)

The Health and Safety (First Aid) Regulations 1981 require employers to provide equipment and facilities which are adequate and appropriate in the circumstances for administering first aid to their employees. Remember that any first-aid materials used from the kit must be replaced as soon as possible. All accidents and emergency aid given within the salon must be documented in the accident book.

Activity

Contents of the first-aid box

Complete the missing information in the table below by using the reference points shown above. Keep the completed table information in your portfolio for future use.

Contents of first-aid box	No. of employees		
	1–5	6–10	11–50
First-aid guidance notes			
Individual sterile adhesive dressings			
Sterile eye pads			
Sterile triangular bandages			
Safety pins			
Medium size sterile unmediated dressings			
Large size sterile unmediated dressings			
Extra-large size sterile unmediated dressings			

Recording accidents and illness

All accidents must be recorded in the accident book. The recording system should always be kept readily available for use and inspection. When you are recording accidents, you will need to document the following details:

- date, time and place of incident or treatment
- name, and job of injured or ill person
- details of the injury/ill person and the treatment given
- what happened to the person immediately afterwards (e.g. went home, hospital)
- name and signature of the person providing the treatment and entry.

General guidance on first aid

The following basic information is available in leaflet form from HSE ISBN 0 7176 1070 5.

Basic rules for first aiders

REMEMBER: YOU SHOULD NOT ATTEMPT TO GIVE ANYTHING MORE THAN BASIC FIRST AID!

When giving first aid it is vital that you assess the situation and that you:

- take care not to become a casualty yourself while administering first aid (use protective clothing and equipment where necessary)
- send for help where necessary
- follow this advice from the HSE.

What to do in an emergency

Check whether the casualty is conscious. If the casualty is unconscious or semi-conscious:

- check the mouth for any obstruction
- *open the airway* by tilting the head back and lifting the chin using the tips of two fingers.

If the casualty has stopped breathing and you are competent to give artificial ventilation, do so. Otherwise send for help without delay.

Unconsciousness

In most workplaces expert help should be available fairly quickly, but if you have an unconscious casualty it is vital that his or her airway is kept clear. If you cannot keep the airway open as described above, you may need to turn the casualty into the recovery position. The priority is an open airway.

Reporting of Injuries, Diseases and Dangerous Occurrences Regulations 1995 (RIDDOR)

Under these regulations there are certain diseases and groups of infections that if sustained at work are notifiable by law. So if any employees suffer a personal injury at work which results in either:

- death
- major injury
- more than 24 hours in hospital
- an incapacity to work for more than three calendar days.

You must report them to the incident contact centre. In addition to this, if a member of the public or salon visitor is injured within the salon and taken to hospital, this is also reportable.

Certain industrial diseases are reportable using form F5208A and these include occupational dermatitis (a condition connected with hairdressing/barbering industry).

Other accidents that occur within the salon must also be recorded. Entries must be kept up to date within the accident record book.

Health and Safety (Information for Employees) Regulations 1989

The regulations require the employer to make available to all employees, notices, posters and leaflets in either the approved format or those actually published by the Health and Safety Executive (HSE).

The *Health and Safety Law* leaflet is available in packs of 50 from HSE Books Box 1999, Sudbury, Suffolk CO16 6FS tel. 01787 881165. Other useful HSE publications are:

- *Essentials of Health and Safety at Work* (ISBN 0 7176 0716)
- *Writing your Health and Safety Policy Statement* (ISBN 0 7176 0425)
- *Successful Health and Safety Management* (ISBN 0 7176 0425)
- *A Guide to RIDDOR* (ISBN 0 7176 0432 2)
- *Step by Step Guide to COSHH Assessment* (ISBN 0 11886379 7) or online information at www.cosh-essentials.org.uk
- *First Aid at Work* (ISBN 0 7176 0426 8)

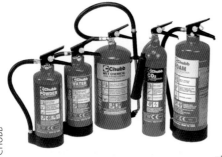

CHUBB

Fire Precautions Act 1971

The Act is concerned with fire prevention and the emergency evacuation escape routes from premises. Your employer is responsible for fire safety in the workplace and that it complies with fire regulations.

A building needs a fire certificate when:

- 20 or more people are working on the premises at one time
- more than 10 people work on floors other than the ground floor.

Fire Precautions (Workplace) Regulations (Amendment) 1999

The employer is responsible for undertaking a fire risk assessment, to produce an emergency evacuation plan and to inform and provide adequate training about the fire safety arrangements in your workplace.

Diversion (See Appendix 2 for more information.)

Your employer may also nominate a designated person to help them.

Health and Safety (Display Screen Equipment) Regulations 1992

These regulations cover the use of computers and similar equipment in the workplace. Although not generally a high risk, prolonged use can lead to eye strain, mental stress and possible muscular pain. As more hairdressing salons now use information technology it is becoming a consideration for employees.

It is the employer's duty to assess display screen equipment and reduce the risks that are discovered. They will need to plan the scheduling of work so that there are regular breaks or changes in activity and provide information training for the equipment users. Computer users will also be entitled to eyesight tests which will be paid for by the employer.

> **Good practice/Health and safety: PUWER**
> - Is all salon equipment checked regularly?
> - Are maintenance logs kept for items of equipment?
> - Has introduced secondhand equipment been checked?
> - Have all the staff been trained to use the equipment?

Manual Handling Operations Regulations 1992

These regulations apply in all occupations where manual lifting occurs. They require employers to carry out a risk assessment of the work processes and activities that involve lifting. The risk assessment should address detailed aspects:

- any risk of injury
- the manual movement that is involved in the task
- the physical constraints that the loads incur
- the work environmental constraints that are incurred
- the worker's individual capabilities
- steps and/or remedial action to take in order to minimise the risk.

Diversion (See Appendix 2 for more information.)

Provision and Use of Work Equipment Regulations (PUWER) 1998

These regulations refer to the regular maintenance and monitoring of work equipment. Any equipment, new or secondhand, must be suitable for the purpose that it is intended. In addition to this they require that anyone using this equipment must be adequately trained.

Environmental Protection Act 1990

These regulations refer to the safe disposal of waste products including chemicals. All salon waste should be disposed of in a manner that does not pollute the environment or cause harm to others.

The employer's responsibilities are to:

- dispose of all waste in a safe manner
- provide adequate training for all employees for safe disposal
- contact product manufacturers for information regarding safe disposal.

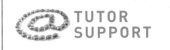

TUTOR SUPPORT

Discussion 15.1: Health and safety complying

An example of a local bye-law (South Yorkshire)

All hairdressers and barbers are subject to various pieces of legislation paramount among which are the Health and Safety at Work Act 1974, South Yorkshire Act 1974, South Yorkshire Act 1980 (registration) and the bye-laws. This code is intended as a guidance to fulfilling these obligations.

General

1   All premises must be kept in a clean condition.

2   All fixtures and fittings should be of such material as to be easily cleanable, e.g. fabric-covered chairs not suitable. All surfaces should be wiped down with a disinfectant regularly throughout the day.

3   All tools or instruments which come into contact with a customer must be sterilised before use on each customer (see below for appropriate methods).

4   All towels and other items which come into contact with customers must be clean and used only once before being washed on a high temperature cycle.

5   All gowns should be washed regularly and should any contamination or soiling with blood etc. occur that gown should not be reused until it has been washed on a high temperature cycle.

6   Solid soap, powder puffs, alum blocks or sponges should not be used.

7   A shaving brush must only be used for the first lather, once shaving has commenced the brush cannot be used.

8   Styptics should only be applied using disposable pads, e.g. cotton wool or swabs.

9   Powder should be applied using a spray.

10 Where clippers are used they must be sterilised between customers and if the skin is cut the clipper blades must be removed immediately, washed carefully and then sterilised.

11 The use of razors should be restricted to either disposable or cut-throat razors with disposable blades (e.g. Magic or Alcoso). The blades must be discarded after each customer and the holder washed and sterilised.

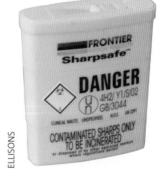

ELLISONS

Sharps box

- Electric razors should not be used because of sterilisation difficulties.

- Cut-throat razors with integral blades must not be used.

- The disposable razors and blades must be discarded in an approved 'sharps disposal' box clearly marked 'Danger: Contaminated Needles'.

- These boxes must be disposed of only to an authorised incinerator.

- Details of a suitable collection service are available from the Environmental Services Directorate.

Personal hygiene

1   Hands should be washed before every client.

2   Any skin problems, cuts or boils must be covered with a waterproof, impervious dressing. Dermatitis or similar condition on the hands or arms should be covered using disposable seamless gloves changed for each customer.

3   Clean, washable overalls must be worn and must be changed if contaminated or soiled by any blood or other body fluid. Dirty overalls should be washed on a high-temperature programme.

Disinfection and sterilisation procedures

1   All equipment once used should be disinfected or sterilised (according to contamination) before reuse and should be divided into plastic items – combs, brushes, etc. – and metal items – scissors, razors, etc.

2   The plastic items should be rinsed and all hair removed. Any items contaminated by blood or body fluid must be handled with care to ensure that the contaminated area does not come into contact with any broken skin.

3 These should then be placed in a solution of hypochlorite until required.

4 The metal equipment should be sterilised, ideally in an autoclave.

Autoclaves may be automatic and go through a cycle with appropriate holding times, otherwise the times and temperatures shown in the table must be achieved.

Temperature	Holding times
121°C	15 minutes
126°C	10 minutes
134°C	3 minutes

An alternative to an autoclave is to boil all equipment for 30 minutes in a boiler specially designed for instruments.

The third alternative method for dealing with metal instruments is to rinse away visible contamination. Care must be taken to avoid touching any contamination, especially with areas of broken skin. The instruments must then be placed in a solution of glutaraldehyde for at least 30 minutes. It is advisable to use disposable razors.

Disinfectants

The two most commonly used disinfectants are hypochlorite and glutaraldehyde. These do not sterilise, i.e. kill all known germs, but do reduce the number to the extent that there is very little danger of infection.

Hypochlorite (sold commercially as Milton or bleach) is corrosive to metals and therefore can only be used for wiping down work surfaces, chairs, etc. and for soaking combs, brushes, etc. The solution should be made up freshly each day with a dilution of one part Milton to ten parts water or one part good quality bleach to one hundred parts water.

Glutaraldehyde (sold commercially as Cidex or Totacide) can be used for wiping down all surfaces including metals and for soaking metal implements. The solution can be made up weekly according to manufacturers' instructions.

G22.2	Make sure that risks are controlled safely and effectively

Hazard and risk

Almost anything may be a hazard, but may or may not become a risk. For example: a trailing electric cable from a piece of equipment is a hazard, if it is trailing across a passageway, presents a high risk of someone tripping over it, but if it is along a wall out of the way, the risk is much less.

Poisonous or flammable chemicals are hazards and may present a high risk. However, if they are kept in a properly designed secure store and handled by properly trained and equipped people, the risk is much less than if they are left about for anyone to use.

A failed light bulb is a hazard. If it is just one of many in a room it presents very little risk, but if it is the only light on a stairwell, it is a very high risk. Changing the bulb may be a high risk, if it is up high or if the power has been left on, or a low risk if it is in a table lamp which has been unplugged.

A box of heavy material is a hazard. It presents a higher risk to someone who lifts it incorrectly, rather than someone who uses the correct manual handling techniques.

EKU *statement*

G22 (eku5) The difference between a hazard and a risk

EKU *statement*

G22 (eku7) Why you should remain alert to the presence of hazards in the workplace

Activity

Hazard and risk

For this activity, think of examples of hazards that could exist within your workplace. For each one, specify the risk involved and the measures that should be taken to control the risk.

Here is an example to start you off.

Identify the hazard	What is the risk?	How can this be controlled?
Hair clippings on the floor	Slipping	Make sure that they are swept up and put in the bin

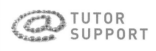

TUTOR SUPPORT

Discussion 15.2: Risk assessment

Potential hazards in workplace

Working with equipment

What could be a potential hazard?	What is the risk?	What action should I take?	**Relevant legislation** (other than) Management of Health and Safety at Work Regulations 1999
Razor blades, scissors	Injury – cuts and abrasions	1 Inform staff of the correct ways to handle sharps 2 Ensure that a sharps box is available for safe disposal 3 Check with local authority for bye laws affecting your premises	Health and Safety (First Aid) Regulations 1981
Loose plugs or coiled leads on blow-dryers, tongs straighteners	Electric shock	1 Inform staff on how to check for faults before plugging into the mains 2 Show staff how to put equipment away safely 3 Regular maintenance of equipment test records	Electricity at Work Regulations 1989
Faulty or worn equipment	Electric shock Accidental injuries	1 Visually check equipment regularly 2 Report findings to management 3 Stop others from using equipment until replaced or mended	Workplace (Health Safety and Welfare) Regulations 1992 The Provision and Use of Work Equipment Regulations 1992 Electricity at Work Regulations 1989

Handling chemicals

What could be a potential hazard?	What is the risk?	What action should I take?	Relevant legislation (other than) Management of Health and Safety at Work Regulations 1999
Handling hydrogen peroxide	Burns Contact dermatitis	1 Check manufacturer instructions 2 Inform/show staff the correct ways to handle chemical products 3 Check storage arrangements 4 Monitor staff for safe handling	Control of Substances Hazardous to Health 1999 RIDDOR 1995 (re. occupational dermatitis) Personal Protective Equipment at Work Regulations 1992
Inhalation of powder lighteners	Asthma or respiratory conditions		
Chemical spillage	Injury Slipping		

Process for undertaking COSHH risk assessment

The following table is the guidance from HSE for undertaking COSHH risk assessment. If your employer designates *you* to undertake this assessment, you should follow these steps.

Step 1	Assess the risks	Assess the risks to health from hazardous substances used in or created by your workplace activities.
Step 2	Decide what precautions are needed	You must not carry out work which could expose your employees to hazardous substances without first considering the risks and the necessary precautions, and what else you need to do to comply with COSHH.
Step 3	Prevent or adequately control exposure	You must prevent your employees being exposed to hazardous substances. Where preventing exposure is not reasonably practicable, then you must adequately control it (e.g. shampooing – wear vinyl gloves).
Step 4	Ensure that control measures are used and maintained	Ensure that control measures are maintained properly and that safety procedures are followed.
Step 5	Monitor the exposure	Monitor the exposure of employees to hazardous substances, if necessary.
Step 6	Carry out appropriate health surveillance	Carry out appropriate health surveillance where your assessment has shown this is necessary or where COSHH sets specific requirements.
Step 7	Prepare plans and procedures to deal with accidents, incidents and emergencies	Prepare plans and procedures to deal with accidents, incidents and emergencies involving hazardous substances, where necessary.
Step 8	Ensure employees are properly informed, trained and supervised	You should provide your employees with suitable and sufficient information, instruction and training.

Working environment

What could be a potential hazard?	What is the risk?	What action should I take?	Relevant legislation (other than) Management of Health and Safety at Work Regulations 1999
Hair clippings on the floor	Slipping	1 Inform staff of the risks of leaving floors unswept 2 Monitor staff in the work environment	Workplace (Health Safety and Welfare) Regulations 1992
Obstructions	Slips or trips Injury	1 Inform staff of the risks of leaving obstructions in work areas 2 Check staff knowledge for safe handling methods 3 Identify training needs 4 Inform management of staff training needs	Manual Handling Operations Regulations 1992 Workplace (Health Safety and Welfare) Regulations 1992
Poor hygiene, cleaning, and maintenance of salon resources	Cross-infection Cross-infestation	1 Inform staff of the risks of poor salon/shop maintenance. 2 Show staff methods of disinfecting and sterilising surfaces, tools, equipment 3 Monitor staff in the work environment	Workplace (Health Safety and Welfare) Regulations 1992 Personal Protective Equipment at Work Regulations 1992
Poor personal hygiene	Cross-infection Cross-infestation	1 Inform staff of the risks of poor personal hygiene 2 Monitor staff in the work environment	
Computers	Eye strain Repetitive strain injury	1 Inform staff of the risks of using computers for long periods of time 2 Monitor staff ensure that they take regular breaks	Health and Safety (Display Screen Equipment) Regulations 1992

Controlling risks in the workplace

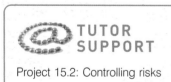

TUTOR SUPPORT

Project 15.2: Controlling risks

The following aspects look at the ways in which you can control risks within the workplace.

Sterilisation

The salon equipment and tools must be clean and well maintained at all times and one way of doing this is by sterilisation. Sterilisation is the eradication of all living organisms which will prevent cross-infection. All tools and equipment should be cleaned before sterilising to remove dirt, grease and particles of hair. Combs, brushes, rollers and curlers need to be washed in hot soapy water. Scissors and razors should be carefully wiped with alcohol or spirit.

Chemical sterilisers Chemical sterilisers should be handled only with suitable personal protective equipment, as many of the solutions used are hazardous to health and should not come into contact with the skin. The most effective form of salon sterilisation is achieved by the total immersion of the contaminated implements into a jar of fluid.

Ultraviolet radiation Ultraviolet (UV) radiation provides an alternative sterilising option. Items should be cleaned to remove grease and dirt and placed in wall- or worktop-mounted cabinets fitted with UV-emitting light bulbs and exposed to the radiation for at least 15 minutes. If your scissors or combs are sterilised in a UV cabinet, remember to turn them over to make sure both sides have been done.

Autoclave The autoclave is a very effective method for the sterilisation of metal or glass items. It works by superheating water under pressure in the same way that a pressure cooker does; heating the water to 120°C. This very high temperature kills all organisms within 20 minutes.

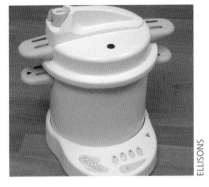

ELLISONS

An autoclave

Lifting and handling large objects

The incorrect handling of large and/or heavy items can result in low back pain/problems, repetitive strain injuries and strain disorders.

Think about the situations that can occur in a salon environment i.e.

- moving stock into storage
- unpacking heavy or awkward items
- lifting equipment and moving salon furniture
- working heights – chairs, trolleys driers etc.

The regulations require employers to:

- *avoid* the need for hazardous manual handling, so far as is reasonably practicable;
- *assess* the risk of injury from any hazardous manual handling that can't be avoided; and
- *reduce* the risk of injury from hazardous manual handling, so far as is reasonably practicable.

Diversion (See Appendix 2 for more details about manual handling techniques.)

Avoid contact dermatitis

Fact: Up to 70 per cent of hairdressers suffer from skin damage. Keep your hands healthy and wave goodbye to bad hand days.

Cut out dermatitis: many trainee hairdressers have to give up hairdressing because of this common occupational health hazard. You can avoid this condition by making sure that you always use disposable vinyl gloves. Always dry your hands thoroughly after and moisturise to keep your hands healthy.

Five steps to prevent dermatitis

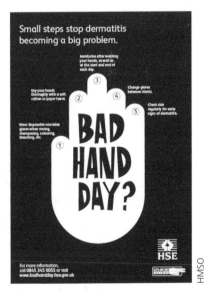

Small steps stop dermatitis becoming a big problem.

BAD HAND DAY?

For more information, call 0845 345 0055 or visit www.badhandday.hse.gov.uk

HSE

HMSO

Bad hand day poster

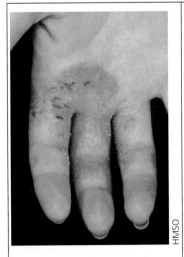

HMSO

What does dermatitis look like?

Step 1. Wear disposable vinyl gloves when rinsing, shampooing, colouring, bleaching, etc.

Step 2. Dry your hands thoroughly with a soft cotton or paper towel.

Step 3. Moisturise after washing your hands, as well as at the start and end of each day. It's easy to miss fingertips, finger webs and wrists.

Step 4. Change gloves between clients. Make sure you don't contaminate your hands when you take them off.

Step 5. Check skin regularly for early signs of dermatitis.

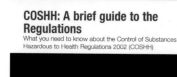

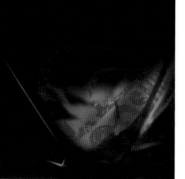

COSHH: A brief guide to the Regulations
What you need to know about the Control of Substances Hazardous to Health Regulations 2002 (COSHH)

COSHH leaflet

Hazard signs

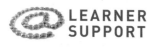

Handling chemicals

Many of the hairdressing services involve some contact with chemicals and salons have safe ways of dealing with this. Employers have a legal obligation to control the exposure of hazardous substances in the workplace and you are protected by the **C**ontrol **O**f **S**ubstances **H**azardous to **H**ealth Regulations (2003) *COSHH*. Most hairdressing chemicals are safe and only propose a risk to health at the point when they are handled and used.

COSHH precautions Risk assessments will indicate the types of chemicals available within the salon and the safe ways in which they may be handled or used. These chemical products will vary from cleaning items, such as washing materials, bleach and polish, to the more typical salon-specific items such as colours, lighteners, hydrogen peroxide and general styling materials.

Make sure that all staff are aware of the assessments, they will indicate the level of risk that each of the chemical products presents to you i.e. a hazard rating and details on how they can be handled safely with the PPE provided by your employer.

Keep floors clean and thoroughfares clear

The most common cause of injuries at work is the slip or trip. Resulting falls can be serious and a busy salon means lots of people and the more clients there are, the more hair clippings there will be. Loose clippings left on the salon floor present a hazard to staff and clients alike.

Both wet and dry hair clippings are easily slipped on, make sure that working areas are swept regularly, and don't wait for stylists to finish: get rid of clippings before they build up. Clear them away from areas where people are working or walking and then brush them into a dustpan and put them into the waste bin.

Keep thoroughfares clear of obstructions, move any hazards away from busy traffic areas. (See Appendix 2, Manual handling section.)

Working with computers

Using a computer for long periods of time can give rise to back problems, repetitive strain injury or other musculoskeletal disorders. These health problems may become serious if no action is taken. They can be caused by poor design of workstations (and associated equipment such as chairs), insufficient space, lack of training or not taking breaks from display screen work.

Work with a screen does not cause eye damage, but many users experience temporary eye strain or stress. This can lead to reduced work efficiency or taking time off work.

Working with electricity

Electricity can kill. Although deaths from electric shocks are very rare in hairdressing salons, even a non-fatal shock can cause severe and permanent injury. An electric shock from faulty or damaged electrical equipment may lead to a fall (e.g. down a stairwell.)

Those using electricity may not be the only ones at risk. Poor electrical installations and faulty electrical appliances can lead to fires which can also result in death or injury to others.

Get into the habit of looking for loose cables and plugs on tongs, straighteners and hand dryers *before* plugging them in for use. If you think that a piece of electrical equipment is faulty or damaged, tell your supervisor immediately. Make sure that no-one else tries to use it.

Personal health and hygiene

Hairdressing, beauty therapy and nail craft are all personal services, and as such are very different to trades such as retail, joinery or engineering in the way that practitioners communicate with and handle their clients. Salon staff and their clients can have quite a close relationship, which has both advantages and disadvantages.

Poor personal hygiene can lead to cross-infection to the client, your fellow staff needs to be aware of this hazard to public health and demonstrate their professionalism in this, by making it a major personal priority.

TUTOR SUPPORT

Short answer test

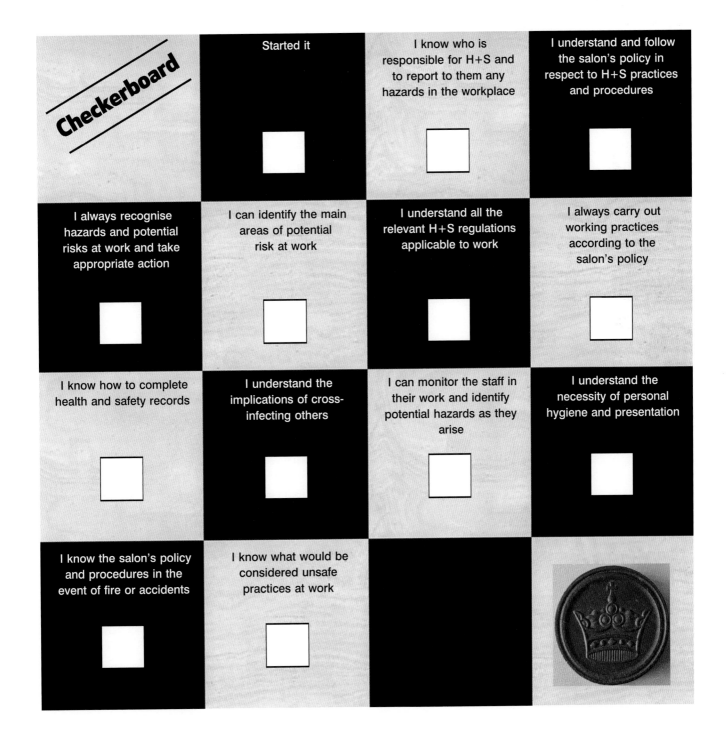

Assessment of knowledge and understanding

Revision questions

Quick quiz: a selection of different types of questions to check your knowledge.

Q1 A _____ is something with potential to cause harm.   Fill in the blank

Q2 Risk assessment is a process of evaluation to ensure safe working practices.   True or false

Q3 Select all that apply.   Multi selection
Which of the following are hazards:

Shampooing with disposable gloves on	☐ 1
Hair clippings on the floor	☐ 2
Wet or slippery floors	☐ 3
Shampooing products	☐ 4
Styling mirrors	☐ 5
Trailing flexes from electrical equipment	☐ 6

Q4 A standard first-aid kit should contain Paracetamol tablets.   True or false

Q5 Which of the following regulations relate to the safe handling of chemicals?   Multi choice

PPE	○ a
RIDDOR	○ b
COSHH	○ c
OSRPA	○ d

Q6 All salons must have a written health and safety policy.   True or false

Q7 Which of the following records must a salon keep up to date by law: Multi selection

Stock records	☐ 1
Accident book	☐ 2
Appointment book	☐ 3
Electrical equipment annual test records	☐ 4
Health and safety at work checklist	☐ 5
Fire drill records	☐ 6

Q8 Safety regulations require employers to provide adequate equipment and facilities in case of a _____ occurring.   Fill in the blank

Q9 What sign/poster is required by law to be displayed on the premises?   Multi choice

Latest hairstyles	○ a
Health and safety information	○ b
Employer's name, address and contact details	○ c
Forthcoming events	○ d

Q10 Contact dermatitis is an occupational health hazard.   True or false

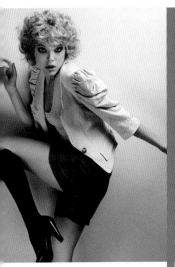

Chapter**sixteen**
Being effective in your work

G11

G11.1

G11.2

CREDIT VALUE
FOR UNIT G11
4 Credits

Diversion See Health and safety chapter, Unit G22, and the appendices for information on:

- COSHH legislation G11 (eku2)
- RIDDOR G11 (eku2)
- Manual Handling Regulations G11 (eku2)
- Cosmetic product Regulations G11 (eku2)
- Electricity at Work Regulations G11 (eku2)

Personal effectiveness: quick overview

Unit title

G11 Contribute to the financial effectiveness of the business

This is an **optional** unit for both hairdressing and barbering at level 3, it is made up of two main outcomes

Main outcomes

G11.1 Contribute to the effective use and monitoring of resources

G11.2 Meet productivity and development targets

What do I need to do for G11.1?

- You need to monitor the use of resources within the salon
- Gather stock control information and check deliveries when they arrive
- Notify management of any discrepancies
- Identify problems with salon resources and try to rectify them
- Make recommendations for improvements to resources to management
- Maintain salon records to support resources

What do I need to do for G11.2?

- Agree personal productivity targets with your supervisor
- Look for ways in which you can improve productivity
- Make sure that others work collectively to achieve better productivity
- Review progress towards achieving targets
- Consistently achieve your personal targets

Keywords

Productivity

The levels of output achieved in a work setting

Effectiveness

The quality of output achieved in a work setting

Resources

The variety of means available to a business that can be utilised or employed within any given task or project: time, money, people etc.

Appraisal

A process of reviewing work performance over a period of time

Information covered in this chapter

- How to make the best of the salon's resources
- How to achieve personal productivity targets
- How to communicate effectively

Other aspects of legislation covered within this chapter

- Health and safety legislation (see pp. 411–412)
- Consumer and retail legislation
- Data Protection Act
- Working time directives
- Equal opportunities
- Disability discrimination

What aspects do I need to cover for G11.1 and G11.2?

- A variety of salon's resources that are human, stock and equipment and relate to time
- Personal productivity targets for retail, technical services and personal development

What do I need to know for G11.1 and G11.2?

- Your salon's requirements to targets, productivity and personal development
- A range of legislation covering health and safety, data protection, employment and consumers
- How to use resources effectively and the sorts of problems that you may encounter
- Salon stock control systems
- The importance of effective communication
- How to be positive and present clear accurate information
- The principles of time management
- How you can reach personal productivity targets
- How you can review your progress towards achieving your targets

Introduction

Being effective in our work is essential. The way in which we use salon resources and maintain productivity has a direct impact on the viability of the business. We will be looking at these two aspects in closer detail:

- resources
- productivity.

The resources are the key aspects that are available to the business. The way they are utilised and controlled enables the business to function properly and refers to the salon staff, salon materials, equipment and time. Productivity refers to the effective usefulness of your efforts whilst you are at work.

This chapter describes how you can contribute to the financial effectiveness of the business. It focuses upon the use of the salon's resources, human, stock, tools and equipment, as well as making the best use of your time whilst you are there. If you do make the most of these resources, you will be going a long way towards your own self-improvement and the achievement of your personal targets.

G11.1 Contribute to the effective use and monitoring of resources

Hairdressing is a labour-intensive service industry. It relies solely on the profits generated from the sales of services and treatments to clients. The people that work within a hairdressing salon are therefore an essential part of the business. Many people are involved in the process. The receptionist meets and greets the clients, handles bookings over the telephone, operates the till and assists in the selling of retail products. The stylists tend to their clients, providing them with services and treatments. The junior staff undergoes training to add to the skill base of the salon. They also tend to the clients by providing customer services. The manager delegates the tasks, collects information and makes decisions in order for the business to function. The cleaners ensure that all areas are fit for their purpose and hygienically safe. They are all part of one team and work together collectively in order to make the business work.

The way that the team is orchestrated, i.e. managed, really counts. Each and every member of staff has a duty to perform and personal targets to achieve.

EKU *statement*

G11 (eku7) How the effective use of resources contributes to the profitability of the business

Remember

To find out what your salon's policies are in relation to the use of salon's resources.

Human resources

The people employed within the salon are its human resources (HR) and they are the most important asset that a well run business can utilise. During induction, new staff are familiarised with the role that they must perform. It is important that this is formalised in a staff member's *job description*. It details their role, the duties involved with their role and the responsibilities associated to the role by carrying out those duties.

Each member of staff will have targets; these are the personal productivity and/or development targets that will be monitored and reviewed at regular intervals over time. These targets are set and mutually agreed by the staff member and their supervisor, so that staff know what is expected of them whilst they are at work.

There should be a grievance and disciplinary procedure provided to each employee, this will emphasis the importance of staff discipline and is essential in the case of complaint, poor performances, staffing issues and misconduct.

Remember

Be positive in the way that you receive feedback on performance, even if it is negative.

EKU *statement*

G11 (eku1) Your salon's requirements relating to the use of the resources in the range

G11 (eku13) The common problems associated with salon resources (e.g. staffing, stock control, tools and equipment breakdowns, time overruns, etc.) and how to resolve them

---

Arbitration and Conciliation Advisory Service (ACAS)

Helpline 08457 47 47 47

Working conditions

A *contract of employment* (written statement of the terms of employment) should be given to an employee within two months of starting. The written statement is not a contract in itself, but in the case of a dispute it can be used as evidence of an employee's terms and conditions.

EKU *statement*

G11 (eku4) Your own limits of authority in relation to the use of resources

The principal statement

The employee's written statement can be set out in one or more documents. However, either that document or one of those documents – known as the *principal statement* – must contain, at the very least, all the information listed below:

- The legal name of the employer company – it is a good idea also to include the trading name, if different.
- The legal name of the employee.
- The date the current employment began.
- Any earlier date upon which employment with a previous employer began which is treated as 'continuous' with the current employment.
- The employee's pay, or how it is calculated, and the intervals at which it will be paid – e.g. weekly or monthly.
- The employee's hours of work.
- Entitlement to holidays – including public holidays – and holiday pay. The information must be accurate enough to allow precise calculation of accrued entitlement.
- Job title or a brief description of the work.
- The address of the employee's place of work. If they will be working in more than one place then this should be indicated along with the employer's address.

The rules about hours of work under Working Time Regulations 1998

In general, **workers aged 18 and over** are entitled to:

- 4.8 weeks' holiday a year (previously four weeks' holiday a year)
- work no more than six days out of every seven, or 12 out of every 14
- take a 20-minute break if they work more than six hours
- work a maximum 48-hour average week

and **workers aged 16 and 17** should:

- take at least 30 minutes' break if they work more than four-and-a-half hours
- work no more than eight hours a day and 40 hours a week
- have 12 hours' rest between working days and two days off every week.

Working hours

Workers aged 18 or over cannot be forced to work for more than 48 hours a week on average. The employer will calculate employee's hours as an average over 17 weeks. This will include:

- work-related training
- travel as part of a worker's duties
- working lunches.

Rest breaks during the working day

Employees are entitled to regular breaks in the working day.

- Workers aged 18 or over should be offered a minimum 20-minute break for every shift lasting more than six hours. (The break cannot be taken at the start or the end of a work shift.) It is the employer's duty to ensure that your workers can take their breaks.
- Young workers, aged 16 and 17, should take at least 30 minutes' break if they work more than 4.5 hours.

Holiday entitlement

Under the Working Time Regulations 1998 most workers are entitled to paid holidays or annual leave.

A full-time worker is entitled to holiday from their first day of employment and the entitlement is 4.8 weeks (or 24 days) annually. Pay is based on a normal week's pay. Part-time workers are entitled to the same holidays as full-time workers but this is calculated on a pro rata basis.

Payment for leave

A worker's entitlement to paid holiday or leave starts on the first day of employment and is not subject to a minimum period of employment.

For each week of leave, workers are entitled to a week's pay. A week's pay is calculated according to the type of work performed:

- for workers on fixed hours and pay it equals the amount due for a week's work
- for workers on variable hours and pay (piece work, bonus or commission workers) it equals the average hourly rate multiplied by the normal working hours in a week
- for shift workers it equals the average weekly hours of work in the preceding 12 weeks at the average hourly rate.

However, if an employee requests payment in place of taking the time off, the employer will point out that an arrangement like that is unlawful.

Public and bank holidays

When the Christmas and New Year public holidays fall at a weekend, other week days are declared public holidays.

Paid time off does not legally have to be given for public holidays, and if it is it can be included in the employee's minimum leave entitlement.

Part-time workers have the same entitlement to leave as full-time workers, so if full-time workers are given paid leave for bank holidays, part-time workers should also be granted payment on a pro rata basis.

Employment of young workers between the ages of 13 and school leaving age

National law

In England, Wales and Scotland young people aged between 13 and the minimum school-leaving age may not do any work, paid or unpaid:

- before 7 am or after 7 pm
- for more than two hours on a school day or Sunday
- before the close of school hours (however, local authority by e-laws may allow young people to work for one hour before school)
- for more than 12 hours a week during term time
- for more than five hours (13- to 14-year-olds) or eight hours (15- to 16-year-olds) on Saturdays and during school holidays on weekdays
- for more than 25 hours in total a week – 35 hours if aged 15 or over – during school holidays
- for more than four hours without taking a break of at least one hour
- in any occupations prohibited by local bye-laws or other legislation, for example in any industrial setting, pubs, betting shops, or in any work that may be harmful to their health, well-being or education.

In addition, young people must have a two-week break from any work during the school holiday in each calendar year.

Diplomas for 14- to 19-year-olds

The Diploma in Hair and Beauty Studies is one of the seventeen new qualifications for 14- to 19-year-olds, which was introduced in England in September 2009. It offers young people a more practical, hands-on way of learning and gaining generic, transferable skills employers and universities look for.

Designed in partnership with employers and universities, the Diploma involves practical, hands-on experience related to the six industries in the hair and beauty sector as well as classroom learning. It's a combination aimed at encouraging students to develop broad, sector-related skills – along with their abilities in English, Maths and ICT – in an applied and enjoyable way.

Employers can get involved with consortia delivering the Diploma in Hair and Beauty Studies by:

- offering (around ten days') work experience places for students or work shadowing for teachers
- providing access to resources, equipment and use of premises
- setting actual/realistic business problems for students to solve in their projects
- giving talks and lectures to enrich the curriculum with real business experience.

Staff training

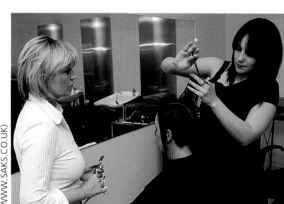

COURTESY OF SAKS HAIR AND BEAUTY (WWW.SAKS.CO.UK)

The employer makes the investment in staff training; so that it will eventually, repay the business in the form of:

- increased productivity
- improved services and treatments
- better financial performance.

The lack of staff training will affect all of these goals. If staff carries out technical services in which they are inexperienced, the results will show through:

- client dissatisfaction
- lack of confidence and poor self-esteem
- eventual loss of business through lost clients.

Good technical skills and sound product knowledge are the way of combating these negative aspects and retaining clients.

Good working relationships have a lot to do with these factors too. The relationships between staff in the work are vitally important to the overall success of the business. Every member of staff needs to feel part of the team; each one plays and important role in ensuring that success.

Poor working relationships create an unpleasant working environment for the staff and the clients and one way of controlling this is through good effective communication.

EKU *statement*

G11 (eku14) Why it is important to communicate effectively

G11 (eku15) How to present the benefits of recommendations in a positive manner

G11 (eku17) How to give clear, accurate and timely instructions to those who may be assisting you

G11 (eku18) How to encourage others to work effectively on your behalf

Good communication

Effective communication takes place when information is passed from one to another with a clear, unambiguous message. The technique of communication could be oral, written or inferred.

The oral and written styles of communication are generally more reliable in conveying intention whereas the inferred is generally the most problematic.

Oral communication

Oral communication occurs when you speak to clients over the telephone or during consultation or during the service. As a more senior member of staff it also occurs when you instruct junior staff, handle complaints and deal with external bodies such as trade suppliers.

Oral communication is a good technique for providing information quickly. When you communicate orally with others remember:

- that the tone of your voice will also be taken into account by the listener
- that where you provide the information may affect the listener's response
- that clear information will not be misunderstood.

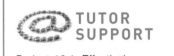

TUTOR SUPPORT

Project 16.1: Effectively managing resources

Written communication

Written communication may not be as quick as oral at providing information, but the results of it are much longer lasting. And in certain situations a detailed or documented record is far more useful than 'I thought you said I could ... '

The most obvious forms of written salon communication will relate to:

- formal instructions to staff
- reports prepared for management
- formal details or instructions to external bodies
- details of treatments, tests and responses from clients
- records of complaint.

There are times when information has to be recorded. Client records, taking messages and stock procedures are typical examples of this.

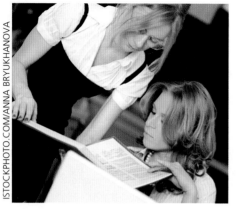

ISTOCKPHOTO.COM/ANNA BRYUKHANOVA

Client records can be manual or computerised; in either event they will contain similar information:

- client name, title, address and contact information
- previous service, treatment, tests and product information
- date, costs and timings of previous visits
- stylist/operator details and any other additional memos
- Detailed responses from clients during consultation for potentially; more problematic services e.g. hair extensions, hair patterning and design.

Written communication: taking memos and notes An effective memo is clear and includes the following:

- for whom it is intended
- who took the message
- the date and time
- its purpose
- clear details or instructions.

Body language

It's not what you say that counts; it's the expression that your body makes that punctuates the sentences.

For more information on positive and negative body language see Chapter 1 Unit G21 Provide hairdressing consultation services pp. 4–43.

Generally accepted code of conduct at work

Be polite and courteous with colleagues (and clients) at all times.

Specifically:

- Never talk down to staff members – treat them in a way that you would wish to be handled.
- Never lose your temper with staff members in front of clients – if you do need to amplify your comments, do it away from the salon floor. (If the matter is serious you may need a witness to your instructions.)
- Never, never ridicule a member of staff in front of clients or other staff.
- If you do have a contentious situation or personal issues with a colleague, do not let your professionalism fail. Settle grievances as soon as possible and move on.

Dealing with client complaints

A client has every right to expect the service that were agreed and paid for and when an unexpected result occurs the client has every right to complain. Dealing with a dissatisfied client is not easy and should therefore be handled with consideration and care.

If a client approaches you with a complaint you should move your client away to a quieter area of the salon.

The complaint may then be resolved by:

- finding out exactly what the problem is
- assess the validity of the complaint
- mutually agree on a suitable course of action (seek a second opinion if needed)
- carry out/organise any corrective work
- recording the occurrence and the remedial action that was taken.

People's rights and consumer legislation

Equal opportunities

The Equal Opportunities Commission (EOC) has the statutory duty to:

- work towards the elimination of discrimination
- promote equality of opportunity between men and women (and in relation to persons undergoing gender reassignment)
- keep the relevant legislation under review.

The legislation within the remit of the EOC is wide ranging; however, the main considerations are:

- equal pay
- sex discrimination
- disability discrimination (summary below).

In general, the *Sex Discrimination Act* (SDA) requires goods, facilities and services, whether for payment or not, which are offered to the public to be provided on the same basis for both sexes. The SDA prohibits direct and indirect sex discrimination.

Direct sex discrimination is treating a woman less favourably than a man (or vice versa) because of her sex.

Indirect sex discrimination occurs when a condition or requirement is applied equally to both women and men but, in fact, it affects more women than men (or vice versa) and is not justifiable on objective grounds unrelated to sex.

The Act provides for exceptions but unless a relevant exception to the requirements of the SDA can be used, facilities and services should be open to both sexes in the same way.

Disability Discrimination Act 2005 (DDA 2005)

The Act makes it unlawful to discriminate against disabled persons in connection with employment, the provision of goods, facilities and services or the disposal or management of premises; to make provision about the employment of disabled persons; and to establish a National Disability Council.

EKU *statement*

G11 (eku2) The critical aspects of current legal requirements relevant to hairdressing salons relating to the use of resources in the range (e.g. use of personal protective equipment, use of products, tools and equipment, disposal of waste and sharps, staff working times and break entitlements etc. linked to current Health and Safety At Work legislation, COSHH Regulations, Manual Handling Operations Regulations, Electricity at Work Regulations, RIDDOR, Workplace Regulations, Data Protection Act, Working Time Directives and Cosmetic Products Regulations)

Diversion For more information visit: www.eoc.org.uk/index.asp.

Diversion For more information on this or accessibility issues visit www.disability.gov.uk/legislation.

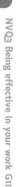

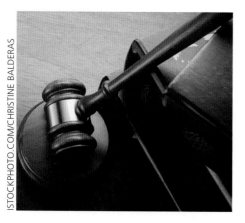

ISTOCKPHOTO.COM/CHRISTINE BALDERAS

The Act protects the rights of disabled people and new revisions in 2005 have particular relevance to the business proprietor.

Data Protection Act (1998)

Your clients have the following rights which can be enforced through any county court:

- *Right of subject access* – This is the right to find out what information about them is held on computer and in some paper records.
- *Correcting inaccurate data* – They have the right to have inaccurate personal data rectified, blocked, erased, or destroyed. If your client believes that they have suffered damage or distress as a result of the processing of inaccurate data they can ask the court to award compensation.
- *Preventing junk mail* (from salons that market to their customer base) – Your client has the right to request in writing that a data controller does not use your personal data for direct marketing by post (sometimes known as 'junk mail'), by telephone or by fax.

Diversion For more information on consumer rights in relation to the Data Protection Act visit www. informationcommissioner.gov.uk/

Data Protection Act 1998

The Data Protection Act (DPA) applies to any business that uses computers or paper-based systems for storing personal information about its clients and staff.

It places obligations on the person holding the information (data controller) to deal with it properly.

It gives the person that the information concerns (data subject) rights regarding the data held about them.

The duties of the data controller

There are eight principles put in place by the DPA to make sure that data is handled correctly. By law, the data controller must keep to these principles. The principles say that the data must be:

1 fairly and lawfully processed
2 processed for limited purposes
3 adequate, relevant and not excessive
4 accurate
5 not kept for longer than is necessary
6 processed in line with your rights
7 secure
8 not transferred to other countries without adequate protection.

for more information see http://www.ico.gov.uk/

EKU *statement*

G11 (eku3) Current legal requirements relating to the sale of retail goods (e.g. Sale of Goods Act)

The Sale of Goods Act (1979) and Sale and Supply of Goods Act (1994)

The Sale of Goods Act 1979 and the later Sale and Supply of Goods Act (1994) are the main legal instruments helping buyers to obtain redress when their purchases go wrong. It is in the interest of anyone who sells goods or services to understand the implications of these Acts and the responsibilities they have under them. Essentially, these Acts state that what you sell must fit its description, be fit for its purpose and be of satisfactory quality. If not, you – as the supplier – are obliged to sort out the problem.

Briefly these Acts require the vendor:

- To make sure that goods *'conform to contract'*. This means that they must be as you describe them e.g. highlight shampoo stops your highlights from fading.
- The goods must also be of *satisfactory quality*, meaning they should be safe, work properly and have no defects.
- You must also ensure the goods are *'fit for purpose'*. This means they should be capable of doing what they're meant for. For example, in the case of a brush it shouldn't fall apart when it is first used.

The Consumer Protection Act (1987)

This Act follows European laws to protect the buyer in the following areas:

- *product liability* – a customer may claim compensation for a product that doesn't reach general standards of safety
- *general safety requirements* – it is a criminal offence to sell goods that are unsafe; traders that breach this conduct may face fines or even imprisonment
- *misleading prices* – misleading consumers with wrongly displayed prices is also an offence.

The Act is designed to help safeguard the consumer from products that do not reach reasonable levels of safety. Your salon will take adequate precautions in procuring, using and supplying reputable products and maintaining them so that they remain in good condition.

The Prices Act (1974)

The price of products has to be displayed in order to prevent a false impression to the buyer.

The Trades Descriptions Act (1968 and 1972)

Products must not be falsely or misleadingly described in relation to their quality, fitness, price or purpose, by advertisements, orally, displays or descriptions. And since 1972 it has also been a requirement to label a product clearly, so that the buyer can see where the product was made.

Briefly, a retailer cannot:

- mislead consumers by making false statements about products
- offer sale products at half price unless they have been offered at the actual price for a reasonable length of time.

The Resale Prices Act (1964 and 1976)

The manufacturers can supply a recommended price (MRRP or manufacturers' recommended retail price), but the seller is not obliged to sell at the recommended price.

EKU statement

G11 (eku6) Your salon's procedures for monitoring the use of resources

G11 (eku8) Principles of stock control

G11 (eku10) How salon ordering systems work and how to interpret them

G11 (eku11) The importance of keeping accurate records for the use and monitoring of resources

G11 (eku12) The resource records for which you are responsible

Stock and stock control

Stock is a valuable resource of the business and at any one time; the business may have large amounts of money tied up in it. It is essential that stock; is used appropriately, that wastage is kept at an absolute minimum and that it is kept secure whilst on the premises.

Stock levels can only be maintained if accurate records are kept of how much stock the business has. Stock records should be able to accurately show:

- the minimum holding levels of each product line that the business needs
- the current levels of each of those product lines
- the items that need to be reordered.

Good stock-keeping practice

Monitor the usage of products against the minimum holding levels, so that stock needs are anticipated and reordered before the business runs out. Quite simply, good practice would be placing orders when stock levels run low.

Check deliveries when they arrive against the delivery note. The delivery note is not necessarily a copy of what has been ordered, it is a list of what has been dispatched by the supplier.

The order specified is not always what has been delivered; this can be different if:

- the products ordered are out-of-stock at the suppliers, or
- the products delivered do not tally with the delivery note and are therefore missing.

And in cases where the delivery not does tally with the stock delivered, the stock should always be checked to see that it is not damaged or that it has not deteriorated.

Stock control

The systems that your salon uses will provide management with up-to-date information for controlling stock. You can support your salon by helping to maintain stock control. These systems will deal with:

- reordering stock
- movements of stock
- usage of stock
- shortages of stock
- the safety and security of stock.

Consumables may be used in the salon or sold to clients for home use. Either way the salon must have enough stock or it won't be able to function. Products are purchased by the salon in varying quantities, for short-term or long-term availability. To ensure that the products remain usable or saleable, the stock controller must monitor them and will therefore need to be aware of:

- shelf life
- handling
- losses
- damage.

Stock held in store is a valuable asset to the company. The stock controller is responsible for its safe storage between delivery and use or sale.

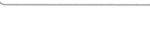

TUTOR SUPPORT

Project 16.2: Stock levels

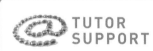

TUTOR SUPPORT

Discussion 16.5: Stock the products required to deliver services

TUTOR SUPPORT

Discussion 16.6: Stock control

Activity

Dealing with resources

This activity looks at the problems associated with shortages, surpluses and breakdowns of salon resources. Complete the table below with the missing information and keep a copy for use in your own portfolio.

Resource issue	What are the possible reasons for this problem?	What could happen if this is not addressed?	Suggest possible ways to resolve the issue.
Stock shortages			
Stock excess			
Stylist overbooked			
Stylist 'off' ill			
Stylist running late			
Equipment breakdowns			
Backlog of clients waiting for a basin			

Stocktaking

Items for use such as tools, small pieces of equipment and potentially hazardous chemicals should be kept in a locked store, the size of which will depend on the salon and its needs. Individual items are accounted for by stocktaking.

Stocktaking at regular intervals provides management with up-to-date information of stock movement. Without regular stocktaking, individual items and product lines could run out, creating a situation in which services and treatments normally offered were not available. This would mean lost profit to the salon, both at the time and later through a damaged reputation. Every business requires accurate, reliable accounting systems which:

- categorise products
- monitor usage
- identify shortages
- report damages or defects
- update records.

These guidelines provide the basis for a simple yet effective stock management system.

Product coding

Many salons now use the technology of personal computers to produce management information. Stock control is one of the facilities available in software systems for salon management. Salons turning over large quantities of stock find it helpful to devise coding systems for the products they use and sell.

The product's manufacturer, its category, name and size can all be stored as a single alpha numerical code, the product code. These codes can streamline the processes of stock control, monitoring, pricing and tax calculation.

Remember

Stock rotation
When new stock is placed on shelves for sale or use, ensure that old products are brought forward so that they may be sold first.

EKU statement

G11 (eku9) The stocking levels for your salon

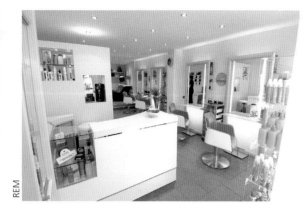

REM

Products received into storage are individually itemised and allocated the relevant product code. The information is then fed into the computer, as is the information that a product has been used or sold. The computer continually recalculates the stock levels, providing management with automated stock control information and printouts for use in manual stocktaking checks. This coded system is one form of point-of-sale (POS) management; another system uses barcoding. The principle here is exactly the same, but the product information is converted into a series of stripes printed on labels or directly on to the product. The barcodes can be read directly by the computer via a scanning barcode reader, which recognises the product and makes the necessary stock control adjustments.

Remember

If your salon uses tubes of permanent colour, encourage staff to replace part-tubes in original packaging with a clear indication of how much is left.

Ordering stock

Products are purchased either directly from the manufacturer or via a wholesaler, on a credit- or cash-based agreement. Credit account terms are arranged with the supplier, usually on a monthly payment system.

Stock records and recording stock movements

Placing an order

A salon's order may be placed with a company representative, who completes a purchase order on the salon's behalf. The purchase order is a paper system documenting all the manufacturer's product listings and categories. This is returned to the company so that the order can be processed and despatched.

Taking delivery

When the stock order arrives at the salon it will be accompanied by a delivery note that will list the items so far despatched and any that are to follow, such as items temporarily out of stock. The delivery note must be checked against the contents of the consignment and discrepancies or damages in transit identified before countersigning the order and confirming the delivery. Any discrepancies between the documents should be referred to the management for later adjustment. The incoming stock should be moved immediately from reception to a secure location away from the working area of the salon. At a convenient time the salon stock systems can be updated and stock put into storage.

After a period of time the supplier will send an invoice, a request for payment. Details of the invoice must be checked against the delivery note and the stock actually received.

Choice of stock supplier

Wholesalers carry stock from a wide range of manufacturers, providing the salon owner with a choice of products and differing prices to suit various budgets. When orders are placed through a manufacturer's representative, the salon is restricted to buying the products available from that manufacturer.

Activity
A manual stock recording system

This activity will provide you with a working system for operating a small, but effective manual stock record system.

Keep copies of the stock control sheets that you create over an 8–12-week period so that you can collect a reasonable amount of data for use in your portfolio.

The example shown in the figure below provides a simple format for a paper-based stock recording system. We can see that in the first column there is a range of product types: each family of products – shampoos, conditioners etc. – is grouped together. In the next column the product's unit size is identified.

The next two columns are each repeated several times. These contain space to enter the date product minimum holding levels, amount in stock and quantities for order. Stock is then ordered when the amounts fall below the minimum holding levels. When repeated over several columns it is easy to identify faster moving products and trends or patterns.

Stock Master		Date 12/Sept /10			Date			Date		
Salon retail products	Size	Minimum Holding Level	In Stock	Order	Minimum Holding Level	In Stock	Order	Minimum Holding Level	In Stock	Order
Shampoos										
Moisturising	250ml	4	3	1 box						
Enriching	250ml	4	4	0						
Revitalising	250ml	3	7	0						
Oil control										
Conditioners										
Protein	250ml	4	2	1 box						
Colour care	250ml	4	2	1 box						
Moisturising	400ml	2	4	0						
Frequent Use	400ml	2	4	0						

You may be able to visit a nearby wholesale cash-and-carry warehouse. Such warehouses provide an alternative service to the salon, holding stocks ranging from consumable product lines to sundry items such as towels, gowns and hair ornaments, and even coffee and washing powders.

Wholesalers like this provide the salon with a one-stop shopping facility.

Stock handling

Most products used by salons are packaged and many are chemicals. Movements of stock into or within the salon may involve lifting, stacking, dispensing, displaying or pricing, all of which are subject to stringent legislation (see Manual Handling Regulations 1992). The Health and Safety at Work Act 1974 relates to all workplace health and safety, although the Act has specific requirements for the employer.

Employees have a duty under the law not to endanger their own health or safety, or that of other people who may be affected by their actions. The responsibilities of the employer are summarised below:

- Ensure that the building and the people within it are as safe as possible.
- Train staff in safe working practices and the use of equipment.
- Maintain an accident book and provide first-aid facilities.
- Maintain all equipment and tools.
- Provide safe systems for the handling, transit and storage of all materials.
- Implement immediate action when any hazard is reported.
- If the salon employs more than five staff, provide a written health and safety policy describing arrangements for employees.

All cosmetic products come under strict legislation (Cosmetic Products Regulations 1989) and a specific guide to health and safety in the salon relating to the control of substances hazardous to health (the COSHH regulations) has been written by the Cosmetic, Toiletry and Perfumery Association (CTPA) with the cooperation of the Hairdressing and Beauty Suppliers' Association (HBSA).

This guide assesses substances potentially hazardous to health and provides information to employers about exercising adequate controls.

Apart from basic rules for hairdressers relating to hair product and salon safety, substances are categorised as 'potential' or 'unlikely' hazards. Each type of product identified is specified by:

- name – including ingredients and a general description
- health hazard – from inhalation, ingestion, absorption, contact or injection
- precautions – during work activity, storage, and disposal or spillage
- first aid – in relation to eyes, skin or ingestion
- fire risk – if applicable.

Security

Stock in storage is a valuable asset to the company. Thieves are often opportunist, not always planning their activities. They will seize opportunities as they arise – money left around, products on display, unlocked doors and open windows. You should take all necessary precautions to maintain a secure working environment.

Remember

If you are unsure about the contents of your salon's products, contact your supplier for relevant COSHH information.

Science

Good practice/Health and safety

Don't:
- leave keys in locks or lying around
- leave products or valuables unattended
- allow unauthorised entry, even by friends or family, to staff-only areas.

Do:
- report to management any items that appear to be missing
- ensure that materials and equipment are returned to safe areas
- make available company policy with regard to theft, loss, or damages.

Avoiding waste and damage

Regular checks on goods through careful stock control will assist in minimising short-ages, but shortages can still occur if items are neglectfully wasted, such as preparing a colour using a whole tube of colour where half would have been enough. Applications should be carefully measured. Manufacturers' recommendations can be found on all products.

Utilities   Staff should be given clear guidelines about the efficient use of utilities as wastage will increase costs for the salon. For example, taps should not be left on between shampoos. Hood dryers should not be left running after the client has finished. Personal calls should not be made from the salon telephones.

Tools and equipment   Regular checks on tools and equipment will help minimise problems. These may still occur, however, if items are misused. Using tools for purposes other than those intended could be negligent, if not dangerous. Think of the risks involved in changing a plug using a pair of scissors instead of a screwdriver. Staff must know how to use and maintain tools and equipment in the proper manner and should be given relevant health and safety training.

Main reasons for monitoring tools and equipment:

- to maintain the correct numbers of working items that are needed to provide an uninterrupted, smooth salon operation should any damages or broken items occur
- to identify which items need replacing or updating to maintain the levels of service.

Space   Effective use of space should also be monitored. Turnover can be measured against the square metre to gauge the productivity of a given area; for example, retail sales.

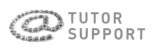

TUTOR SUPPORT

Discussion 16.4: How equipment contributes to the effectiveness and profitability of the salon

EKU *statement*

G11 (eku20) General principles of time management applicable to the delivery of salon services

Time and time management

The resource that once lost, can never be replaced

Time is a resource that, although not tangible, is of importance to the financial effec-tiveness of the business. It affects issues such as pricing structure and staff training. As the financial income of the salon is largely based on client service, the price structure will reflect on the length of time a service takes. For example, a cut and blow dry may have a time allowance of 45 minutes, while a highlighting service may have an allowance of two hours and will therefore be correspondingly more expensive, irrespective of other resources that have been used, i.e. light and heat, laundered items, equipment and products.

TUTOR SUPPORT

Project 16.3: Time management and productivity

Ineffective use of time comes from not doing the right job at the right time. Wasted or what we can now call lost time cannot be made back up in the normal allocation of work. So therefore by having to spend extra time clawing back to where we were before, we expend more efforts and usually more money in the process. This ineffective work method is directly linked to inefficiency and is a burden on all those other people pulling together to try to work as a team.

Activity
Work study

Ask your fellow work colleagues if they mind taking part in a work survey.

Over a period of six observations, see how long it takes them to complete the following services:

- Cut and blow-dry (short hair including shampoo/conditioning, etc.)
- Cut and blow-dry (shoulder length hair including shampoo/conditioning, etc.)
- Blow-dry (short hair including shampoo/conditioning, etc.)
- Blow-dry (shoulder length hair including shampoo/conditioning, etc.)

Now make your evaluation of the work study by answering these questions:

1   What was the average time taken for each service?
2   What was the longest and shortest time taken in each case?

In answering questions 1 and 2 now draw your conclusions by answering these final questions:

a)   Have you any suggestions how the results of (Q2) can be improved?
b)   What did the stylists feel about the time available for each instance?
c)   How does this fit in with the salon's expected timescales?

Keep the results of your survey in your portfolio for future use.

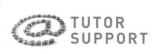

TUTOR SUPPORT

Discussion 16.2: How managing time contributes to the effectiveness and profitability of the salon

Time management

We could probably think that as hairdressers we are good managers of time, particularly when our total working life insists that we work and keep to time. We may never keep clients waiting, not even five minutes, but it doesn't end there. It's not just how we manage our time in our work that counts. It's a lot more to do with how much impact does our work have on other's time. Do we shine purely by eroding other people's time? Quite simply, putting it another way, do we achieve our goals at someone else's expense? If you are busy in constant turmoil, other staff will be affected in the same way and in turn this will affect someone's clients, if not your own.

Get organised

If you don't take control and organise your time, you'll never have time for anything. After people, time is the most important asset to the business so it must be used constructively. You have to take control of the time at your disposal and decide how you want to spend it.

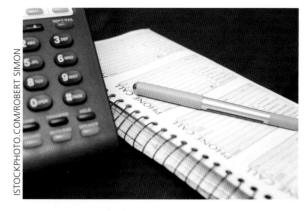

ISTOCKPHOTO.COM/ROBERT SIMON

Prioritising things to do

Tasks need to be graded in order of priority. For example, it may be your job to check the stock levels on a weekly basis. If this is not done at the right time, what happens? Don't waste time dealing with non-urgent tasks. Make a list of things to do. Once you have a complete list of everything to do, you can set about prioritising the content. (This list could be tabulated, see below.) Lists are very useful time management tools, but they only work if you stick to them rigidly. Find a system that works for you and a way of keeping your list to hand so that you can work with it, add to it and finally cross things off when completed.

Write things down

People are neither computers nor infallible. If you don't write things down you may forget some of them, only remembering at the last minute or too late. Build list-writing into a daily routine and set aside time to review the items on the list on a regular basis. There is a saying: 'Never handle a piece of paper more than once.' Attend to the important issues as soon as possible. We could all spend our lives putting them off until tomorrow so if we get those annoying little things done straight away we could save so much time.

People who are really in control of their time plan their activities, remembering that social and leisure time are just as important as their working life.

Activity
Create a things to do list
Writing things down is a very easy and effective way of remembering what has to be done and is a major contribution to effective time management.

Create your own things to do list by copying an example of the table below. You can then complete the activity by writing down the things that you need to do and when they have to be done by.

Cross them off when you have completed them and you also benefit from seeing what you have achieved.

My things to do list

Things to do today	Things to do this week	Things to do this month

G11.2   Meet productivity and development targets

Fierce competition is the driver for improvement and in order to keep ahead of the competition, it is essential that you strive to improve your own skills and learn new things. Learning new things means changing what you do now to meet the expectations of the clients tomorrow.

Your employer already has a plan of how they will take the business forward or keep abreast of the competition. You might be able to see gaps in the range of services that your salon delivers to its clients, or think of ways in which there is room for improvement; if you do have ideas report them to your line manager.

Ideally, you should be able to analyse your own performance in the salon and identify areas where there are weaknesses; which provides you with room to improve.

Maintaining productivity

Low productivity is the result of poor service, lack of training and ineffective use of materials and time. The guaranteed outcome of this is easy to forecast. It also signifies a failure of management. If people are not given the time, skills and materials in the first place, they can not achieve anyway.

Good productivity is the result of achievement, so it is easy to see that in order to achieve there must be clear objectives. Targets should be clearly understood and attainable. Virtually all salons work on the basis that stylists earn a basic salary with commission incentive scheme. Commission is payable as a bonus on top of wages when individual or group targets have been achieved.

Targets

We may not like the thought of targets, but we all need them. We all like the benefits that come with achievement: credit and praise, higher self-esteem, increased confidence, an ability to please others and, last but not least, rewards. All these are positive outcomes for doing what is expected of us. They are the food on which we all thrive. Collectively, well-defined targets forge a unity within a working team that acts as a motivator for everyone involved.

Targets should be an incentive though. In order for people to respond to the challenge, the targets should be realistic, achievable and tailored to the individual. Unrealistic targets, which from the outset are perceived as unrealistic and unachievable, will have a very negative impact. The result will be a reduction in the bond of the working team and demotivation in the struggling individual.

Targets are not just about selling though. The targets that you will encounter at work can also be relevant to personal learning.

Activity
Strengths and weaknesses chart
This activity provides a way for you to study and assess your strengths and weaknesses at work and to provide a course of action for the future.

When you have filled in the table below ask your supervisor to check your responses.

Personal skill	My strengths	My weaknesses	Action to take
Dealing with clients			
Dealing with complaints			
Communicating with work colleagues			
Organising work for others			
Helping others in their work			
Sorting out problems			

SMART productivity

For a hairdressing business to be successful, the salon owner has to take an overall view of productivity. As we have established the business to be mainly labour intensive, there needs to be a continuous analysis of personal performance which can only be measured against a target figure.

First, the salon owner has to set an overall salon target. This figure can then be divided between departments of stylists, technical and retail. Each person in each department then has a personal target which they understand and agree with. The personal target can be worked out as follows:

Target = service price × number of clients

For example, if stylist Kerry charges £30 for a cut and blow-dry and can take ten clients a day, her daily takings for this service would be £300 and her weekly takings would be £1500 (based upon a five-day week). This may be adjusted to allow for different daily performances. We cannot ensure consistent bookings, although through analysis we can establish high and low points. In addition to the styling takings we would also expect some retail sales, so the overall personal target would include this. Target setting should follow the SMART principle and should be:

- **S**pecific – clearly defined
- **M**easurable – quantifiable in some way
- **A**greed – between both parties
- **R**ealistic – able to be achieved
- **T**imed – for the duration of a fixed time period

Targets may be confidential between the manager and employee, in which case salon procedures relating to confidentiality must be observed. Personal reviews or appraisals provide an opportunity for management to establish an employee's performance level, to compare it against her target and to discuss ways of improving productivity. Most hairdressing businesses work on an incentive payment scheme. This can have a major impact on the overall salary rates. The salon owner needs to establish fixed costs and variable costs and the wage percentage needs to be established in order for the necessary profit margins to be maintained. From the overall wage portion of income, an individual target is set for each stylist. See Chapter 16 for more on setting SMART objectives.

Recognise achievement

It's really about developing people's confidence and creating an environment of encouragement, but this has to be translated in the right way. Individuals should not only be allowed to make mistakes, but also given praise and recognition. There should be both financial targets and learning targets. Training is a major incentive – with relevant rewards.

Evaluating results

The benefits must suit individuals and prove worthwhile. Typical amounts spent vary from 3 to 5 per cent of turnover on training budgets, to 30 per cent salary equivalent on total packages. Measuring the return is notoriously difficult since incentives can have a ripple effect. But health care benefits (check-ups, dental treatments, counselling) are also tangibly cost effective.

EKU *statement*

G11 (eku21) How to plan and reschedule your own work and that of those who may assist you in order to maximise any opportunities to meet your targets

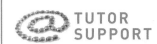 TUTOR
SUPPORT

Discussion 16.3: How products
contribute to the effectiveness
and profitability of the salon

Working together

Always remember that your work colleagues also need your help to meet their targets. Sharing the workload is working as a team and can be achieved by:

- providing support
- anticipating the needs of others
- maintaining harmony
- communicating effectively.

In some salons, you might see some staff busy attending to their clients while others hang about around reception, flicking through magazines or disappearing off to the staffroom for a coffee. Teamwork is about making an active contribution, seeking to assist others even if only by passing up rollers. It is good for staff morale and presents a good image to the clients. In short, make yourself useful and contribute to the team effort by assisting your fellow workers.

Anticipating the needs of others follows on from providing support. Clean and prepare the work areas ready for use, locate and prepare products as and when they are required. This will help the smooth operation of the salon. Cooperate with your colleagues. Make a positive contribution to your team by assisting them to provide a well-managed and coordinated quality service. Be self-motivated and keep yourself busy. Don't wait to be asked to do things. Maintain harmony and try to minimise possible conflicts. Most good working relationships develop easily. However, others may need to be worked at. Whatever your personal feelings about your fellow work associates, the clients must never sense a bad atmosphere within the salon caused by a friction between staff. You will spend a lot of time in the company of people you work with, but you will not always like everyone you meet. At work, in order to maintain teamwork, a mutual respect for others is more important than close friendships. So remember, treat others with respect and be sensitive and responsive to other's feelings. Show concern and care for others.

Personal development

Managers of people use *performance appraisal* or *progress reviews* to evaluate the effectiveness of the work team. An appraisal is a system whereby you and your manager, in an interview situation, review and evaluate your personal contribution and/or progress over a predetermined period of time, as measured against expected targets or standards.

A similar process would take place at suitable points within a personal programme of training in order to review progress and training effectiveness, measured against specific training objectives.

Measuring effectiveness

To measure progress towards overall work contributions as well as training targets, there need to be clear stated expectations of the performance required.

These standards should show:

- what tasks need to be performed
- what training activities will take place
- what standards are expected to be reached

- when assessment should be expected
- when a review of progress towards the agreed targets is to take place.

In normal, ongoing work situations, performance appraisal will be based on the following factors:

- results achieved against targets and job requirements
- additional accomplishments and contribution
- contribution made by the individual compared with those of other staff members.

The job requirements are outlined in the employee's job description. A job description is a written specification of the main purposes and functions expected within a given job. Good job descriptions will include the following:

- job title
- work locations
- responsibility (to whom and for what)
- the job purpose
- main functions (listed)
- standards expected
- any special conditions.

Standards expected from the job holder will often include behaviour and appearance. If these have been stated from the outset, the job holder will know what is expected of them.

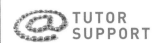

TUTOR SUPPORT

Short answer test

Activity

Identify strengths and weaknesses

Use this self-check-system before your appraisal as a way of appraising your own performance.

Keep a record for use in your portfolio.

Area of work	I am strong in this	I am not so good at this	Supervisor's comments
Consultation			
Communication			
Customer care			
Retailing			
Cutting			
Colouring			
Perming			
Styling and dressing			
Long hair-ups			
Extensions			
Health and safety			
Barbering			
Shaving			
Creative development			

TUTOR SUPPORT

Project 16.4: Job description and contract of employment

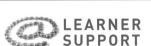

LEARNER SUPPORT

Contribute to financial effectiveness quiz

An example of job description

Job description – stylist	
Location:	Based at salon as advised
Main purpose of job:	To ensure customer care is provided at all times
	To maintain a good standard of technical and client care, ensuring that up-to-date methods and techniques are used following the salon training practices and procedures
Responsible to:	Salon manager
Requirements:	To maintain the company's standards in respect of hairdressing/beauty services
	To ensure that all clients receive service of the best possible quality
	To advise clients on services and treatments
	To advise clients on products and aftercare
	To achieve designated performance targets
	To participate in self-development or to assist with the development of others
	To maintain company policy in respect of:
	• personal standards of health/hygiene
	• personal standards of appearance/conduct
	• operating safety whilst at work
	• public promotion
	• corporate image
	as laid out in employee handbook
	To carry out client consultation in accordance with company policy
	To maintain company security practices and procedures
	To assist your manager in the provision of salon resources
	To undertake additional tasks and duties required by your manager from time to time

The appraisal process

At the beginning of the appraisal period, the manager and employee discuss jointly, develop, and mutually agree the objectives and performance measures for that period. An *action plan* will then be drafted, outlining the expected outcomes.

During the appraisal period, should there be any significant changes in factors such as objectives or performance measures, these will be discussed between the manager and employee and any amendments will be appended to the action plan.

At the end of the appraisal period, the results are discussed by the employee and the manager, and both manager and employee sign the appraisal. A copy is prepared for the employee and the original is kept on file.

An appraisal of performance will contain the following information:

- employee's name
- appraisal period
- appraiser's name and title
- performance objectives
- job title
- work location
- results achieved
- identified areas of strength and weakness
- ongoing action plan
- overall performance grading (optional).

Dealing with negative feedback

It is difficult for any conscientious person to take criticism. But negative feedback can be positive, particularly, if it is seen as an opportunity to improve.

It is not always easy to respond in a positive manner, especially when you have been given bad news about your performance and your initial feelings are of hurt or despair.

However, it is important that you try to remain positive and look upon it as a snapshot or part of something with a far bigger importance. Use it as a learning experience that you use, like a tool, to move onwards and upwards.

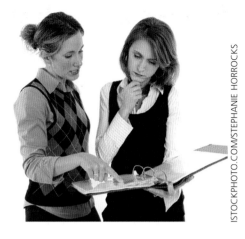

Self-appraisal

In order for you to manage yourself within the job role, you need to identify the areas where you meet the expectations of your job and also the areas where there is room for improvement. Measuring your own strengths and weaknesses against laid-down performance criteria (as found in the NVQ level 3 standards of competence) is one way of monitoring your own progress. Simply use the performance criteria set out within the standards as a checklist. This will help you to:

- identify areas where further training is required
- identify areas where further practice is needed
- identify areas where competence can be achieved.

Remember

When receiving negative feedback; it's not just what you say that counts, your body language may be screaming something else too.

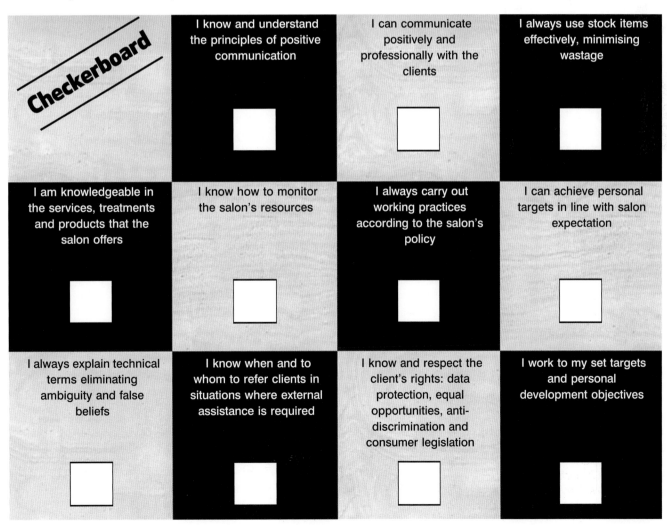

Checkerboard

I know and understand the principles of positive communication	I can communicate positively and professionally with the clients	I always use stock items effectively, minimising wastage
I am knowledgeable in the services, treatments and products that the salon offers	I know how to monitor the salon's resources	I always carry out working practices according to the salon's policy	I can achieve personal targets in line with salon expectation
I always explain technical terms eliminating ambiguity and false beliefs	I know when and to whom to refer clients in situations where external assistance is required	I know and respect the client's rights: data protection, equal opportunities, anti-discrimination and consumer legislation	I work to my set targets and personal development objectives

Assessment of knowledge and understanding

Revision questions

Quick quiz: a selection of different types of questions to check your knowledge.

Q1 A worker aged 18 or over cannot be forced to work for more than _____ hours a week (on average).

Fill in the blank

Q2 A key feature of good customer service is being customer focused.

True or false

Q3 Which of the following would be considered as an indication of poor communication?

Multi selection

Avoiding eye to eye contact	☐ 1
Smiling	☐ 2
Standing over the client and talking to them through the styling mirror	☐ 3
Talking with your hand covering your mouth	☐ 4
Being polite	☐ 5
Being courteous	☐ 6

Q4 Employees are entitled to regular breaks in the working day.

True or false

Q5 Which of these laws has specific relevance to holding peoples private information on computer?

Multi choice

Equal opportunities	○ a
Disability Discrimination Act (2005)	○ b
Data Protection Act (1998)	○ c
The Prices Act (1974)	○ d

Q6 Stock rotation means turning products around on the shelves so they don't get too dusty.

True or false

Q7 Which of the following are advisable when dealing with a client's complaint?

Multi selection

Find out what the problem is	☐ 1
Keep them waiting so that they cool off	☐ 2
Assess the validity of the complaint	☐ 3
Let them have a rant then you can retaliate	☐ 4
Move them to a quieter part of the salon	☐ 5
Let someone else deal with it	☐ 6

Q8 A _____ note should accompany ordered stock when it arrives at the salon.

Fill in the blank

Q9 Which legislation protects the clients from defective purchases?

Multi choice

Data Protection Act (1998)	○ a
The Sale of Goods Act (1979)	○ b
Disability Discrimination Act (DDA 2005)	○ c
The Prices Act (1974)	○ d

Q10 A barcode is the same as having a personal ID card.

True or false

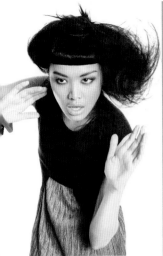

H32

H32.1
H32.2
H32.3

**CREDIT VALUE
FOR UNIT H32**
5 Credits

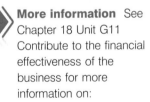
More information See
Chapter 18 Unit G11
Contribute to the financial
effectiveness of the
business for more
information on:

● Consumer rights and
products sales
legislation

● Data Protection Act

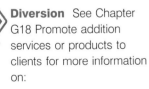
Diversion See Chapter
G18 Promote addition
services or products to
clients for more information
on:

● Selling skills
EKU H32.21,
EKU H32.22 and
EKU H32.23

● Features and benefits
of services and
products

Chapter**seventeen**
Planning promotional activities

Promotional activities: quick overview

Unit title

H32   Contribute to the planning and implementation of promotional activities

This is an **optional** unit for hairdressing and barbering at level 3, it is made up of three main outcomes

Main outcomes

H32.1   Contribute to the planning and preparation of promotional activities

H32.2   Implement promotional activities

H32.3   Participate in the evaluation of promotional activities

What do I need to do for H32.1?

● Make recommendations for promotional activities to management

● Agree activity objectives with the relevant person

● Produce a detailed plan of the promotional activity

● Ensure that planned activities comply with legislation

What do I need to do for H32.2?

● Carry out the planned promotional activity

● Use the available resources in an effective way

● Communicate the features and benefits to the target group in a suitable way

● Encourage participation by prompting the target group to ask questions

● Encourage the target group to take advantage of promoted services or treatments

Keywords

Features

The aspects of a product or service that state its functions; i.e. what it does

Benefits

The ways in which the functions provide advantages

SMART

An acronym used for setting objectives i.e. **S**pecific, **M**easurable, **A**chievable, **R**ealistic and **T**imed

Information covered in this chapter

- The planning considerations for implementing a promotional event
- How to create a detailed plan
- How to present information to others
- How to communicate effectively
- How to identify the objectives of a promotional event
- How to work collectively to achieve the business goals
- Other useful reference information

What do I need to do for H32.3?

- Gain feedback from your promotional activity and collate the findings
- Evaluate the effectiveness of the activity and summarise a report
- Make recommendations for future promotional activities

What aspects do I need to cover for H32.1, H32.2 and H32.3?

- Demonstrations, promotional displays and advertising campaigns
- Ways of enhancing the image of the salon and increase business

What do I need to know for H32.1, H32.2 and H32.3?

- The restrictions that need to be considered at the planning stage; i.e legal issues, available size/space, health and safety and contractual obligations
- The hazards that could arise in implementing the promotional activity
- The reasons for creating a clear, detailed plan for the event
- How to write SMART objectives
- The importance of working to a budget
- How to present clear accurate information to all concerned
- The importance of delegation in team activities
- How to present features and benefits to a target group
- How to recognise buying opportunities and tailor presentation information to specific individuals
- The skills of professional communication in promotional contexts
- How to evaluate the outcomes of the event

Introduction

Salon promotional activities have a simple purpose; they are designed to stimulate interest and generate revenue. The interest is not just for the target group though; as the staff involved in these sorts of events, will be motivated by their participation too. It promotes a sense of renewal, a break from the general day to day routines, which is exciting in itself.

You will need to work with other people as part of a team and like any team sport; you all have a role to play. You need to develop your skills; in thorough planning, careful research and a close attention to detail.

Get it right and everyone wins; get it wrong and it could be GAME OVER.

Initial preparation

There are all sorts of promotional events that you can get involved with; some of them will be internal others may be external. The bigger the ideas are, the more complex it becomes. If this is something that you find really exciting, then the table below sets out the initial things that you must consider first.

Planning a promotion overview

What type of event do you want to put on?
What is the purpose of the event?

Is it an internal event?	Is it an external event?
-1 Window displays **0** Internal product promotion **1** Internal display **2** Demonstration	**1** Demonstration **2** Hair show **3** Seminar

What is the budget?
What resources will you need?
When will it take place?
Who will be involved?
What preparation or training is needed for participating staff?
What advance notification, publicity or advertising is needed?
How will you get the message across to the target group?
What advantages will there be by implementing the event?
How will you evaluate the event?

EKU *statement*

H32 (eku7) The purpose and value of detailed and accurate planning

H32 (eku8) The type of resourcing requirements necessary for promotional activities (e.g. individuals, tools and equipment, materials, time, venue)

H32 (eku9) How the nature of the target group can influence the choice of promotional activity

H32 (eku10) How to match types of promotional activities to objectives

H32 (eku11) How to present a plan for promotional activities

H32 (eku12) Why it is important to consider methods of evaluation at the planning stage

H32 (eku13) How to write objectives that are Specific, Measurable, Achievable, Realistic and Time Bound (i.e. SMART objectives)

H32 (eku14) The importance of working to a budget

H32 (eku15) Where and how to obtain resources

H32 (eku16) The importance of clearly defining roles and responsibilities of those involved in promotional activities

This model provides a quick overview of the information that you need to consider before you start, make a copy so that you can cover the answers to all the questions before you put it before management.

Finding a comprehensive answer to all of those questions may take you a lot of time, particularly if you haven't had any experience in planning an event before. But unless you can be convincing with your proposition to management, your plans are likely to come to grief!

EKU *statement*

H32 (eku20) The features and benefits of the products and/or services being promoted

If planning is a new experience to you, don't panic, you need to rationalise your thoughts into something that gives you the framework of a plan and management something to go on.

The first things to consider are the *five servants* (shown in the activity below). If you want to put forward an idea to management for a promotional activity, you need to be clear in your own mind why the event is useful at all.

Activity
Preparing your promotional ideas

Useful suggestions for finding ways of stimulating business are always going to be allowed to get an airing.

So what ideas do you have?

As a way of initially looking at possible ideas, try assembling your thoughts by filling in the table below. This will help you to get a more balanced view of the essential basic information.

WHAT?	WHY?	WHERE?	WHO?	HOW?

With that exercise completed you can now consider the following before making your pitch.

Working to a budget

One of the biggest considerations that you have to make is: will the outcomes or objectives be sufficient to warrant the cost of the event?

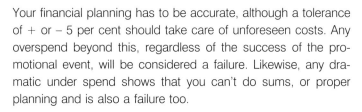

M. BALFRE

Your financial planning has to be accurate, although a tolerance of + or − 5 per cent should take care of unforeseen costs. Any overspend beyond this, regardless of the success of the pro-motional event, will be considered a failure. Likewise, any dra-matic under spend shows that you can't do sums, or proper planning and is also a failure too.

Getting the sums right means that you have planned down to the last photocopied leaflet or product used within the event. If you involve external suppliers, make sure that you get written quotes to back-up your plans. If they change the rules at some later time at least you have given management something to bargain with.

If several people are involved with the financial side then you will need regular reports from them to check on progress.

Decide on the type of promotion

There are many possibilities and here are a few examples:

- themed window display for general salon promotion
- in-salon display to promote a new range of products

- introductory offers – offering a free retail conditioner for permed hair with each perm treatment
- carnival float – a general salon promotion through taking part in a local external event
- demonstration 'hair show'; either as an internal evening seminar, or as an external event at a venue suitable for the target group.

Setting your objectives

Your objectives should fulfil the business objectives; quite simply, they will be ways of:

- increasing salon business and
- enhancing the salon's image.

So as an acid test you can test your plans against the main overarching aspirations of the business and there are many ways in which those objectives can be met. For example, you could create an in-salon campaign to promote a new product range. Or, run a seminar to specific clients (who are not yet colour clients) on the range of effects that can be achieved through new partial colouring techniques.

When you set objectives you should follow the SMART principle. Your objectives should be:

- **S**pecific – clearly defined stating what it is that you want to achieve
- **M**easurable – have some form of evaluation that can measure the success
- **A**chievable – do you have the resources to attain the objectives
- **R**ealistic – relate to something that is achievable
- **T**imed – set within a fixed timeframe without over-running.

Most importantly, focus upon your target market or group: is your plan something that they *would or could* benefit from?

If you can honestly say yes to this question, you have a starting point.

Activity
Features and benefits
With your colleagues, select six of the services provided by your salon and jointly consider what the features and benefits to the client are in each case. Make a record of the collective opinions and keep this within your portfolio for future reference.

Remember

When running a salon promotion, everyone needs to be informed about the campaign. Make sure before the promotion is rolled out that there are sufficient staff meetings to make everyone aware of what is going on.

Define your target market

Different promotions or campaigns are going to suitable for different client (or potential client) groups. For example, what would be the point of planning an in-salon promotion for a new treatment for male pattern baldness if the majority of clients are female? Similarly, what would be the expected attendance if you planned an external event over the August bank holiday?

You need to look closely at the target group that you are trying to aim at and focus upon their needs and social patterns.

If you were planning a catwalk show case of new looks, say for example, at a local night club, what time would be preferable to maximise the audience?

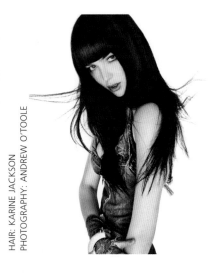

When you have defined the target group and the age range that it relates to, you need to think about the visual content of your programme.

- Is it going to be stimulating to the audience?
- Is it going to promote feedback from the audience?
- How will you respond to the feedback from the audience?
- Is it going to enhance the salon's name?

Pitch your idea

The term 'pitch' is marketing jargon for attempting to gain interest or business. An advertising agency *pitches* its ideas to prospective clients in the hope that their detailed outline plan is *bought* by the client. If the agency is successful, it produces an agreement that the newly acquired client signs and this confirms the business arrangement for the campaign, or agency services over a set period of time.

You might think, what's that got to do with me?

In a way, you are doing exactly the same. It may not be for the same scale of campaign, it may not involve anything like the same sorts of budget. But in essence, you are putting your neck on the block. If you get it right, you might find that your work role and respect takes off like a rocket!

In a pitch at an advertising or PR agency, the presenter will use the industry standard tools for conveying their ideas. These are:

- PowerPoint – for digital presentation
- a Flip Chart – for writing ideas on.

Ideally, if you want to make the most of your pitch to management, you would use one or both of these too. Being able to stand up and present ideas to others is a major attribute and as a hairdresser you might be finding it similar to what you already do with your clients every day.

Checklist for making your presentation

✔	Have you created an outline plan?
✔	Have you timed your presentation?
✔	Are your objectives clearly defined?
✔	Have you costed out your promotional activity?
✔	Have you provided any copies for management to take away?

Produce a detailed plan

The previous topics have given you the basics for:

- the initial preparation
- setting your objectives
- working to a budget
- defining your target market
- deciding on the type of promotion
- pitching your idea.

This is the starting point. It is pointless to 'put the flesh on the bones' at these stages until you have had the go-ahead from management. But the initial planning was worth it because it enabled you to get to this point and get the 'Yes, in principle' response.

Now this is where the work really starts, because you have to hone down on each aspect of the promotion to produce an expanded, detailed plan that would still be acceptable to management.

Activity

Detailed planning

This activity will help you to produce a detailed plan for your selected promotional event. Any materials that are produced such as; designs, photographs, storyboards, checklists, copies of invoices and quotations, should all be kept for final compilation in your portfolio.

First of all, go back to the beginning, to the section covering initial preparation, then.

1   For each aspect covered on the promotional blueprint produce a new sheet of paper and put them into a ring binder or presenter.

2   Label each sheet of paper with a title from the blueprint.

3   Now, on each sheet mark out the page with a table with the following headings.

Event element: .... (What is it?)

How does it fit into the plan?	Who needs to be involved?	When does it need to be done by?	What does it cost?	Done √

4   Complete each section with as much information that you have at this stage.

5   Now add into each of these sections any pictures, magazine snippings, drawings etc. to illustrate your ideas as a storyboard.

6   Now create your Master list (a composite document) that will go at the front of the binder; it will be a table or list that covers all the pages and components of your plan listed in chronological (timed) order.

Event master list

Item	Date	Event element	Running total £	Done √	Page
1					
2					
3					

The size of the list of items will depend on the scale of the event, but by doing this you will have a detailed binder that you can use to show to management as a progress report and finally presentation folder that has documented evidence of your planning abilities.

Other things to consider

Order stock and promotional materials

You may need to have leaflets printed or place an advertisement to inform potential clients. You may need additional materials: for instance, for a perm promotion you will need to order additional perms. Most product houses will provide advice and merchandising support.

Inform staff

Ensure that all staff is fully aware of the promotion. This may require refresher training, for example, in product knowledge, new skills or treatments. You cannot ask people to take part in an event if they don't have the skills to carry it off.

Your presentation to the staff needs to make them enthusiastic, they need to feel part of a team event and they too need to have the same positive outlook so that you all pull together on a united front. Only when they have the correct skills and advance knowledge, will they then be able to sell the concept on to clients.

Advertise the event

Select the best medium of communication. You may inform clients verbally. You may try a mailshot, distribute leaflets, display posters or notices, or advertise in local papers or selected magazines. In any written literature, remember to highlight the features and benefits of the service.

Evaluate and record the results

To make full use of the results, you need to keep a permanent record of the facts. This record can then be referred to later. Gradually you will identify strengths and weaknesses and be able to repeat or amend the promotion, depending upon the results.

Promotional outline: ....

Date .... Leaflets mailshot (No.)...

.... Posters (No.)..

.... Advertisement (type/place): ....

Leaflets returned: Week ending: .... No.: ....

Week ending: .... No.: ....

Week ending: .... No.: ....

Week ending: .... No.: ....

New clients recorded:

Revenue increases: Cutting: ....%

Cutting: ....%

Perm: ....%

Sales: ....%

Beauty: ....%

Comments: ....

Hairdressing demonstration

Hairdressing demonstrations form a very important part in training and promotion. Displays, both of the skill of the hairdresser's technique and the finished style that they can produce, provide opportunities for increasing sales. Informally, of course, every person working in the salon is continually demonstrating their skills from shampooing through to technical services, but there is also a place for the formal demonstration. To organise a demonstration, you again need to keep to a structure in your planning.

Select the venue

Is the demonstration going to be carried out in the salon, or at a local hall or hotel?

- Will the audience be able to see the demonstration area? Are lighting and sound provided? Can you make use of a raised platform or stage, panoramic mirrors, or revolving hydraulic chairs?
- Are shampooing and dressing facilities available?
- Do you need to arrange transport to the venue for your models and equipment?
- Is the venue easily accessible to your audience by public transport? Are there parking facilities?
- Will you offer refreshments?

The requirements and restrictions of any external locations are far more problematic than running an event on the premises. You will also have to consider the following aspects:

- *Accessibility* – How will your audience get in, where do they park?
- *Health and safety* – Who is responsible for public and staff safety?
- *First aid/emergencies* – What facilities are provided for emergencies?
- *Insurance* – Has the venue got a public liability policy?
- *Risk assessment* – Commercial venues have assessments they can show you. However, if your activity presents a different use; you need to do an assessment too.
- *Legislation* – Are there any local or national laws affecting your proposal?
- *Contracts* – Are there any contractual obligations with external contacts that tie you into timescales, cancellation clauses, hidden costs or penalties?

Plan the demonstration

Consider the model, the content, the method and the explanation. Depending on the scale of the demonstration, you may need to build in opportunities for the audience to participate and ask questions. This is not possible when demonstrating to a very large number of people, but good communication skills are always essential in creating a rapport with your audience.

Remember

Create a plan
- Identify the objectives. What is the purpose of the demonstration? Is it, for example, staff training or salon promotion?
- Prepare the resources. What resources do you need? How many people do you expect to attend?

Remember

Storyboarding
Be professional. Always create a storyboard of the event processes and actions, starting with the listings of equipment and resources, people, contact information and other external factors, right through to the expected running pattern of the event.

During the planning of the promotion, always remember to update your storyboard in line with any changes.

EKU *statement*

H32 (eku19) The types of foreseeable problems that occur and ways of resolving them

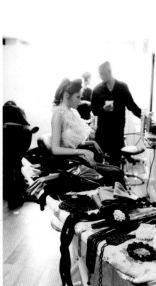

Remember

Planning ahead ensures smooth running.

Expect the unexpected

To maintain control of the event, your preparation needs to include contingency plans in the event of things going wrong.

For example, what would you do:

- if your models did not arrive on time
- if your guest artist was delayed
- if there was a power failure
- if there was a emergency evacuation
- if you do not achieve your desired result?

Give thought to each component of the event and be mentally prepared for any eventuality. You will then feel confident and your demonstration will be a success.

Make a time schedule

Once you have planned the event, it is advisable to make a checklist with a time schedule. To do this, start with the event time and work backwards, for example:

6.00 pm	The event. Guest artist will demonstrate the latest long hair fashion.
5.30 pm	Facility open to the audience.
5.00 pm	Final check: platform, demonstration chair, lighting, microphone/sound. Feed models and platform artist.
4.30 pm	Check platform tools and equipment. Prepare tray: this should contain everything that the artist will use during their demonstration. Check that all sprays work. (For a cutting demonstration it is a good idea to include a plaster – even the best hairdressers cut their fingers occasionally.)
3.30 pm	Model to be made up.
3.00 pm	Arrival of make-up artist.
2.00 pm	Arrival of model and guest artist.
12.00 noon	Organiser to arrive at venue. Arrange eating, erect display material. Check preparation area.

Alongside this schedule, make a checklist of each item needed or the event.

Communicating the message

The style of communication that you use is going to depend upon the promotional event.

For example, if you are running an in-salon promotion then you will probably be dealing with your potential purchaser on a one-to-one basis. There is enough material within this book to take you through the selling skills needed to make the most of your selling opportunity. See Chapter 2, Unit G18 Promote additional services to clients.

However, if you are conducting an in-salon seminar or an external event, you will now be dealing with a one-to-many situation. The style of communication in this scenario is completely different.

Presentation and demonstration skills

Regardless of how interesting the content of your presentation is; you need to remember that your audience will only have an attention span of 20 minutes at best! So with this in mind you need to schedule the content of your event in a way that it re-awakes your audience with something interesting and different. Your audiences are not hairdressers and barbers; so to watch a technical seminar with your leading hairstylists banging on about precision layering and weight positioning at the occipital will not necessarily have much impact.

But people are really impressed with visual magic. The elements of surprise, wonder and vibrant colour are psychologically very stimulating. So showcases of hair work teamed with current seasons clothes are always a winner. Similarly, makeovers are really popular and visually stimulating; so if you really want to impress, *turn a frog into a princess.*

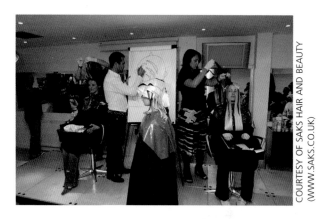

COURTESY OF SAKS HAIR AND BEAUTY (WWW.SAKS.CO.UK)

The most impressive makeover done to a large TV audience was initially, by Vidal Sassoon (for *The Generation Game* in 1973) and it was then copied by Lee Stafford in a live show 30 years later. The response to the original 1970s TV programme was huge. It made an already successful, professionally respected hairdressing company into a national household name, and the no longer practising Vidal Sassoon into a legend.

The makeover took 60 seconds! Vidal Sassoon is sitting talking with the game show host, the host asks to see a demonstration of his expertise. So a tall, beautiful, blonde model with beyond-the-shoulder, one-length hair is brought onto stage. She kneels on the stage facing the studio audience. VS asks her to put her head forwards and then carefully brushes all of her hair into a single ponytail, about a hands width away from a position just above the forehead. He then asks the model to reach up and hold the pony above his hand and then takes a pair of scissors from his suit top pocket and cuts the whole pony off, just above his hand and below hers!

She stands up and shakes her head, her hair then falls into a beautifully layered, graduated transformation and she holds up the pony to the audience. The whole thing takes less than a minute and has the visual imagery of a religious execution. The visual impact was stunning and it produced the first ever live makeover. Lee did the same show live but with a young child, not quite the same impact as with an adult but still impressive.

The point that is being made here is that:

'It's not about great hairdressing it's about showmanship.'

This story is an example of magic and you too can create the same long lasting impressions and be talked about for years *if* you can pull off the same sort of stunt. *But remember: ask your model if they want that much cut off first!*

When you are demonstrating or presenting remember this checklist:

Presenting points to remember

✔	Be clear about what it is that you want to sell
✔	Break down your presentation into a sequence of logical parts or steps
✔	Keep the presentation at a steady pace; don't rush, take your time

EKU *statement*

H32 (eku28) How and when to make openings to encourage others to ask questions

H32 (eku29) How to answer questions and manage queries in a way likely to maintain goodwill

✔	Encourage your audience to participate in some way; questions, volunteers etc.
✔	Keep lengthy technical processes to 20 min (or have other things going on too)
✔	Be professional, confident and assertive (*no shrinking violets*)
✔	Provide answers to audience questions in a way that everyone will understand
✔	If there are too many questions, say that you will make yourself available in the foyer afterwards so that the amount of feedback doesn't de-rail your programme
✔	If there isn't a flow of questions, then you can *fish* for a few by asking the obvious ones, like 'Does anyone here tonight, find that their hair lacks volume?'

Activity

Handling problems

Even the best planners can't plan for every eventuality. You can try to build contingencies into your planning, but there will always be the unexpected. What you can do though is work together with the team during the planning stage to brainstorm the sorts of things that could go wrong.

If you create a list from the brainstorming event work together with a flip chart to find solutions to the ones that you have found.

Try to cover a range of issues; here are a few to start you off:

1   How do you go about releasing a member of the audience who is in the toilet and can't get out?

2   You are halfway through the hair show and the lighting rig fuses and the stage lighting goes out.

3   You have one member of the audience that is becoming difficult and keeps asking questions and is stopping others from getting their points across.

4   Someone lets off the fire extinguisher in the reception area.

5   Progress through the programme is slow and the team are starting to seriously run over on time.

Advertising, PR and the Press

Advertising

Advertising is always a useful way of promoting your salon's services. It is important to define the purpose of the advertisement so that you can choose the most appropriate form of advertising:

- Do you want to attract new customers?
- Do you want to advertise a new service?
- Do you want to increase the salon's profile?
- Do you want to increase retail sales?
- Do you want to maintain loyalty with regular customers?
- Do you want to draw customers' attention to other services on offer?

Activity

Local research

Make a list of all the venues that can accommodate a seated audience of over 100 people in your local area.

What additional facilities do they have to offer?

Venue/size	Accessibility/parking	Facilities available

There are many different forms of advertising, including:

- magazines
- leaflets/posters
- newspapers
- local radio
- directories
- calendars.

Advertising can be very expensive. Therefore, the form of advertising you choose will also depend on the budget available. If you decide to advertise your business through printed media, careful consideration must be given to the content of the message you wish to convey. As this is a very special and important form of promotion you do need to consider whether the content as well as the origination is handled by the professionals.

Local newspapers and business directories provide comprehensive advertising services, hence combining all of the individual considerations listed below. However, their ability to get to know the needs of your particular business are poor. Here is a simplified overview of the different processes involved:

- *Commercial artist* – responsible for creating graphical illustrations through image manipulation and typography.
- *PR consultant/agency* – responsible for content and media management.
- *Reprographics* – the intermediaries, between the originators and printer, who create the film or digital output.
- *Printer* – the company employed to produce the finished material.

Public relations

Public relations (PR) is an effective tool with which to promote the business or product. It targets the media best suited to the company image or product profile, hence bringing the finished package to the eye of the consumer and thus increasing your business potential. Salons can opt to handle their own PR or employ the services of a PR constancy.

DIY PR With the right contacts and more importantly the time, it is possible to promote the business effectively as a team. However, be aware that dealing with the press is not necessarily a simple case of a phone call and then a letter. It is a question of knowing whom to contact, working on them and then how to get your message across. E-mail is

Remember

If you make contact with any representative of the local press, remember to get their direct e-mail address for swift access to the 'right' pair of eyes!

EKU statement

H32 (eku24) How and when to participate in discussions

H32 (eku25) How to give a short presentation (e.g. timing, pace, use of voice, use of graphics, etc.)

H32 (eku26) Methods of presenting information (e.g. pictorially, graphically, verbally)

H32 (eku27) Methods of creating a visual impact

H32 (eku28) How and when to make openings to encourage others to ask questions

H32 (eku29) How to answer questions and manage queries in a way likely to maintain goodwill

H32 (eku30) The purpose of evaluation activities

H32 (eku31) The areas of the promotional activity which should be evaluated

H32 (eku32) The most suitable methods of gaining feedback for the promotional activities in the range

H32 (eku33) How to collate, analyse and summarise evaluation feedback in a clear and concise way

H32 (eku34) Suitable ways of formatting and producing an evaluation report.

particularly useful medium for putting information on to the right desk and in front of the right eyes. However, it is also a question of degree: How much promotion do you want? Is it for one specific project or is it ongoing? If the latter, then be prepared for PR to take up a lot of your time.

The press

Trade and consumer press are completely different so it is therefore essential that they are each approached in the appropriate manner.

Trade press Aimed at other businesses within the same industry, the trade press is interested in news items within the trade (e.g. new salons, trends, techniques, etc., plus charity events and product launches). It is also very warm to launching new photographic collections, showcasing salon interiors and conducting business profiles. On the whole, trade journalists tend to be easier to deal with and more accessible. After all, they are already sympathetic to your salon's product and require your salon's help to fill their pages.

Consumer press Aimed at the general public, consumer magazines reach a great number of people who may never have heard of you or your product, but are about to do so through effective PR. Public relations is about editorial endorsement. This is quite different from advertising. It means the journalist is giving your salon magazine space without expecting any payment for it. Such editorial endorsement can be much harder to secure, but the benefits can be huge. The consumer press is not interested in new staff appointments, but it does want to know about innovative techniques, upcoming seasonal trends, latest product advancements and new salons. Happily, more and more consumer magazines are coming round to the idea that the consumer is interested in her hair, and, through increased hairdressing standards and higher stylist profiles, are becoming increasingly confident in our industry. Magazines now have hair supplements banded to their issues and these have to be filled.

Hair salons and product companies with effective PR are the ones who are helping to fill these supplements and hair features, supplying press releases to the appropriate journalists outlining new techniques and products, photographic material, seasonal trends and quotes.

H32.3 Participate in the evaluation of promotional activities

LEARNER SUPPORT

Promote Additional Services puzzle

Why do an evaluation? If we look at a definition and the purpose of doing evaluation, the benefits should be apparent.

An evaluation is:

1 the systematic collection, analysis and reporting of information

2 about an audience's knowledge, attitudes, skills, intentions and/or behaviours

3 regarding specific content, experiences or issues

4 for the purpose of making informed decisions about future services and products.

The purpose of your evaluation

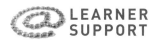
The purpose of your evaluation is to provide the decision-makers with enough information to help them make decisions about service design and delivery without overwhelming them with details.

From your evaluation you could:

- learn about your customers' needs, knowledge, abilities, current practices, etc.
- improve services so it matches staff abilities and resources while meeting your customers' needs, abilities, etc.

Either

- determine if your customers are satisfied/content with existing service/product arrangements

or

- determine the impact of your promotion.

Evaluating your promotional response

How will you know if the event was a success? By people telling you that they enjoyed it? That's good feedback but it hasn't necessarily turned into a sale yet, so how useful is it?

Unless you find some sort of mechanism for evaluating the impact and subsequent success, then the event will have little or no meaning at all.

A complete evaluation must be built in during the planning stage to measure the effectiveness of the investment. Yes, investment. The time used, the resources used, the people involved, all of these aspects are an investment made by the business for building on and into the future.

The methods that you use to evaluate the success of the event will depend on the type of event that you arrange. For example, it's relatively straightforward to distribute questionnaires in a small seminar scenario, but how do you get a town hall audience to fill in questionnaires before they dash home?

You need to tailor the mechanism of response to suit the needs of your event. The table below provides a list of the sorts of things that you can use.

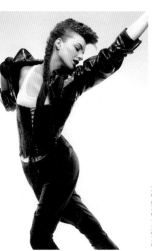

RUSH LONDON

Evaluation systems

- A written questionnaire (simplest standard evaluation system)
- Telephone follow-up (pre-prepared standard questionnaire)
- Pre-paid business reply service (mailshot to attendees or left on seats in the event)
- Focus group feedback (invite a sample of the audience to attend a meeting)
- Sales reports, sales summaries
- Increase of clients within the salon database

Collect, collate and analyse the information

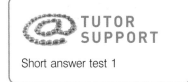
If you have collected the information in a multiple choice or standardised way; it would be easier to analyse the responses into a computerised way. (By means of spreadsheet

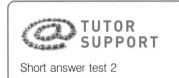

or database searches.) That way you can let the power of computing draw the conclusions from the patterns of response, rather than having to manually count each type of reply.

Ideally, for future data handling and easy reporting the replies would be contained within a database. This provides the most useful way of *interrogating data* and of *data mining*.

If this is not possible then, as second best, a spreadsheet will suffice. Your data from this can quickly be managed to provide charts and reports to show trends, likes and dislikes. Again, if this is not available or beyond your current limitations, you can tabulate the results in a Word document.

When compiling your data, be honest with the response. If you find that the results are not what you expected, don't be too concerned as any negative results or general indicators are all indicative of people's feelings. This will help management to tailor their offerings in future promotional events, so that they are closer to meeting the needs of your customers in the future.

Presenting an evaluation report

When the analysis has been done and you have created a presentation from the data you can arrange a time and date to feedback your findings to management. Your detailing needs to be clear and concise; you should present information 'as is' without providing speculative comments. The whole idea is to provide the information to others so that they can draw *their own* conclusions from the data, don't try to put a 'spin' on the findings as you may find yourself in 'hot water'.

The report should provide facts that are (hopefully) positive; the facts should raise issues which can then be discussed.

Be prepared to provide answers to the attendee's questions; where you do know the answer, be clear and concise, where you haven't got an answer, say so.

Finally, make notes of what has been said and if there are questions that still need to be answered; you can re-evaluate your data to find your response.

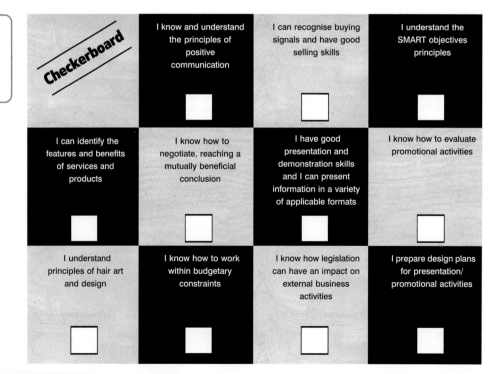

Revision questions

Quick quiz: a selection of different types of questions to check your knowledge.

Q1   Selling opportunities will occur when the features and
_____ of products are explained to the client.

Fill in the blank

Q2   A budget for a promotion can normally be ignored.

True or false

Q3   Which of the following are not parts of setting objectives?

Multi selection

Specialise	☐	1
Spontaneous	☐	2
Specific	☐	3
Metered	☐	4
Measurable	☐	5
Achievable	☐	6

Q4   Objectives should be set within a timeframe.

True or false

Q5   When pitching your ideas to management, which of the following
should you *never* do?

Multi selection

Have an outline plan	☐	a
Time your presentation	☐	b
Have your objectives clearly defined	☐	c
Make a guess at the costings	☐	d

Q6   An external event should be stimulating for the audience.

True or false

Q7   Which of the following are essential to an effective, external
presentation?

Multi selection

Being clear about what you want to sell	☐	1
Skipping over difficult questions	☐	2
Ignoring problems encountered by the team	☐	3
Rest breaks	☐	4
Encouraging the audience to participate	☐	5
Being professional and confident	☐	6

Q8   A smooth event should always _____ to time.

Fill in the blank

Q9   If, during an external demonstration there isn't a good flow of
questions. What should you do?

Multi choice

Forget it and finish early	○	1
Drag out the presentation to fill the time	○	2
Prompt for questions by cautious 'fishing'	○	3
Just say 'have you lot lost your tongues?'	○	4

Q10   The success of an external event is evenly 'weighted' throughout the
whole participating team?

True or false

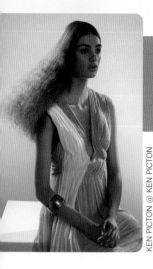

Appendix 1 Useful addresses and websites

Business

Arbitration, Conciliation and Advisory Service (ACAS)

Head Office Brandon House
180 Borough High Street
London, SE1 1LW

T: 020 7210 3613

www.acas.org.uk
Helpline 08457 47 47 47

Hairdressing Employers Association (HEA)

10 Coldbath Square
London, EC1R 5HL

T: 020 7833 0633

Training and education

Hairdressing and Beauty Industry Authority (HABIA)

Oxford House
Sixth Avenue
Sky Business Park
Robin Hood Airport
Doncaster, DN9 3GG

T: 08452 306080

www.habia.org

Association of Hairdressing Teachers (AHT)

5 Viscount Gardens
Byfleet
Surrey, KT14 6HE

City & Guilds (C & G)

1 Giltspur Street
London, EC1A 9DD

T: 020 7294 2800

www.city-and-guilds.co.uk

Department for Education and Skills

www.dfes.gov.uk

Lifelong Learning

www.lifelonglearning.co.uk

The Institute of Trichologists

Ground floor office
24 Langroyd Road
London, SW17 7PL

T: 08706 070602

www.trichologists.org.uk

Vocational Training Charitable Trust (VTCT)

Third Floor
Eastleigh House
Upper Market Street
Eastleigh
Hampshire, SO50 9FD

World Federation of Hairdressing Schools

73 Marlpit Lane
Coulsdon
Surrey, CR5 2HF

Publication

Hairdressers Journal International (HJ)

Quadrant House
The Quadrant, Sutton
Surrey, SM2 5AS

T: 020 8652 3500

www.reedbusiness.com

Creative Head

Mallan House
Bridge End
Hexham
Northumberland, NE46 4DQ

www.head1st.net

Black Beauty and Hair

Culvert House
Culvert Road
London, SW11 5DH

T: 020 7720 2108

www.blackbeauty.co.uk

Trade associations

British Association of Beauty Therapy and Cosmetology Limited (BABTAC)

Meteor Court
Barnett Way
Barnwood
Gloucester, GL4 3GG

Caribbean and Afro Society of Hairdressers (CASH)

42 North Cross Road
East Dulwich
London, SE22 8PY

T: 020 8299 2859

Commission for Racial Equality

Elliot House
10–12 Allington Street
London, SW1E 5EH

T: 020 7828 7022

www.cre.gov.uk

Cosmetic, Toiletry and Perfumery Association (CTPA)

Josaron House
5–7 John Princes Street
London, W1G 0JN

T: 020 7491 8891

www.ctpa.org.uk

Fellowship for British Hairdressing

Bloxham Mill
Barford Road
Bloxham
Banbury
Oxon, OX15 4FF

T: 01295 724579

Freelance Hair and Beauty Federation

6 Warleigh Road
Brighton
East Sussex, BN1 4TN

T: 01273 604556

www.fhbf.org.uk

Guild of Hairdressers (GUILD)

Unit 1E
Redbrook Business Park
Wilthorpe Road
Barnsley, S75 1JN

T: 01226 730112

Hairdressing and Beauty Suppliers' Association (HBSA)

Bedford Chambers
The Piazza,
Covent Garden
London, WC2E 8HA

T: 020 7836 4008

Hairdressing and Beauty Suppliers Association

1st Floor, Manfield House
1 Southampton Street
Covent Garden
London, WC2R OLR

Hairdressing Council (HC)

12 David House
45 High Street
South Norwood
London, SE25 6HJ

T: 020 8771 6205

www.haircouncil.org.uk

Health and Beauty Employers Federation (part of the Federation of Holistic Therapists)

18 Shakespeare Business Centre
Hathaway Close
Eastleigh Hampshire, SO50 4SR

www.fht.org.uk

Incorporated Guild of Hairdressers, Wigmakers and Perfumers

Unit 8, Vulcan Road
M1 Distribution Centre
Meadowhall
Sheffield, S9 1EW

National Hairdressers' Federation (NHF)

One Abbey Court
Fraser Road
Priory Business Park
Bedford, MK44 3WH

www.the-nhf.org

Legal and regulatory

Health and Safety Executive

Publications
PO Box 1999
Sudbury
Suffolk, CO10 6FS
(HSE) Infoline

T: 0845 345 0055

www.hse.gov.uk

Equal Opportunities Commission

Arndale House
Arndale Centre
Manchester, M4 3EQ

T: 0161 833 9244

Union of Shop, Distributive and Allied Workers (USDAW)

188 Wilmslow Road
Fallowfield
Manchester, M14 6LJ

T: 0161 224 2804

Appendix 2 Accidents, emergencies and manual handling

FELLOWSHIP FOR BRITISH HAIRDRESSING F.A.M.E. TEAM 2008

Fire

Fires occurring in salons are more likely to arise from electrical faults, gas leaks, or smoking. Faulty or badly maintained electrical equipment, such as hand dryers or hood dryers, may malfunction and overheat, and even ignite! Gas appliances, such as ovens or hobs, present a possible risk if they are left unattended. Staff cooking facilities need to be closely monitored to prevent gas being left on, whether lit or not. Your salon will have set fire safety procedures, which must always be followed.

Your salon premises will have been assessed for fire risk and a written policy will exist if five or more people are employed there. The fire risk assessment will take into account all other people on the premises, clients and visitors as well as other entities on a shared occupancy basis, if other firms occupy other parts of the building.

Emergency evacuation

All premises must have a designated means of escape from fire. This route must be kept clear of obstructions at all times and during working hours the fire doors must remain unlocked. The escape route must be easily identifiable, with clearly visible signs. In buildings with emergency lighting, these lighting systems automatically illuminate the escape route in the event of a power failure and are operated by an independent battery back-up.

In the event of fire breaking out the main consideration is to get everybody out:

- *Raising the alarm* – Anyone discovering a fire must immediately raise the alarm by operating the nearest alarm. Staff and customers must be warned and the premises must be evacuated.

- *On hearing the alarm* – All people must exit the building via the designated fire exits and proceed to the designated assembly point. Doors should be closed on exiting the building and designated staff may assist less able customers.

- *Assembly point(s)* – Everyone must remain at the assembly point, away from danger whilst awaiting further instruction

- *Call the fire brigade* – After exiting the building, call the emergency services. Dial 999, ask the operator for the fire service and give your telephone/mobile number. Wait for the transfer to the fire service and then tell them your name and the address of the premises that are on fire. Do this even if you believe that someone else has already phoned.

Firefighting

Under the Regulatory Reform (Fire Safety) Order 2005, all premises are required to have firefighting equipment, which must be suitably maintained in good working order. However, *only* those people with adequate training can attempt to put a fire out.

Extinguisher	Type	Colour	Used on	Must not be used on
Non-electrical fires	Water	Red marking	For wood, paper and textiles and other similar materials	On burning liquids and flammable metal fires
	Foam	Cream marking	On burning liquids	On electrical fires or flammable metal fires
Electrical fires	Dry powder	Blue marking	For burning liquid, electrical fires and flammable liquids	On flammable metal fires
	Carbon dioxide	Black marking	Safe on electrical fires and burning and flammable liquids	On flammable metal fires
	Vaporising liquids	Green marking	Safe on electrical fires and burning and flammable liquids	On flammable metal fires

Fire safety training

It is essential for staff to know the following fire procedures:

- fire prevention
- evacuation during a fire
- raising the alarm
- assembly points following evacuation.

Training is given to new members of staff during their induction period. This training must be regularly updated for all staff, and fire drills must be held at regular intervals.

Accidents (first aid)

The Health and Safety (First Aid) Regulations 1981 require the employer to provide equipment and facilities which are adequate and appropriate for providing first aid. In the event of an accident the 'Appointed Person' should be notified. This person takes control in these situations and will, if necessary, call an ambulance. There is also an appointed first aider who is qualified to administer first aid within the salon.

What is an Appointed Person?

An Appointed Person is someone who:

- takes charge if someone is injured or falls ill including calling an ambulance if required
- looks after the first aid equipment, e.g. restocking the first-aid box.

They should not attempt to provide first aid unless they have received appropriate training.

Every salon must have a first-aid kit in accordance with the regulations and, in the event that materials have been used, they must be replaced as soon as possible. All accidents and emergency aid given within the salon must be documented in the accident book.

Minimum contents of a typical first-aid box

1 First-aid guidance notes (HSE leaflet *Basic Advice on First Aid at Work*)

20 Individually wrapped sterile adhesive dressings

2 Sterile eye pads

4 Individually wrapped sterile triangular bandages

6 Safety pins

6 Medium size (12 cm × 12 cm approx) sterile unmedicated dressings

2 Large size (18 cm × 18 cm approx) sterile unmedicated dressings

1 Pair of disposable gloves

What is a first aider?

A first aider is someone who has undergone a training course in administering first aid at work and holds a current first aid at work certificate. A first aider can undertake the duties of an appointed person. (Lists of approved first-aid training organisations in your area are available from HSE.)

Recording accidents and illness

All accidents must be recorded in the accident book. The recording system should always be kept readily available for use and inspection. When you are recording accidents, you will need to document following details:

- date, time and place of incident or treatment
- name and job of injured or ill person
- details of the injury/of ill person and what treatment given
- what happened to the person immediately afterwards (e.g. went home, or went to hospital); was she taken in an ambulance?
- name and signature of the person providing the treatment and record entry.

The Reporting of Injuries, Diseases and Dangerous Occurrences Regulations 1995 (RIDDOR)

Under these regulations there are certain diseases and groups of infections that, if sustained at work, are noticeable by law. So if any employees suffer a personal injury at work which results in one of the following:

- death
- major injuries including fractures (not fingers and toes) amputation, dislocation, loss of sight and other eye injuries
- more than 24 hours in hospital
- an incapacity to work for more than three calendar days

they must be reported to the appropriate authority.

General guidance on first aid

The following basic information is available in leaflet form from HSE, ISBN 0 7176 1070 5 in priced packs of 20.

Remember

You should not attempt to give anything more than basic first aid!

What to do in an emergency

Priorities

Your priorities are to:

- assess the situation – do not put yourself in danger;
- make the area safe;
- assess all casualties and attend first to any unconscious casualties;
- send for help – do not delay.

Check for a response

Gently shake the casualty's shoulders and ask loudly, 'Are you all right?' If there is no response, your priorities are to:

- shout for help;
- open the airway;
- check for normal breathing;
- take appropriate action.

Unconsciousness

In most workplaces expert help should be available fairly quickly, but if you have an unconscious casualty it is vital that their airway is kept clear. If you cannot keep the airway open as described above, you may need to move the casualty into the recovery position. *The priority is an open airway.*

A = Airway To open the airway:

- place your hand on the casualty's forehead and gently tilt the head back;
- lift the chin with two fingertips.

B = Breathing Look, listen and feel for normal breathing for no more than 10 seconds:

- look for chest movement;
- listen at the casualty's mouth for breath sounds;
- feel for air on your cheek.

If the casualty is breathing normally:

- place in the recovery position;
- get help;
- check for continued breathing.

If the casualty is *not* breathing normally:

- get help;
- start chest compressions (see CPR).

C = CPR To start chest compressions:

- lean over the casualty and with your arms straight, press down on the centre of the breastbone 4–5 cm, then release the pressure;
- repeat at a rate of about 100 times a minute;
- after 30 compressions open the airway again;
- pinch the casualty's nose closed and allow the mouth to open;
- take a normal breath and place your mouth around the casualty's mouth, making a good seal;
- blow steadily into the mouth while watching for the chest rising;

- remove your mouth from the casualty and watch for the chest falling;
- give a second breath and then start 30 compressions again without delay;
- continue with chest compressions and rescue breaths in a ratio of 30:2 until qualified help takes over or the casualty starts breathing normally.

Wounds and bleeding

Open wounds should be covered – *after putting on sterile gloves*. Apply a dressing from the first-aid box over the wound and press firmly on top of it with your hands or fingers. The pad should be tied firmly in place. If bleeding continues another dressing should be applied on top. *Do not remove the original dressing.* Seek appropriate help.

Severe bleeding If there is severe bleeding:

- apply direct pressure to the wound;
- raise and support the injured part (unless broken);
- apply a dressing and bandage firmly in place.

Minor injuries

Minor injuries, of the sort which the injured person would treat themselves at home, can be treated from the contents of the first-aid box. The casualty should wash their hands and apply a dressing to protect the wound and prevent infection. In the workplace special metallic and/or coloured or waterproof dressings may be supplied according to the circumstances. Wounds should be kept dry and clean.

Broken bones and spinal injuries

If a broken bone or spinal injury is suspected, obtain expert help. Do not move casualties unless they are in immediate danger.

Burns

Burns can be serious – if in doubt seek medical help. Cool the part of the body affected with cold water until the pain is relieved. Thorough cooling may take ten minutes or more, but this must not delay taking the casualty to hospital.

Certain chemicals may seriously irritate or damage the skin. Avoid contaminating yourself with the chemical. Treat in the same way as for other burns but flood the affected area with water for 20 minutes. Continue treatment even on the way to hospital, if necessary. Remove any contaminated clothing which is not stuck to the skin.

Eye injuries

All eye injuries are potentially serious. If there is something in the eye, wash out the eye with clean water or sterile fluid from a sealed container, to remove loose material. Do not attempt to remove anything that is embedded in the eye.

If chemicals are involved, flush the eye with water or sterile fluid for at least 10 minutes, while gently holding the eyelids open. Ask the casualty to hold a pad over the injured eye and send them to hospital.

Suggested numbers of first-aid personnel

Category of risk	Number employed at one location	Suggested number of first aid personnel
Low risk: shops, offices	Fewer than 50	At least one Appointed Person
	50–100	At least one first aider
	100+	One additional first aider for every 100 people employed

Note. Under the Management of Health and Safety at Work Regulations 1999, the employer is responsible for ensuring that a risk assessment to determine the requirement and sufficiency of 'first aiders' within the workplace is implemented.

Special hazards

Electrical and gassing accidents can occur in the workplace. You must assess the danger to yourself and not attempt assistance until you are sure it is safe to do so. If the casualty has stopped breathing and you are competent to give artificial ventilation and cardiac resuscitation, do so. Otherwise send for help without delay.

Manual handling

As manual handling is an everyday part of salon processes, it is covered here. A range of skeletal and muscular disorders can occur if safe lifting procedures are not observed.

The bad posture of incorrect handling of large and/or heavy items can result in low back pain/problems, repetitive strain injuries and strain disorders.

Think about the situations involving manual handling which can occur in a salon environment i.e.

- moving stock into storage
- unpacking heavy or awkward items
- lifting equipment and moving salon furniture
- working heights – chairs, trolleys, dryers etc.

EKU statement

G20 i) The safe working practices for your own job

The Regulations require employers to:

- *avoid* the need for hazardous manual handling, so far as is reasonably practicable;
- *assess* the risk of injury from any hazardous manual handling that can't be avoided; and
- *reduce* the risk of injury from hazardous manual handling, so far as is reasonably practicable.

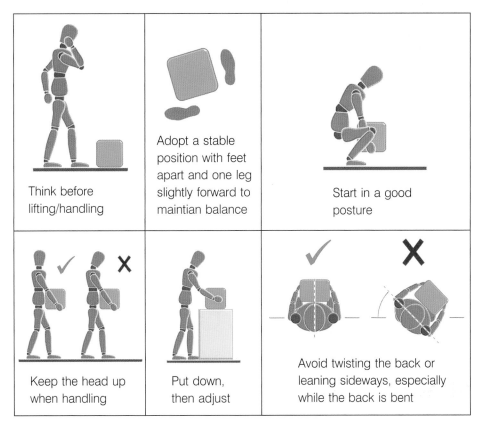

Think before lifting/handling

Adopt a stable position with feet apart and one leg slightly forward to maintian balance

Start in a good posture

Keep the head up when handling

Put down, then adjust

Avoid twisting the back or leaning sideways, especially while the back is bent

Manual handling

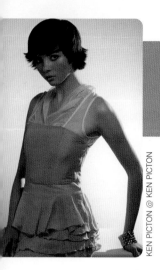

Chapter**one**

Consultation and advice quiz p. 43

Q1 Catagen
Q2 False
Q3 1,2,4
Q4 False
Q5 d
Q6 False
Q7 2,5
Q8 Germinal
Q9 c
Q10 True

Chapter**two**

Promote services and products quiz p. 54

Q1 Features
Q2 True
Q3 2,5
Q4 True
Q5 b
Q6 False
Q7 1,2,6
Q8 Listening
Q9 b
Q10 True

Chapter**three**

Customer services quiz pp. 68–69

Q1 Closed
Q2 True
Q3 1,2
Q4 True
Q5 c
Q6 False
Q7 1,2
Q8 Suggestion
Q9 d
Q10 True

Chapter**four**

Creative cutting quiz p. 103

Q1 Holding
Q2 False
Q3 3,5,6
Q4 True
Q5 d
Q6 False
Q7 4,6
Q8 Base
Q9 3
Q10 True

Chapter**five**

Cutting men's hair quiz p. 128

Q1 Holding
Q2 False
Q3 3,5,6
Q4 True

Q5 d
Q6 False
Q7 4,6
Q8 Fading
Q9 3
Q10 True

Chapter**six**

Styling beards and moustaches quiz p. 145

Q1 Steriliser
Q2 True
Q3 2,5
Q4 True
Q5 4
Q6 True
Q7 1,2,4
Q8 Flexible
Q9 2
Q10 False

Chapter**seven**

Shaving quiz p. 159

Q1 Autoclave
Q2 True
Q3 2,4
Q4 True
Q5 5
Q6 True
Q7 1,3,4
Q8 Sponge
Q9 1
Q10 False

Chaptereight

Creatively style and dress hair quiz p. 186

Q1 Velcro
Q2 False
Q3 3,4
Q4 True
Q5 b
Q6 False
Q7 1,5
Q8 Spiral
Q9 b
Q10 False

Chapternine

Creatively dress long hair p. 213

Q1 French
Q2 True
Q3 2,4,6
Q4 True
Q5 c
Q6 True
Q7 3,5
Q8 Knot
Q9 a
Q10 False

Chapterten

Hair extensions quiz p. 248

Q1 Root
Q2 False
Q3 3,4,5
Q4 True
Q5 b
Q6 True

Q7 5,6
Q8 First
Q9 c
Q10 True

Chaptereleven

Colouring hair quiz p. 290

Q1 Skin
Q2 True
Q3 4,5
Q4 False
Q5 d
Q6 True
Q7 2,4,5
Q8 Red/gold
Q9 b
Q10 True

Chaptertwelve

Colour correction quiz p. 319

Q1 Strand
Q2 False
Q3 1,2,3
Q4 False
Q5 d
Q6 False
Q7 1,3,6
Q8 Mauve ash
Q9 b
Q10 False

Chapterthirteen

Perming hair quiz p. 351

Q1 Curl
Q2 True

Q3 1,4,5
Q4 False
Q5 c
Q6 True
Q7 1,3
Q8 Cortex
Q9 c
Q10 True

Chapterfourteen

Develop your creativity quiz p. 371

Q1 Optimisation
Q2 True
Q3 3,6
Q4 False
Q5 c
Q6 False
Q7 2,4
Q8 NHF
Q9 d
Q10 False

Chapterfifteen

Health and safety quiz p. 396

Q1 Hazard
Q2 True
Q3 2,3,6
Q4 False
Q5 c
Q6 False
Q7 2,4
Q8 Fire
Q9 b
Q10 True

Chapter**sixteen**

Being effective in your work quiz p. 422

Q1   48

Q2   True

Q3   1,3,4

Q4   True

Q5   c

Q6   False

Q7   1,3,5

Q8   Delivery

Q9   b

Q10   False

Chapter**seventeen**

Planning promotional activities quiz p. 439

Q1   Benefits

Q2   False

Q3   1,2,4

Q4   True

Q5   d

Q6   True

Q7   1,5,6

Q8   Run

Q9   3

Q10   True

Appendix 4 People's rights and consumer legislation

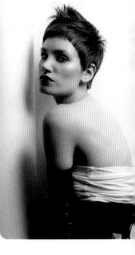

SHARON COX @ SANRIZZ

Equal opportunities

The Equal Opportunities Commission (EOC) has the statutory duty to:

- work towards the elimination of discrimination
- promote equality of opportunity between men and women (and in relation to persons undergoing gender reassignment)
- keep the relevant legislation under review.

The legislation within the remit of the EOC is wide ranging; however, the main considerations are:

- equal pay
- sex discrimination
- disability discrimination (summary below).

In general, the Sex Discrimination Act (SDA) requires goods, facilities and services, whether for payment or not, which are offered to the public to be provided on the same basis for both sexes. The SDA prohibits direct and indirect sex discrimination.

Direct sex discrimination is treating a woman less favourably than a man (or vice versa) because of her sex.

Indirect sex discrimination occurs when a condition or requirement is applied equally to both women and men but, in fact, it affects more women than men (or vice versa) and is not justifiable on objective grounds unrelated to sex. The Act provides for exceptions but unless a relevant exception to the requirements of the SDA can be used, facilities and services should be open to both sexes in the same way.

Diversion For more information visit www.eoc.org.uk/index.asp.

Disability Discrimination Act 2005 (DDA 2005)

The Act makes it unlawful to discriminate against disabled persons in connection with employment, the provision of goods, facilities and services or the disposal or management of premises; to make provision about the employment of disabled persons; and to establish a National Disability Council.

The Act protects the rights of disabled people and revisions introduced in 2005 have particular relevance to the business proprietor. For more information on this or accessibility issues visit www.disability.gov.uk/legislation.

Data Protection Act (1998)

Your clients have the following rights which can be enforced through any county court:

- *Right of subject access* – This is the right to find out what information about them is held on computer and in some paper records.

Diversion For more information on consumer rights in relation to the Data Protection Act visit www. informationcommissioner. gov.uk/

- *Correcting inaccurate data* – They have the right to have inaccurate personal data rectified, blocked, erased, or destroyed. If your client believes that they have suffered damage or distress as a result of the processing of inaccurate data they can ask the court to award compensation.

- *Preventing junk mail* (from salons that market to their customer base) – Your client has the right to request in writing that a data controller does not use your personal data for direct marketing by post (sometimes known as 'junk mail'), by telephone or by fax.

Data Protection Act 1998

The Data Protection Act (DPA) applies to any business that uses computers or paper-based systems for storing personal information about its clients and staff.

It places obligations on the person holding the information (data controller) to deal with it properly.

It gives the person that the information concerns (data subject) rights regarding the data held about them.

The duties of the data controller

There are eight principles put in place by the DPA to make sure that data is handled correctly. By law, the data controller must keep to these principles. The principles say that the data must be:

1 fairly and lawfully processed
2 processed for limited purposes
3 adequate, relevant and not excessive
4 accurate
5 not kept for longer than is necessary
6 processed in line with your rights
7 secure
8 not transferred to other countries without adequate protection.

For more information see http://www.ico.gov.uk/

The Sale of Goods Act (1979) and Sale and Supply of Goods Act (1994)

The Sale of Goods Act 1979 and the later Sale and Supply of Goods Act (1994) are the main legal instruments helping buyers to obtain redress when their purchases go wrong. It is in the interest of anyone who sells goods or services to understand the implications of these Acts and the responsibilities they have under them. Essentially, these Acts state that what you sell must fit its description, be fit for its purpose and be of satisfactory quality. If not, you – as the supplier – are obliged to sort out the problem.

Briefly these Acts requires the vendor:

- To make sure that goods '*conform to contract*'. This means that they must be as you describe them e.g. highlight shampoo stops your highlights from fading.

- The goods must also be of *satisfactory quality*, meaning they should be safe, work properly, and have no defects.

- You must also ensure the goods are '*fit for purpose*'. This means they should be capable of doing what they're meant for. For example, in the case of a brush it shouldn't fall apart when it is first used.

The Consumer Protection Act (1987)

This Act follows European laws to protect the buyer in the following areas:

- product liability – a customer may claim compensation for a product that doesn't reach general standards of safety
- general safety requirements – it is a criminal offence to sell goods that are unsafe; traders that breach this conduct may face fines or even imprisonment
- misleading prices – misleading consumers with wrongly displayed prices is also an offence

The Act is designed to help safeguard the consumer from products that do not reach reasonable levels of safety. Your salon will take adequate precautions in procuring, using and supplying reputable products and maintaining them so that they remain in good condition.

The Prices Act (1974)

The price of products has to be displayed in order to prevent a false impression to the buyer.

The Trades Descriptions Act (1968 and 1972)

Products must not be falsely or misleadingly described in relation to their quality, fitness, price or purpose, by advertisements, orally, displays or descriptions. And since 1972 it has also been a requirement to label a product clearly, so that the buyer can see where the product was made.

Briefly, a retailer cannot:

- mislead consumers by making false statements about products
- offer sale products at half price unless they have been offered at the actual price for a reasonable length of time.

The Resale Prices Act (1964 and 1976)

The manufacturers can supply a recommended price (MRRP or manufacturers' recommended retail price), but the seller is not obliged to sell at the recommended price.

Glossary

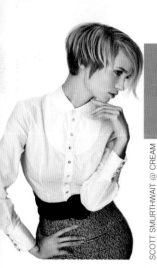

accelerator A machine that produces radiant heat (infrared radiation); can speed up chemical hair processes such as colouring or condition.

acid A substance that gives hydrogen ions in water and produces a solution with a pH below 7.

activator A chemical used in bleaches or some perm lotions to start or boost its action.

added hair A general term that covers the addition of hair pieces, wefts and extensions.

adverse hair and scalp condition In hairdressing terms: a condition which indicates a contra-indication.

alkali A substance that gives hydroxide ions in water and produces a solution with a pH above 7.

alopecia Baldness.

alpha keratin Hair in its natural state

anagen The stage of hair growth during which the hair is actively growing.

appraisal A process of reviewing work performance over a period of time.

arrector pili The muscles that raise the hair (in humans they are very feeble).

astringent A substance applied after shaving to close the pores.

asymmetrical Unevenly balanced, without an equal distribution of hair on either side.

artificial colour The term refers to any form of colour that is not a naturally occurring pigment also called synthetic colour.

autoclave A device for sterilising items in high temperature steam.

avant garde A genre of fashion that is considered progressive or exaggerated.

backcombing/backbrushing Pushing hair back to bind or lift the hair using a comb or brush.

backhand razoring A method of razoring where the cutting action occurs with a backhand technique.

banding An unwanted effect that appears as distinct bands of uneven colour.

benefits The ways in which the functions of products or services provide advantages.

beta keratin Hair in its moulded shape i.e. curly hair that has been dried straight.

blending A technique for mixing different colours of hair extension fibres to create: more naturally occurring effects, multi-toned effects, highlighted effects.

block colouring Colouring areas of hair in a way that is intended to enhance the cut style.

blunt cutting See club cutting.

brick cutting A way of point cutting into a held section of hair in different positions to create the 'scatter' pattern like brick work.

canities Hair that is without pigment and therefore grey or white.

catagen The stage of hair growth during which the hair stops growing, but the hair papilla is still active.

cleanser Removes dead skin cells, sebum and debris from the skin.

clipper over comb A technique of cutting hair with electric clippers, using the back of the comb as a guide, especially on very short hair and hairline profiles.

club cutting Cutting a hair section straight across, producing blunt ends.

colour stripper A colouring product that is specially formulated to remove synthetic/artificial colour from previously coloured hair.

colouring back A process of re-colouring previously lightened hair (e.g. highlights) back to the hair's natural hair depth and tone.

concave A concave perimeter slopes inwards.

confidential Private information, not for general use.

consumer protection The legislation protecting customers from unlawful sales practices and mishandling of personal information.

contra-indication A reason why a proposed course of action or treatment should not be pursued because it may be inadvisable or harmful.

control The ways in which risks identified are eliminated or reduced to an acceptable level.

convex Sloping outwards.

corn row Fine plaits running continuously across the scalp.

croquignole winding Winding a curl from point to root.

customer feedback The information retrieved by a variety of methods, used as a mechanism for evaluating the customer's experiences.

Data Protection Act 1984 Legislation designed to protect the client's right to privacy and confidentiality.

databank A manual or computerised store of data or records.

decolouring Removing synthetic colour from hair.

demonstration A display and explanation of a physical instruction.

depilatory A hair-removing compound.

discolouration Unwanted colour produced by a chemical.

disconnection An area within a hair cut where there is a distinct difference between two levels within the layering patterns or perimeter baselines.

double wind A variation of a weave wind – where the hair left out of the rod is wound on another rod.

dreadlocks The naturally occurring looking of hair aided by twisting to create a matted effect.

effectiveness The quality of output achieved in a work setting.

effleurage A light stroking massage movement applied with either the fingers or the palms of the hands.

eumelanin Black and brown pigment in the skin and hair.

exfoliation The removal or shedding of a thin outer layer of skin from the epidermis.

fading A cutting term that refers to the blending of short layered hair, usually from a neck outline into the graduated shape.

features The aspects of a product or service that state its functions, i.e. what it does.

fish hook A point of hair that has been bent back during rollering or winding.

folliculitis Inflammation of the hair follicles; may be caused by bacterial infection.

forehand razoring A method of razoring where the cutting action occurs with a forehand technique.

fragilitas crinium Splitting of the hairs at their ends.

franchise A business which is licensed to operate under the branding and reputation of another.

freehand cutting A method of cutting without holding between the fingers, or below or above a comb.

graduation A sloping variation from long hair to short, or from short to long, produced by cutting the hair ends at a particular angle.

hair extension Real or synthetic fibre added to existing hair.

HASAWA Health and Safety at Work Act 1974.

hazard Something with a potential to cause harm.

humidity The levels of moisture within the air.

hygroscopic Readily absorbing moisture from the atmosphere.

incompatible Causing a chemical reaction on mixing; as between a chemical being added to the hair and another chemical already on the hair.

incompatibility In hair science terms: A chemical process that is unable to co-exist with previously applied processes/treatments.

inversed clippering A way of holding the clippers to produce outlines necklines and detail within a design.

keratin The principal protein of hair, nails and skin.

knot The effect produced when long hair is wound, positioned and secured to take on a tied or knotted rope like effect.

melanins The pigments that give colour to skin and hair.

merchandise Goods for sale.

moisturising balms Cooling, soothing and moisture replenishing lotions applied after shaving to counteract the abrasive effects of the process

monilethrix Beaded hair.

monitoring Being responsible for checking incorrect practices.

non-conventional styling materials Items that can be used to style hair other than rollers and pin clips such as rags, chopsticks, straws, rik-rak etc.

occipital bone Bone forming the back of the head.

oxidation Reaction with oxygen, as in the neutralising of a perm.

para-dyes A term that refers to permanent colours containing paraphenylenediamine or PPD.

personalising A term which refers to a variety of cutting techniques applied to a style dependent on the client's specific needs.

petrissage A kneading massage movement of the skin that lifts and compresses underlying structures of the skin

pheomelanin A natural hair pigment.

piggy back wind A technique of winding curlers/rods into hair to create a multi textured effect that has curls/ movement of differing diameters

pleat A visual description of hair that is folded e.g. a 'French pleat'.

point cutting A texturising technique for using the point ends of the scissors to remove hair nearer the root area.

pointing See **point cutting.**

postiche A dressed hairpiece.

pre-pigmentation Applying a preliminary colouring of red to hair so that new colour will adhere.

Pre- and post-perm/colour treatments These are special products that can even out the porosity before perming or colouring.

pre-softening A process of softening resistant white hair with hydrogen peroxide.

productivity The levels of output achieved in a work context.

quasi-permanent A colour that is mixed with a developer for a longer-lasting effect.

real hair extensions Naturally occurring hair types derived from organic proteins found in humans and animals used for extending hair.

referral The situations where you need to re-direct people to other sources of treatment or service.

resources The variety of means available to a business that can be utilised or employed within any given task or project: time, money, people etc.

risk The likelihood of the harm occurring.

risk assessment A careful examination of what could cause harm to people in the workplace.

roll A visual description of hair that is rolled to create a bulked, rounded shape. This can be aided by using a 'bun ring' or similar styling aid.

root perm A technique for winding perming rods near the root area to produce lift without end movement.

scissor over comb A technique of cutting hair with scissors, using the back of the comb as a guide (usually when the hair is at a length that cannot be held between the fingers).

skin test A test done prior to colouring to establish whether a client has a sensitivity or reaction to chemical products.

slicing A texturising technique for cutting hair using the sharp blades of scissors (without open and closing) like using a razor/shaper.

SMART An acronym used for setting objectives i.e. **S**pecific, **M**easurable, **A**chievable, **R**ealistic and **T**imed.

spiral wind A perming technique of winding longer hair from root to point.

storyboard A way of pictorially and verbally collating ideas and concepts into a visual flow chart or schedule of events.

straightener An ammonium-based lotion similar to perms that can be used to remove wave in hair.

straightening Reducing the curl or wave in hair.

symmetrical Balanced by means of an even and equal distribution of hair on either side.

synthetic colour Another professional term that can be used instead of **artificial colour**.

synthetic fibre extensions A range of alternative, fibrous materials (nylon, acrylic, kerakalon etc.) used for extending hair.

'T' liner A type of clipper with a different blade type to standard clippers, enabling closer cut outlines around ears, necklines and facial hair shapes.

T section highlights A partial highlighting technique around the hairline and along the parting only.

tapering Cutting a hair section to a tapered point (i.e. a point like that of a sharpened pencil).

tapotement A brisk tapping or slapping massage movement (also known as percussion).

tariff A displayed list of fixed charges.

telogen The period during which a hair ceases to grow before it is shed.

temporal Bones forming the lower sides of the head.

temporary bonds The hydrogen bonds within the hair that are modified and fix the style into shape.

texturising A term which refers to a variety of cutting techniques.

tinting back See **colouring back**.

total look A term that is often used to describe a visual themed effect that incorporates hair, clothes, accessories and make-up.

toning Adding colour to bleached hair.

traction alopecia An area of baldness resulting from the stress or pull applied to hair.

tramliner A specialist clipper with a tapered, narrow blade for detailing designs on hair.

trichologist An expert specialising in the treatment of diseases affecting the hair and scalp.

trichology The study and treatment of hair and its diseases.

twist A technique of styling hair (or multiple stems of hair) by twisting together.

weave wind A perming technique for winding rods into the hair so that part of the mesh taken leaves hair out providing a multi textured effect.

whorls Hair growth patterns.

Index

accidents 444
  accident book 445
  broken bones/spinal injuries 447
  burns 447
  CPR 446–7
  eye injuries 447
  minor injuries 447
  recording of 385
  special hazards 448
  wounds and bleeding 447
  see also first aid
acid wave 327, 337
acne 26
added hair 181–2, 193–4
  see also hair extensions
advertising 434–5
aftercare
  barbering 126
  colour correction 316–17
  colouring 287–9
  cutting 100–1
  extensions 243–6
  facial hair 142–3
  perming 349–50
  shaving 157
  styling/dressing hair 184, 211
age of client 82–3
alopecia (hair loss) 26–7
alpha keratin 16, 172
amino acids 16
anagen 19
animal (parasitic) infestations 25
appointed person 444
appraisal 420–1
arrector pili muscle 19
autoclave 77, 393

backbrushing 180–1
backcombing 181, 199
bad breath (halitosis) 131
bacterial diseases 24
barbering 105
  aftercare 126
  benefits of wet cutting 106
  blending 122
  common cutting problems 121–2
  contemporary short style 125–6
  cutting rules 120
  disposal of waste 108
  finishing products 123–5
  gowning 106–7

hair and scalp 113–16
  hair growth patterns 114–15
  influencing factors 111–16
  male pattern baldness 111–12
  men's face shapes/physical features 112–13
  necklines/outline shapes 121
  points to remember 123
  preventing infection 109
  step-by-step 125
  tools and equipment 116–20
  working with damp hair 120
  see also shaving
barrel curls 204–5
barrel spring curl 176
barrier cream 262
beard 141
  see also facial hair
beehive 206–7
beta keratin 16, 172
bleach 281
bleaching *see* lightening hair
blow drying 178–80
  roots to points 179
  step-by-step 179
blow dryers 168
body language 8–10, 51
body position and gestures 9
British Hairdressing Awards 368–70
brushes 166, 195
burns 447
business growth 57

canites (grey hair) 253, 270–1
catagen 19
chemical damage 17
chemical properties of hair 16
chemical sterilisation 392
chignon 210–11
clay/putty 124
client
  age 82–3
  body shape 32
  bone structure, facial contours 136
  chin and jaw line 137
  complaints 404–5
  ears, nose, mouth 31
  eyes 31
  face shape 30–1, 79–80, 112
  growth/attrition 57–9
  hair growth patterns 29–30

hair type, growth, tendency 82
head shape/physical features 30–1, 80–1, 113, 134–5
lifestyle and personality 32, 81
loyalty 45
positioning 75, 131
quality, quantity, distribution of hair 81–2
records 41
size of mouth and lips 136
client information 59
  client surveys, questionnaires 62
  collection of 59–61
  sharing and collating 64–6
client preparation
  barbering 109
  colouring 261–4, 297
  cutting 74, 76
  facial hair 131–3
  perming 324
  shaving 148, 152
  styling/dressing hair 163
client service *see* customer service
clipper over comb 91
clippers 117, 120
  attachment sizes 138
  attachments 85, 120
  maintenance 118
clockspring curl 176
closed questions 11
cold sore (herpes simplex) 24
cold wave 327, 335
colour chart 255–6
colour correction 293
  applying depth/tone 305–6
  banded colour 308–9
  colour removal 311
  consultation/considerations 297–300
  decolouring 304, 307
  discoloured highlights/lowlights 309–10
  DIY disaster 312–13
  gradated colour 309
  lost definition 313–14
  planning 303
  preparation checklist 297
  pre-pigmentation 303–4, 314–15
  reapplying to natural depth 306, 314–16
  reintroducing colour 304
  removing permanent dyes 304, 307
  step-by-steps 312–16

SCOTT SMURTHWAIT @ CREAM

colouring 252
  bleach 281
  colour chart 34, 255–6
  colour design and selection principles
    269–70, 273–5
  consultation 264–6
  counteract/neutralise unwanted tones 269
  current condition of hair 271–2
  depth and tone 254
  full head lightening 282
  full head colour 275–6
  hair and skin tests 266–8
  harmonising and contrasting 273–5
  high lift 280
  hydrogen peroxide 260–1, 279–80
  lightening 279–85
  men's contemporary 282
  metallic dyes 260
  mixing 253
  natural hair colour 253
  natural vs indoor lighting 265
  permanent colour 259–60
  pre/post treatments 272
  pre-softening 271
  principles of 252–3
  problems 285–7
  quasi-permanent 258
  removal 311
  replace missing natural tones 276
  semi-permanent 256–8
  sensitivity test 21
  slices 277–8
  step-by-steps 275–8, 282–3
  temperature 273
  timing 272
  toning 280
  vegetable-based colour 260
  virgin hair 270
combs 84–5, 192
communication 7, 51
  asking questions 8
  body language 8–10, 404
  conversation skills 8
  create the right impression 9–10
  eye contact 9
  mirroring 10
  non-verbal 51–2
  posture, body position, gestures 9–10
  questioning styles 51
  questioning techniques 11–12
  reading skills 8
  verbal/oral 51, 403
  written 403–4
competitions 367–70
competitor information 57, 61–4
complaints 404–5
computer-generated images 34
computers 394
consultation 6–15, 29
  adapting your style 11–12
  avoid misunderstandings 13
  client records 41

collecting information 59–61
colour charts 34
communication skills 7–8
customising 29
dealing with customer resistance 12
effective body language 10
good practice 11–12
hair and scalp diseases, conditions,
  defects 23–8
hair growth patterns 29–30
hair maintenance advice 37–9
influencing factors and features 28–33
lifestyle, personality, age 32
making recommendations 35–7
manageability 33
questioning techniques 11–12
reaching agreement 39
referrals 36–7
service and product costs/timings 40
taking control/responsibility 14–15
using visual aids 33
consumer legislation 405–7
Consumer Protection Act (1987) 407, 455
contra-indication 21
Control of Substances Hazardous to Health
  Regulations (COSHH) (1999) 382–3
corneocytes 18
cortex 16
cowlick 30, 115
creative cutting see cutting
creative design 355–62
creative styling 161
  see also style and dress hair
creativity see working creatively
crimping irons 184
cross-checking 89
curling techniques see winding techniques
curly hair 82
customer satisfaction 57
customer service 46, 56
  client growth/attrition 57–9
  client loyalty 45, 57–8
  complaints 404–5
  feedback 58–9, 62, 67
  improving and changing 56, 64–6
cuticle 16
  damage 28
cutting
  angles 88
  balance 83
  baselines/perimeter outlines 88
  building on basics 73
  checklist 87, 95–6
  client position 75
  cross-checking 89
  graduated bob 99–100
  guidelines 88–9
  layers 98–9
  long hair 98
  maintaining tools 86
  natural fall of hair 87–8
  necklines 121

preventing infection 76
problems 89–90
quality, quantity, distribution of hair 81–2
sectioning 87
step-by-step 96–100
style suitability 82
styling limitations 79–83
tools 84–7
working creatively 73–4
working position 75, 78–9
working with damp hair 75
cutting techniques
  brick cutting 93
  clipper over comb 91, 140
  club cutting 90
  disconnection 73, 94, 96
  fading 105
  freehand 91
  graduation 97, 99–100
  point cutting 92
  scissor over comb 91, 105
  slicing 93
  texturising 73, 92–4
  thinning 91–2
cutting problems 89–90

damaged cuticle 28
dandruff 26
Data Protection Act (1998) 59, 406, 453–5
decolouring 304, 307
defining crème 124
demonstration 431–4
depth and tone 254
dermatitis 26, 263
dermis 18
development strand test 20
differentiation see USP
difficult hair 81
diffuser 167
Disability Discrimination Act (DDA) (2005)
  405–6, 453
discolouration 309–10
diseases
  animal (parasitic) infestations 25
  bacterial 24
  fungal 25
  infectious 24–5
  non-infectious 26–7
  viral 24
disposal of sharps 77
disulphide bonds 323
disulphide bridges 16
double crown 29, 114
doughnut ring 193, 210
dressing hair see style and dress hair
dry, frizzy hair 81

eczema 26
effectiveness see personal effectiveness/
  development
elasticity test 22–3, 267
Electricity at Work Regulations (1989) 384

emergencies 385, 446–8
   CPR 446–7
   fire 443–4
   first aid box 445
   unconsciousness 446
   see also first aid
employment
   contract of 399–400
   equal opportunities 405, 453
   job description 420
   principle statement 400
   staff training 402–3
   working conditions 399–405
   working hours 400–2
   young workers 380, 402
Environmental Protection Act (1990) 387
epidermis 18
equal opportunities 405, 453
exothermic perming systems 327
extensions 216
   aftercare 243–6
   blending/block colour 228–9
   braided/plaited 217, 242
   cold fusion systems 217, 241–2
   common problems 246
   consultation 222–3, 226–7
   contra-indications 223–4
   cutting 238–9
   hot bonded systems 217, 241
   human hair 220
   length of wefts 220, 225
   maintenance 226, 243–6
   planning and placement 234–8
   pre-bonded step-by-step 233–4
   products and equipment 219–22
   real hair step-by-step 232
   removal 240–2
   removal tools/products 221
   risks/safety considerations 217–18
   sectioning 234–5
   selection of hair 225, 228
   sewn-in 217, 242
   styling 239–40, 245–6
   synthetic fibre step-by-step 230–1
   synthetic hair 220
   timing 226
eye injuries 447

face shape 30–1, 79–80, 112
facial hair 130
   beard shapes 141
   cutting techniques 139–40
   gowning 131
   influencing factors 134–7
   moustache 136
   outline shape 139
   positioning client 131
   size of mouth and lips 136
   step-by-step 142
   width of chin and jaw line 137
   working position 132
   see also shaving

facial piercing 135
fine hair 81
finger waving 177–8
Fire Precautions Act (1971) 386
Fire Precautions (Workplace) Regulations
     (Amendment) (1999) 386
fire safety 443–4
   emergency evacuation 443
   extinguishers 444
   firefighting 443–4
   safety training 444
first aid 385, 444–8
   appointed person 444
   contents of first aid box 445
   CPR 446–7
   first aider 445
   general guidance 446–8
   unconsciousness 446
   see also accidents
fish hooks 349
folliculitis 24
fragilitis crinium (split ends) 28
French plaiting 203
French pleat (vertical roll) 201–2
fringe 90
furunculosis 24

gel/glaze 124
germinal matrix 18
Goldwell 170–1
gowning 74, 262
graduation 97
grey hair (canites) 253, 270–1

HABIA 383
hair
   poor condition 17
   stages of growth 19–20
   texture 20
   growth patterns 82
   testing 20–3, 267–9
   signs of healthy hair 15, 17
hair and scalp
   diseases, conditions, defects 23–8
hair and skin tests
   development strand test 20–1, 268
   elasticity 22–3, 267
   incompatibility 22, 267
   porosity 23, 267
   recording results 268–9
   skin sensitivity test (patch test) 21, 267
   test curl/development test curl 22
   test cutting 22
hair creativity *see* working creatively
hair extensions *see* extensions
hair follicle 18
hair growth stages 19–20
hair growth patterns 29–30, 114–15
hair health and condition 17–18
hair loss (alopecia) 26–7
hair pieces 193–4
hair structure 16

hair ups
   barrel curls 204–5
   beehive 206–7
   chignon 210–11
   contemporary knots 205–6
   plaiting 202–3
   special occasion hair 208–10
   twists 207–8
   vertical roll (French pleat) 201–2
   weaving 203
   see also style and dress hair
hairdressing demonstration 433–4
hairspray 125, 171
hairstyling *see* style and dress hair
halitosis (bad breath) 131
hazard 389
   chemical 391
   equipment 390
   working environment 392
head lice (pediculosis capitis) 25
head shape/physical features 30–1, 80–1,
     113, 134–5
health and safety 375
   bye-laws 388–9
   electricity 394
   employee's responsibilities 378–9
   employer's responsibilities 379–80
   first aid 385
   floors and thoroughfares 394
   handling chemicals 394
   hazard and risk 389, 390–1
   manual handling 393, 448–9
   personal health/hygiene 395
   record keeping 379
   recording accidents 385
   regulations 377–8
   responsibility 375
   risk assessment 379–81, 391–2
   working environment 392–5
   working with computers 394
Health and Safety at Work Act (1974) 376–7
Health and Safety (Display Screen
     Equipment) Regulations (1992) 386–7
Health and Safety (First Aid) Regulations
     (1981) 384, 444
heated styling equipment 182–4
   crimping irons 184
   heated brushes 183
   heated rollers 165, 191
   straightening irons 192
   tongs 183, 191
henna 256
herpes simplex (cold sore) 24
highlights *see* lightening hair
home care advice 101
human extension hair 220
human resources 399–400
humidity 174
hydrogen bonds 16
hydrogen peroxide 260–1, 279–80
hygroscopic 16, 172
hypodermis 18

Index

impetigo 24
incompatibility 5
incompatibility test 22, 267
infectious diseases 24–5
influencing factors and features
    age of client 82–3
    body shape 32
    bone structure, facial contours
        136
    chin and jaw line 137
    ears, nose, mouth 31
    eyes 31
    face shape 30–1, 79–80, 112
    hair growth patterns 29–30
    hair type, growth, tendency 82
    head shape/physical features 30–1, 80–1,
        113, 134–5
    lifestyle and personality 32, 81
    make-up 33
    manageability 33
    neck and shoulders 31
    quality, quantity, distribution
        of hair 81–2
    size of mouth and lips 136
    style suitability 82
ingrowing hairs 86
injuries 447
International Colour Chart (ICC)
    254
ionic styling equipment 168

keratin 16, 18, 172, 323

L'Oréal 196
    Colour Trophy 367
    Majirel shade chart 255–6
lifting see manual handling
lightening hair
    checklist 283–5
    chemistry of 279–80
    emulsion bleach 281
    full head 282
    high lift colour 280
    powder bleach 281
    step-by-steps 282–3
    toning 280
    using hydrogen peroxide
        260–1
Likert scale 61
long hair
    dressing 189–211
    style suitability 198
    see also hair ups

maintaining tools 86
male pattern baldness (MPB) 27,
    111–12
Management of Health and Safety at Work
    Regulations (1999) 377
manual handling 393, 448–9
Manual Handling Operations Regulations
    (1992) 387

medulla 16
melanin 253
melanocytes 18
men's hairstyling see barbering
metallic dyes 260
micro-organisms 76
monilethrix 28
moustache 136
    see also facial hair

nape whorl 29, 114
neck brush 86
necklines 121
neutralising 344
    application 346
    how it works 345
    rebalancing 345
    step-by-step 347
    technique 345–7
non-infectious diseases 26–7
non-verbal communication 8, 51–2

obstructions 392
open questions 11
oral communication 403
oxygen 16

patch test (sensitivity test) 21
payments
    taking deposits 40
pediculosis capitis (head lice) 25
permanent colour 259–60
perming 322
    acid wave 327, 337
    after the perm 348
    alkaline systems 336–7
    application of lotion 337
    basic wind 335–6
    body perms 341
    chemical changes 323–4
    cold wave 327, 335
    contra-indications 327, 330
    direction and degree of movement 340
    exothermic systems 327
    gowning 324
    hair tests 331
    influencing factors 328–30
    pre/post treatments 331–2
    processing and development 337–9
    root perms 341
    sectioning 335
    sensitised hair 332–3
    spiral 339–40
    temperature 338
    tools and equipment 335
    winding techniques 333–4, 339–41
perming problems/solutions
    fish-hooks 349
    hair/scalp damage/breakage 348
    no result 349
    weakens 349
    poor result when dry 349

burn 348
    sore hairline/irritation 348
    straight frizz 348
    straight pieces 349
    too curly 348
    curl 349
personal effectiveness/development 398
    appraisal 420–1
    code of conduct 404
    development targets/productivity
        415–18
    job description 420
    keeping abreast of current fashions 36
    measuring effectiveness 418–21
    oral communication 403
    prioritising 414–15
    promoting ourselves 46
    teamwork 418
    time management 413–15
    written communication 403–4
personal health/hygiene 75, 132, 395
Personal Protective Equipment at Work
    Regulations (PPE) (1992) 381–2
personal qualities
    empathy 13
    working intuitively 14
pH scale 324
photography/photo sessions 362–6
physical hair damage 17
physical properties of hair 16–17
pincurling 176
pins and grips 192
plaiting 202–3
polypeptide chains 16, 323
porosity test 23, 267
PPD (paraphenylenediamine) 259
pre-pigmentation 303–4, 314–15
pre-softening 271
Prices Act (1974) 407, 455
products 169, 196
    clay/putty 124
    defining crème 124, 170
    finishing 169
    gel/glaze 124, 170
    hairspray 125, 171
    heat protection 169, 171
    men's 123–5
    mousse 170
    serum 170
    setting lotion 169–70
    varnish 124
products and services 45–53
    being aware of 46
    features and benefits 47
    informing clients 47–9
    in-salon promotions 48
    promotional materials 50
    providing costs 40
    recommending 101
    window displays 50
    see also promotional activities
professionalism 7

promotional activities 424–38
    advertising 434–5
    budgeting 426
    demonstration skills 433–4
    evaluate results 430, 437–8
    hairdressing demonstrations 431–4
    planning 425–6, 428–9
    press 436
    public relations 435–6
    setting objectives 427
    target market 427–8
    types of 426–7
Provision and Use of Work Equipment
        Regulations (PUWER) (1998) 387
psoriasis 26
putty/clay 124

quasi-permanent colour 258
questioning 51
    leading questions 61
    multiple choice 61
    open/closed questions 60
    techniques 11–2
    styles 60–1

razors 85, 117, 120
    honing 150–1
    open blade 149–50
    stropping 151–2
    testing the edge 151
referrals 36–7
Regulatory Reform (Fire Safety) Order (2005)
        443
Reporting of Injuries, Diseases and
        Dangerous Occurrences Regulations
        (RIDDOR) (1995) 385–6, 445
Resale Prices Act (1964 and 1976) 407, 455
resources
    avoiding waste 413
    monitoring 399
    stock control 408–413
    human 399–400
    salon 408–13
    time 413–14
ringworm (tinea capitis) 25
risk 389
    assessment 391–2
    controlling 392–3
rollering 175–6
rollers 165

Sale of Goods Act (1979) and Sale and
        Supply of Goods Act (1994) 406–7,
        454–5
salon
    working environment 392
    hygiene 394
    promotion 424–38
    security 412
sales promotion see promotional activities
scabies 25
scissor over comb 91, 105

scissors 84, 119
sebaceous cyst 28
sebaceous gland 19
seborrhoea 26
sebum 19
sectioning 86–7
selling 49
    buying signals 50–1
    features and benefits 47
    good and bad selling 52–3
    using the senses 49
    see also promotional activities
semi-permanent colour 256–8
senior stylist 6–7
sensitivity test (patch test) 21
setting hair
    finger waving 177–8
    lotion 169
    physical changes 172
    pincurling 176–7
    rollering 175–6
    techniques 175–8
    winding 175
Sex Discrimination Act (SDA) 405, 453
sharps disposal 77
shaving 148
    aftercare 157
    contra-indications 153
    finishing 155
    first time shave 154–5
    honing 150–1
    lathering 153
    preparation 148, 152
    problems 154, 156
    razors 149–52
    second time shave 155
    sponge shaving 155–6
    stropping 151–2
    tools and equipment 149–50
    waste disposal 156
skin
    structure 18
    sensitivity tests 21, 267
spiral perm 339–40
split ends (fragilitis crinium) 28
sterilisation 77
    autoclave 393
    chemical 392
    ultraviolet (UV) radiation 392–3
stock
    avoiding waste 413
    control 408–9
    handling 411–12
    keeping 408
    ordering 410
    product coding 409–10
    recording 410–11
    security 412
    stocktaking 409
    supplier 410
straight hair 82
straightening hair

    influencing factors 343–4
    method 344
    principles of 342
straightening irons 165, 183, 192
strand test 268
stratum corneum 18
structure of hair 16
structure of skin 18
style and dress hair
    added hair 181–2, 193–4
    agree effect 198
    backbrushing 180–1
    backcombing 181, 199
    barrel curls 204–5
    beehive 206–7
    blow dry 178–80
    building structure/support 199
    checklist 174
    chignon 210–11
    contemporary knots 205–6
    curls and curling 175–7
    doughnut ring 193, 210
    dressing long hair 189–211
    finger waving 177–8
    general rules 198
    heated styling equipment 182–4
    materials and tools 164–7, 191–5
    physical changes 172
    pincurling 176–7
    plaiting 202–3
    principles of 173
    rollering 175–6
    service timings 191
    setting 172, 175–8
    special occasion hair 208–10
    step-by-step 204–11
    style suitability 198
    styling products 169–71, 195–6
    techniques and effects 174–5
    twists 207–8
    vertical roll (French pleat) 201–2
    weaving 203
    winding 175
styling products see products
subcutis 18
sweat gland 19
sycosis 24
synthetic hair 220

target market 427–8
targets 416–17
teamwork 418
telogen 19
texturising 73, 92–4
thinning hair 114
    see also male pattern baldness
thinning scissors 85, 119
time management 413–15
tinea capitis (ringworm) 25
tinting see colouring
tongs 183, 191
toning 280

tools and equipment
  blow dryers 168
  bonding/extension applicator 219
  brushes 166
  clipper attachments 85, 120, 138
  clippers 117, 120
  comb 84–5, 192
  crimping irons 184
  diffuser 167
  grips and pins 165, 192
  heat clamp 219
  heated brushes 183
  heated rollers 191
  maintenance 86
  neck brush 86
  rags 164
  razor 85, 117, 120
  rollers 165, 341–2
  scissors 84, 119
  sectioning clips 86
  straightening irons 165, 183, 192
  tail comb 192
  thinning scissors 85, 119
  tongs 183, 191
  trolley 262
  water spray 86
traction alopecia 26
Trades Descriptions Act (1968 and 1972)
    407, 455
training 402–3
treatments
  pre/post colour 272
  pre/post perm 331–2
trichorrexis nodosa 28
trolley 262

ultraviolet (UV) radiation 77, 392–3
unconsciousness 385, 446
USP (unique selling point) 57

varnish 124
vegetable-based colour 260
verbal communication 51
vertical roll (French pleat) 201–2
virgin hair 270
visual aids
  colour charts 34
  computer-generated images 34
  pictures 33

warts 24
waste
  avoiding 413
  disposal 108
water spray 86
wavy hair 82
wax 123, 170
weathering 17
website 50, 62
wefts 193
white hair 253, 270, 271
widow's peak 30, 115
wigs 194
winding techniques 175
  basic 335–6
  directional 340
  double 341
  piggyback 341
  spiral 339–40
  stack 341
  staggered/brick 341
  weave 341
window displays 50
working conditions 399–405
  holiday entitlement 401
  leave payment 401
  public/bank holidays 401

rest breaks 401
  staff training 402–3
  working hours 400–2
working creatively 73–4, 353–70
  backdrops and lighting 365–6
  clothes and accessories 364–5
  colour depth and tone 360
  competitions 367–70
  creative design 355–62
  design aspects 356–8
  dimension, distribution, abundance
      359–60
  make-up artist 364
  models 363
  photography/photo sessions 362–6
  pictures and images 354–5
  storyboard 365
working efficiently, safely, effectively 77–9
working environment
  controlling risk 392–5
  electricity 394
  floors and thoroughfares 394
  handling chemicals 394
  manual handling 393
  personal health/hygiene 395
  potential hazards 392
  sterilisation 392–3
  working with computers 394
working hours 400–2
Working Time Regulations (1998) 400
Workplace (Health, Safety and Welfare)
    Regulations (1992) 381
written communication 403–4

young workers at risk 380

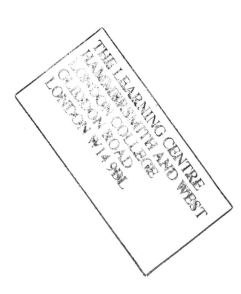